The Changing Visual System

Maturation and Aging in the Central Nervous System

NATO ASI Series

Advanced Science Institutes Series

A series presenting the results of activities sponsored by the NATO Science Committee, which aims at the dissemination of advanced scientific and technological knowledge, with a view to strengthening links between scientific communities.

The series is published by an international board of publishers in conjunction with the NATO Scientific Affairs Division

A	**Life Sciences**	Plenum Publishing Corporation
B	**Physics**	New York and London
C	**Mathematical and Physical Sciences**	Kluwer Academic Publishers
D	**Behavioral and Social Sciences**	Dordrecht, Boston, and London
E	**Applied Sciences**	
F	**Computer and Systems Sciences**	Springer-Verlag
G	**Ecological Sciences**	Berlin, Heidelberg, New York, London,
H	**Cell Biology**	Paris, Tokyo, Hong Kong, and Barcelona
I	**Global Environmental Change**	

Recent Volumes in this Series

Volume 218— Pharmaceutical Applications of Cell and Tissue Culture to Drug Transport
edited by Glynn Wilson, S. S. Davis, L. Illum, and Alain Zweibaum

Volume 219—Atherosclerotic Plaques: Advances in Imaging for Sequential Quantitative Evaluation
edited by Robert W. Wissler

Volume 220—The Superfamily of *ras*-Related Genes
edited by Demetrios A. Spandidos

Volume 221—New Trends in Pharmacokinetics
edited by Aldo Rescigno and Ajit K. Thakur

Volume 222—The Changing Visual System: Maturation and Aging in the Central Nervous System
edited by P. Bagnoli and W. Hodos

Volume 223—Mechanisms in Fibre Carcinogenesis
edited by Robert C. Brown, John A. Hoskins, and Neil F. Johnson

Volume 224—Drug Epidemiology and Post-Marketing Surveillance
edited by Brian L. Strom and Giampaolo P. Velo

Series A: Life Sciences

The Changing
Visual System

Maturation and Aging in the
Central Nervous System

Edited by

P. Bagnoli

University of Tuscia
Viterbo, Italy

and

W. Hodos

University of Maryland
College Park, Maryland

Plenum Press
New York and London
Published in cooperation with NATO Scientific Affairs Division

Proceedings of a NATO Advanced Research Workshop
on the Changing Visual System: From Early to Late Stages of Life—
Maturation and Aging in the Central Nervous System,
held May 26–June 6, 1991,
in San Martino al Cimino (Viterbo), Italy

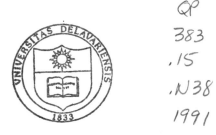

QP
383
.15
.N38
1991

Library of Congress Cataloging-in-Publication Data

NATO Advanced Research Workshop on the Changing Visual System: From
   Early to Late Stages of Life--Maturation and Aging in the Central
   Nervous System (1991 : San Martino al Cimino, Italy)
     The changing visual system : maturation and aging in the central
   nervous system / edited by P. Bagnoli and W. Hodos.
        p.   cm. -- (NATO ASI series. Series A, Life sciences ; v.
   222)
     "Proceedings of a NATO Advanced Research Workshop on the Changing
   Visual System: From Early to Late Stages of Life--Maturation and
   Aging in the Central Nervous System, held May 26-June 6, 1991, in
   San Martino al Cimino (Viterbo), Italy"--T.p. verso.
     "Published in cooperation with NATO Scientific Affairs Division."
     Includes bibliographical references and index.
     ISBN 0-306-44090-3
     1. Visual cortex--Differentiation--Congresses. 2. Visual cortex-
   -Aging--Congresses. 3. Visual pathways--Congresses.   I. Bagnoli,
   P. (Paola), 1945-   . II. Hodos, William. III. North Atlantic
   Treaty Organization. Scientific Affairs Division. IV. Title.
   V. Series.
     [DNLM: 1. Cell Survival--physiology--congresses. 2. Central
   Nervous System--growth & development--congresses. 3. Eye--growth &
   development--congresses.   WW 103 N278c 1991a]
   QP383.15.N38 1991
   618.8'4--dc20
   DNLM/DLC
   for Library of Congress   91-45593
                                                                  CIP

ISBN 0-306-44090-3

© 1991 Plenum Press, New York
A Division of Plenum Publishing Corporation
233 Spring Street, New York, N.Y. 10013

Printed in the United States of America

PREFACE

In late May and early June 1991, a NATO Advanced Study Institute was held at a hotel in the hilltop village of San Martino al Cimino a few kilometers from the city of Viterbo in the Lazio region of Italy. The title of the course was the same as this volume and brought together specialists working at all phases of the life span (embryology, infancy, childhood, middle life and senescence) in both animals and humans to exchange ideas, facts and theories in the search for common principles. Such principles could prove important for understanding developmental changes in the central nervous system and visual behavior within the context of a continuum of life-span processes rather than viewing them as events or mechanisms that occur only in a certain period. For example, changes that are associated with "aging" were considered as extensions or continuations of processes that began at an earlier stage of the life span, rather than being seen as processes that only began late in life.

The visual system has proven extremely useful as an experimental model for studies of early development, plasticity and aging in the nervous system. This Advanced Study Institute represented an important opportunity to review and discuss the considerable amount of data that has been assembled in recent years in order to identify general principles governing developmental changes in the nervous system in a life-span context. As biomedical science progressively increases the human life span, we need to improve the quality of later life. These principles of visual-system development ultimately may assist not only in the prolongation of the integrity of the visual system (including its optical media, retina and central pathways), but also may aid in the improvement of the quality of the progressively lengthening human life-span. The visual system is extremely important in this regard because failing vision can rob the elderly of an important key to an independent life and the enjoyment of their later years.

The meeting began with an opening lecture by Professor Rita Levi-Montalcini entitled "The Role of Environmental Factors on the Development and Function of the Nervous System". We are grateful to Professor Levi-Montalcini for this lecture and her participation in the course. Current research topics that were discussed during subsequent sessions were morphological and functional events such as cell induction, cell proliferation, cell migration, cell differentation, cell death, connectivity and synaptogenesis. Because the theme of the course was to view development as a continuous process throughout life rather than in the traditional "maturation-vs.-aging" context, there was much discussion devoted to plastic events in the immature and adult nervous systems, behavioral changes and their possible relation to the process of aging. In addition, the role of neurotrophic factors and neurotoxic agents in cell death were discussed as well as the protective role of growth factors. These and other topics were discussed not only in the planned topical paper sessions, but in special ad hoc discussion groups that were organized by M. Brunelli, M. B. A. Djamgoz, B. Bagolini and S. Thanos. Although not included in the book, these informal discussions permitted the participants to speculate freely on causes, mechanisms and "cures". The result was a series of lively and wide-ranging discussions that surely will have an impact on the future research of the participants.

The organizers of the course wish to express their profound gratitude to the many persons and institutions that contributed to make this meeting a success. First, we must thank the Scientific Affairs Division of NATO for sponsoring this Advanced Study Institute. We offer our thanks too to the administrators of the Regione Lazio, Amministrazione Provinciale di Viterbo, Amministrazione Communale di Viterbo, USL Vt 13, Ente Provinciale Turismo, Università della Tuscia, Università di Pisa, Consiglio Nazionale delle Ricerche, Cassa di Risparmio della Provincia di Viterbo, Associazione Industriali di Viterbo and Fidia Famaceutici italiani. Finally, we must offer special thanks to the people of San Martino al Cimino and Viterbo as well as the Faculty of Science and students of Università della Tuscia who offered us such a warm welcome and such generous hospitality.

Paola Bagnoli
William Hodos

Viterbo, Italy
August 1, 1991

CONTENTS

Development of the Primate Visual System
Throughout Life 1
P. Rakic

Modern Theories of Aging and their Application
to Ocular Senescence 11
R. A. Weale

Animal Models of Life-span Development 21
W. Hodos

Ontogenetic Clues to the Phylogeny of the
Visual System 33
B. Fritzsch

Are Visual Hierarchies in the Brains of the
Beholders? Constancy and Variability in the
Visual System of Birds and Mammals 51
H. J. Karten and T. Shimizu

The Centrifugal Visual System: What Can
Comparative Studies Tell Us About
Its Evolution and Possible Function? 61
R. Ward, J. Repérant and D. Miceli

Blockade of Proteolytic Activity Retards
Retrograde Degeneration of Axotomized Retinal
Ganglion Cells and Enhances Axonal Regeneration
in Organ Cultures 77
S. Thanos

Organization and Development of Sparsely
Distributed Wide-field Amacrine Cells
in the Rabbit Retina 95
N. C. Brecha, G. Casini and D. Rickman

Aging and Spatial Contrast Sensitivity:
Underlying Mechanisms and Implications for
Everyday Life 119
C. Owsley and K. B. Burton

Life-span Changes in the Visual Acuity and
Retina of Birds 137
W. Hodos, R. F. Miller, K. V. Fite, V. Porciatti,
A. L., Holden, J.-Y. Lee and M. B. A. Djamgoz

Plasticity of Synaptic Connections in the Adult
Vertebrate Retina 149
M. B. A. Djamgoz

New Aspects of Cellular and Molecular Mechanisms
in Learning Processes 171
G. Traina, R. Scuri, D. Cecchetti and M. Brunelli

Maturation and Plasticity of Neuropeptides in
the Visual System 185
P. Bagnoli, S. Di Gregorio, M. Molnar,
C. Romei and G. Fontanesi

Development and Plasticity of the Tectofugal
Visual Pathway in the Zebra Finch 199
H.-J. Bischof, K. Herrmann and J. Engelage

Spatio-temporal Properties of the Pattern ERG
and VEP: Effect of Ageing 209
V. Porciatti, D. C. Burr, A. Fiorentini
and C. Morrone

Methods and Models for Specifying Sites and
Mechanisms of Sensitivity Regulation in the
Aging Visual System 219
J. F. Sturr and D. J. Hannon

Structural Organization and Development of
Identified Projection Neurons in Primary
Visual Cortex 233
J. Bolz, M. Hübener, I. Kehrer and N. Novak

Developmental Status of Intrinsic Connections
in Visual Cortex of Newborn Humans 247
A. Burkhalter

Development of the Visual Cortex Deprived Prenatally
of Retinal Cues 255
R. O. Kuljis

Sensorial and Sensorimotor Phenomena in Strabismus 269
  B. Bagolini

Age, Sex and Light Damage in the Avian Retina:
  A Model System 283
  K. V. Fite, L. Bengston and B. Donaghey

The Damaging Effects of Light on the Eye and
  Implications for Understanding Changes
  in Vision across the Life Span 295
  J. S. Werner

Cellular and Molecular Aspects of Neuronal
  Differentiation 311
  G. Augusti-Tocco, S. Biagioni, M. Plateroti
  G. Scarsella and A. Vignoli

VGF: A Tissue Specific Protein and a Marker of
  NGF-Induced Neuronal Differentiation 319
  A. Levi, N. Canu, E. Trani, M. Benedetti,
  and R. Possenti

Nerve Growth Factor (NGF) Prevents the Effects of
  Monocular Deprivation in the Rat 333
  L. Domenici, N. Berardi, G. Carmignoto,
  T. Pizzurosso, V. Parisi and L. Maffei

Evidence for a Role of NGF in the Visual System 347
  M. C. Comelli, P. Candeo, R. Canella, A. Merighi
  L. Maffei and G. Carmignoto

Ipsilateral Projections During Development and
  Regeneration of the Optic Nerve of the
  Cichlid Fish Haplochromis burtoni 357
  C. Wilm

Abnormal Organization of the Human Retina in a
  Genetic Disorder (Bloch-Sulzberger Syndrome) 361
  A. Silva-Araújo, J. M. Lopes, J. Salgado-Borges
  and M. A. Tavares

Visual System in Some Systemic Diseases 365
  F. F. Demircioglu

Effects of Intraocular Activity Blockade on the
  Morphology of Developing LGN Neurons in
  the Cat 369
  K. Herrmann, R. O. L. Wong and C. J. Shatz

Development of Orientation-Specific Neuronal
    Responses in Ferret Primary Visual Cortex 375
  B. Chapman and M. P. Stryker

Development of the Tyrosine Hydroxylase Immuno-
    reactive Cell Population in the Rabbit
    Retina 379
  G. Casini and N. C. Brecha

Emergence of Visual Cortical Areas: Patterns of
    Development of Neuropeptide-Y Immuno-
    reactivity and Somatostatin-immuno-
    reactivity in the Cat 385
  D. Hogan and N. E. J. Berman

Individual Differences in Contrast Sensitivity
    Functions of Human Adults and Infants:
    A Brief Review 391
  D. Peterzell, J. S. Werner and P. S. Kaplan

A Neural Network Model for Stripe Formation
    in Primate Visual Cortex 397
  W. Cowan and M. J. Zuckermann

Stereo Matching Using Relaxation Labeling
    Based on Edge and Orientation Features 403
  J. S. Jin

Contributors 407

Index 411

DEVELOPMENT OF THE PRIMATE VISUAL SYSTEM THROUGHOUT LIFE

Pasko Rakic

Section of Neurobiology
Yale University
New Haven, CT

Developmental principles derived from experimental analysis of the visual system in nonhuman primates provide insight into the normal and pathological development of vision in man, and reveal some general mechanisms of brain maturation and aging. This overview is based on a series of longitudinal studies in the developing rhesus monkey carried out in my laboratory over the last two decades. This type of work poses extraordinary challenges, as there is no easy and straightforward way to determine how functional circuitry is formed and maintained in a species with a lifespan of more than 30 years. To be meaningful, the research has to be carried out on the entire visual system, rather than focused on its components, and the analysis has to be rigorously quantitative, as many changes may be relatively small. The introduction of computer-aided quantitative methods, and the availability of cell class-specific markers, neurotransmitters and receptors have opened unprecedented opportunities for probing the principles governing the development of functionally dedicated networks even in the large and complex primate brain. I will also include in my presentation our data on the development of binocular as well as color-opponent or broad-band parallel pathways from the retina across the lateral geniculate nucleus to the striate cortex, the formation of cytoarchitectonic maps, as well as the dynamics of synaptic connections and their biochemical maturation in the visual system. Although progress in this field has been possible due to research carried on in many laboratories, this short overview is based exclusively on the studies done in my laboratory. Description of the material and methods, experimental details, factual data and additional relevant literature can be found in the papers listed in the bibliography.

First, we have to address the question of the time of origin of neurons that comprise the visual system in the rhesus monkey. Studies using tritiated thymidine autoradiography revealed that all neurons comprising the primate visual system are generated predominantly before birth, during the first half of gestation, in remarkably precise cell class-specific and area-specific sequences and spatio-temporal gradients. Figure 1A displays graphically the onset, course and cessation of the genesis of retinal ganglion cells as well as all neurons destined for the lateral geniculate nucleus and primary visual cortex. The details of the kinetics of cell proliferation and the rate of daily production of cells can be found in the primary references (La Vail, Rapaport and Rakic, 1991; Rakic, 1974, 1977a). Here, it is sufficient to state that, although neurogenesis of the neurons engaged in the primary visual pathways begins in the retina and then in the lateral geniculate nucleus and finally the cerebral cortex, the completion of neurogenesis in these three structures does not follow this simple hierarchical sequence. For example, photoreceptors situated at the

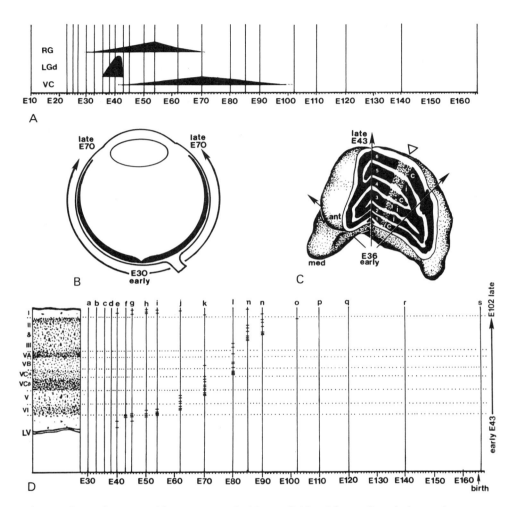

Figure 1. Diagrammatic representation of the time of origin and
neurogenetic gradients in the retina (A,B), lateral
geniculate nucleus (C) and cortical area 17 (D). The series
of over 100 ³H-TdR labeled animals processed for
autoradiography by the partial support of this provided the
only available data of the time of neuron origin in any
primate, and has proven to be invaluable in determining
critical developmental stages in human. The detailed
quantitative data can be found in Rakic, 1974, 1977a,b; La
Vail, Rapaport and Rakic, 1991.

periphery of the retina continue to be generated until birth (La Vail, Rapaport and Rakic, 1991), long after neurogenesis has completely stopped in the lateral geniculate nucleus and cerebral cortex (Rakic, 1974, 1977a). Furthermore, within each structure there is a smooth gradient of neurogenesis which is illustrated graphically by arrows in Figures 1B,C,D. Examination of the direction of these gradients in relation to the pattern of connections reveals clearly that the time of neuron origin is not sufficient to explain the development of either the laminar or areal topography of primary visual projections.

The second problem concerns cell determination and formation of topographic maps within each structure. We recently found that, after settling in their final positions in the fetal retina, various classes of photoreceptors promptly assume both species-specific proportions as well as mosaic-like distribution (Wikler and Rakic, 1990). The emergence of the mosaic of rods and red/green- or blue-sensitive cones as identified by antibody to wave-length sensitive opsins occurs surprisingly early; and we suggested that it may be related to an array of early-maturing, precociously differentiating cones (Wikler and Rakic, 1991). This "protomap" appears in the monkey retina in the first half of gestation, before the photoreceptors have established any synaptic contacts with either horizontal or bipolar cells within the outer plexiform layer (Nishimura and Rakic, 1987). Our finding, therefore, suggests that the basic phenotypic commitment and positional information may be initiated without coordination with neurons in the central structures. On the other hand, at the opposite end of the visual system, neurons in the striate cortex apparently can form their basic laminar and modular organization in the absence of information from the photoreceptors at the periphery. This conclusion has been reached by examining the adult animals in which retinal ablation has been performed *in utero,* before the stage in which photoreceptors begin to make synapses (Rakic, 1988; Rakic et al., 1991; Kuljis and Rakic, 1990). Thus, the cortex, like the retina, contains information for building basic species-specific cytoarchitecture (the protomap, Rakic, 1988). How these protomaps, initially established independently in the retina and visual cortex, become interconnected via a geniculate relay center in the thalamus, and then differentiate into a functionally competent adult form, is the major challenge.

The third issue that needs to be solved is the control of neuronal and synaptic number and their proper ratio at each level of the visual system. Our quantitative electron microscopic analysis provided the timetable of synaptogenesis in the various structures in the rhesus monkey visual system throughout the lifespan. Contrary to prevailing views, our results clearly showed that the pioneer synaptic contacts are formed in the central structures before formation of true line projections that proceed from the photoreceptors via bipolars to ganglion cells (Nishimura and Rakic 1985, 1987). Furthermore, anatomical and ultrastructural analyses demonstrated that neurons, axons and synapses are initially overproduced in all visual structures where the counts have been made (Fig. 2). For example, at midgestation the macaque retina contains close to 3,000,000 ganglion cells. Subsequently, about 60% of these cells are lost (Rakic and Riley, 1983a). Study of the timing, magnitude, and spatial distribution of neuron elimination in the lateral geniculate nucleus shows that, before E60, this thalamic nucleus contains about 2,200,000 neurons, 800,000 of which are eliminated over a 40- to 50-day period during the middle third of gestation (Williams and Rakic, 1988). Just to illustrate the magnitude of this loss, it is sufficient to mention that neurons in the lateral geniculate nucleus are lost at an average rate of 300 an hour between E48 and E60, and at an average rate of 800 an hour between E60 and E100. Very few neurons are lost after E100, and as early as E103 the population falls to the adult average of 1,400,000 (Fig. 2). Degenerating neurons seem to be more common in the magnocellular moiety of the nucleus than in the parvocellular moiety. The period of cell death occurs before the emergence of cell layers in the

lateral geniculate nucleus, before the establishment of geniculocortical
connections and before the formation of ocular dominance columns. Most
important, the loss of neurons in the lateral geniculate nucleus begins
long before the depletion of retinal axons. This finding eliminates
the hypothesis that cell death in the retina plays a major role in
controlling the size of the lateral geniculate and its magno- and
parvocellular moiety. Rather, it suggests that both the total number

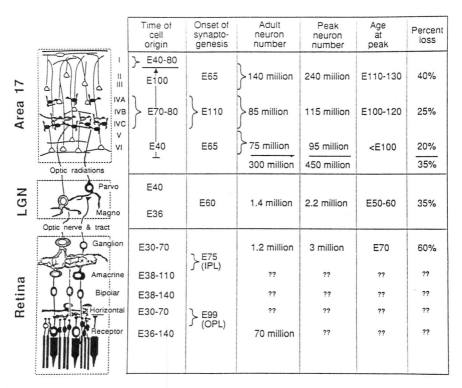

	Time of cell origin	Onset of synapto-genesis	Adult neuron number	Peak neuron number	Age at peak	Percent loss
I	E40-80					
II III	E100	E65	140 miilion	240 miilion	E110-130	40%
IVA IVB IVC	E70-80	E110	85 million	115 million	E100-120	25%
V VI	E40	E65	75 million	95 million	<E100	20%
			300 million	450 million		35%
Parvo	E40					
Magno	E36	E60	1.4 million	2.2 million	E50-60	35%
Ganglion	E30-70	E75 (IPL)	1.2 million	3 million	E70	60%
Amacrine	E38-110		??	??	??	??
Bipolar	E38-140		??	??	??	??
Horizontal	E30-70	E99 (OPL)	??	??	??	??
Receptor	E36-140		70 million	??	??	??

Figure 2.   The total number of various neuronal classes present in
the primary visual pathway of the developing and adult
rhesus monkey. Data on the time of origin, onset of
synaptogenesis, adult neuron number, peak neuron number,
age at the peak and the percent lost are presented for
the retina, LGN and area 17. For further information see
Rakic and Riley, 1983a; Williams and Rakic, 1988; Wikler,
Williams and Rakic, 1990. Data on the cortex are still
preliminary (Ryder, Williams and Rakic, in preparation).
The question marks indicate unavailable data.

and ratio of magno- and parvocellular components are established
intrinsically and that there may be also a species-specific protomap
within the lateral geniculate nucleus.

The fourth broad area of research has been the developmental
mechanisms involved in the formation of neuronal connections. Injections
of radioactive tracers show that terminations of visual projections in the
target structures are transiently overlapping and more diffuse than in
the adult (Rakic, 1976, 1977b, 1986). Subsequent work revealed that the

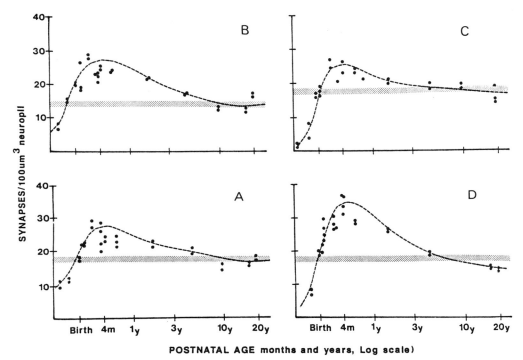

Figure 3. Histograms of the density of synapses per 100 square microns
of neuropil in the primary somatosensory (A), primary motor
(B), prefrontal (C), and primary visual (D) cortices at
various ages. Each black dot represent the value obtained
from an uninterrupted electron microscopic probe consisting
of about 100 photographs across the entire depth of the
cortex. The stippled horizontal stripe denotes the average
synaptic density in the adult monkey for each area. Age in
months (m) and years (y) is presented on a logarithmic scale
in order to fit the entire span of the monkey onto a single
graph (from Rakic et al., 1986).

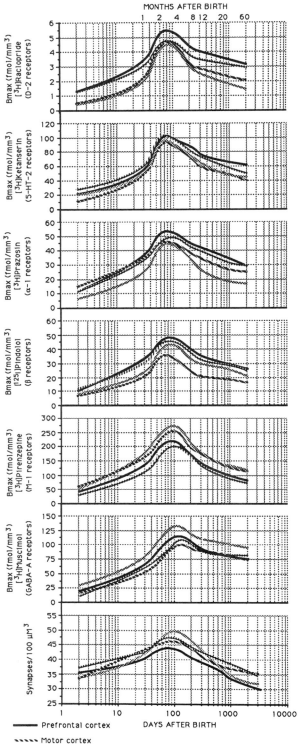

Figure 4. Developmental changes in the overall (across all layers) density of the specific binding of radioligands labeling a representative selection of neurotransmitter receptor subtypes in the prefrontal, primary, motor, somatosensory and primary visual cortical regions. The figure also includes developmental changes in synaptic density in the same regions (adapted from Rakic et al., 1986). For receptor densities, the lines were obtained by locally weighted least square fit with 50% smoothing (KALEIDA GRAPH, Synergy Software, Reading, PA) based on mean B_{max} values obtained from the measurements of the entire cortical thickness in at least two animals at birth, 1,2,4,8,12,36 and 60 months of age. Age is presented in postnatal days on a logarithmic scale (Lidow, Goldman-Rakic and Rakic, 1991).

elimination of the supernumerary neurons, axons, synapses and various molecules involved in transmission occurs during specific time periods (Rakic and Riley, 1983a; Rakic et al., 1986; Lidow, Goldman-Rakic and Rakic, 1992). Their segregation into region-, layer-, column- and cell-specific territories is induced by intracellularly programmed instructions but require further tuning by intercellular competitive interactions (Rakic, 1981; Rakic and Riley, 1983b; Rakic, 1986; Rakic, 1989). The synaptic production in the cortex starts before birth but extends well beyond infancy (Fig. 3). These interactions may involve both spontaneous and induced activity. The phase of high synaptic density, with values above those found in the normal adult, lasts throughout infancy and adolescence and decreases significantly only during sexual maturation (Rakic et al., 1986). Therefore, this phase may provide the opportunity for competitive interaction among various inter- and intracortical connections which comprise the largest fraction of cortical synapses.

The capacity to perform various visual tasks coincides with the time when synaptic density reaches its peak, which suggests that a critical mass of cortical synapses is essential for cognitive functions to emerge. However, the full maturation of such functions may depend upon the elimination of excess synapses that occurs during adolescence. The decline in synaptic density is due primarily to elimination of asymmetrical junctions located on dendritic spines, while synapses on dendritic shafts and cell bodies remain relatively constant during postnatal life (Rakic et al., 1986). It may be significant that the density of all so-far-examined neurotransmitter receptors in the visual cortex also reaches a maximum level between two and four months of age and then declines to the adult level during the period of sexual maturation (Lidow, Goldman-Rakic and Rakic, 1991). For example, this synchronized development of several monoamine receptors occurs *pari pasu* with the course of synaptogenesis (Fig. 4). These findings reveal unusual coordination between biochemical and structural differentiation and supports the hypothesis that these events may be related to maturation of function. In fact, correlative analysis is this structural-functional relationship may provide new insight into cognitive maturation (e.g., Goldman and Rakic, 1978). In addition, this approach may help our understanding of various genetic and acquired developmental disorders.

The fifth major theme is related to competitive interaction and possible molecular mechanisms underlying these changes. In spite of considerable advances made in the past few years, our understanding of the role of synaptic overproduction in the development of vision at the cellular and molecular level is still rather vague. It seems, however, that a simple and straightforward hypothesis will not suffice to explain this enormously complex phenomenon. For example, contrary to our expectation, the phase of ocular-dominance formation, which begins during the last three weeks of gestation and continues during the first two postnatal months, is characterized by an increase rather than decrease in synaptic density. Furthermore, we recently found that premature visual stimulation in infant monkeys delivered before term does not affect the rate of synaptic accretion or the size, topology, and laminar distribution of synapses (Bourgeois, Jastreboff, and Rakic, 1989). Rather, the morphological parameters develop according to the time of conception and are not influenced by the time of birth. These results suggest that visual stimulation in infancy may affect the visual cortex predominantly through strengthening, modifying, and eliminating synapses already formed rather than regulating the rate of their production.

The concept of competitive interactions has been verified by experiments involving the selective destruction of various visual centers and/or pathways in monkey fetuses, neonates and juveniles, and subsequent analysis of the effects of these procedures on the pattern of axonal pathways, architecture of synaptic contacts and distribution of neurotransmitters and their receptors. These interactions may begin before birth, but they clearly extend postnatally and continue until puberty, when most structural and biochemical properties become more stabilized. The steady state seems to last throughout more than two decades of adult life in this species, and only at the end of the lifespan begins to fall again. These statements are, however, made on the basis of a relatively small number of specimens and their significance need to be verified on a larger sample.

Presently, we are studying the stability of neural connections and the modifiability of visual cortical maps by early lesion-induced reduction of afferent input (Rakic, Suner and Williams, 1991). The results indicate that lesion of a synaptically-related structure or reduced input to a given visual center, occurring during a critical developmental period, may exert structurally limited but molecularly significant changes that, in turn, influence subsequent developmental events in other structures and thereby provide the setting for new patterns of neural and synaptic relationships. In-depth analysis of cellular events and the consequences of experimental modification of the visual system set the stage for identification of biological principles and molecular mechanisms involved in synaptic specification of large neuronal populations.

ACKNOWLEDGEMENT

This series of studies have been supported by the United States Public Health Service.

REFERENCES

Bourgeois, J.-P., Jastreboff, P. and Rakic, P., 1989, Synaptogenesis in the visual cortex of normal and preterm monkeys: Evidence for intrinsic regulation of synaptic overproduction, Proc. Nat. Acad. Sci. USA, 86:4297-4301.
Goldman, P.S. and Rakic, P., 1979, Impact of the outside world upon the developing primate brain. Perspective from neurobiology, Bulletin of the Menninger Foundation, 43:20-28.
Kuljis, R.O. and Rakic, P., 1990, Hypercolumns in primate visual cortex develop in the absence of cues from photoreceptors, Proc. Nat. Acad. Sci. USA, 87:5303-5306.
Lidow, M.S., Goldman-Rakic, P.S. and Rakic, P., 1991, Synchronized overproduction of neurotransmitter receptors in diverse regions of the primate cerebral cortex, Proc. Nat. Acad. Sci. USA, in press.
Nishimura, Y. and Rakic, P., 1985, Development of the rhesus monkey retina: I. Emergence of the inner plexiform layer and its synapses, J. Comp. Neurol., 241:420-434.
Nishimura, Y. and Rakic, P., 1987, Development of the rhesus monkey retina: II. A three-dimensional analysis of the sequences of synaptic combinations in the inner plexiform layer, J. Comp. Neurol., 262:290-313.
Rakic, P., 1974, Neurons in the monkey visual cortex: Systematic relation between time of origin and eventual disposition, Science, 183:425-427.
Rakic, P., 1976, Prenatal genesis of connections subserving ocular dominance in the rhesus monkey, Nature 261:467-471.
Rakic, P., 1977a, Genesis of the dorsal lateral geniculate nucleus in the rhesus monkey: site and time of origin, kinetics of proliferation, routes of migration and pattern of distribution of neurons, J. Comp. Neurol., 176:23-52.
Rakic, P., 1977b, Prenatal development of the visual system in the rhesus monkey, Phil. Trans. Roy. Soc. Lond. B. 278:245-260.
Rakic, P., 1981, Development of visual centers in the primate brain depends on binocular competition before birth, Science, 214:928-931.
Rakic, P., 1986, Mechanism of ocular dominance segregation in the lateral geniculate nucleus: competitive elimination hypothesis, Trends in Neuroscience, 9:11-15.

Rakic, P., 1989, Competitive interactions during neural and synaptic development, in: "From Neuron to Reading," A.M. Galaburda, ed., MIT Press, Cambridge.

Rakic, P., Bourgeois, J.-P., Eckenhoff, M.E., Zecevic, N. and Goldman-Rakic, P.S., 1986, Concurrent overproduction of synapses in diverse regions of the primate cerebral cortex, Science, 232:232-235.

Rakic, P., Gallager, D. and Goldman-Rakic, P.S., 1988, Areal and laminar distribution of major neurotransmitter receptors in the monkey visual cortex, J. Neurosci., 8:3670-3690.

Rakic, P. and Riley, K.P., 1983a, Overproduction and elimination of retinal axons in the fetal rhesus monkey, Science, 209:1441-1444.

Rakic, P. and Riley, K.P., 1983b, Regulation of axon numbers in the primate optic nerve by prenatal binocular competition, Nature, 305:135-137.

Rakic, P., Suner, I. and Williams, R.W., 1991, A novel cytoarchitectonic area induced experimentally within the primate visual cortex, Proc. Nat. Acad. Sci. USA, 88:2083-2087.

Wikler, K.C. and Rakic, P., 1990, Distribution of photoreceptor subtypes in the retina of diurnal and nocturnal primates, J. Neurosci., 10:3390-3400.

Wikler, K.C. and Rakic, P., 1991, Emergence of the photoreceptor mosaic from a protomap of early-differentiating cones in the primate retina, Nature, 352:397-400.

Wikler, K.C., Williams, R.W. and Rakic, P., 1990, Photoreceptor mosaic: Number and distribution of rods and cones in the rhesus monkey retina, J. Comp. Neurol., 297:499-508.

Williams, R.W. and Rakic, P., 1988, Elimination of neurons in the rhesus monkey's lateral geniculate nucleus during development, J. Comp. Neurol., 272:424-436.

MODERN THEORIES OF AGING AND THEIR APPLICATION TO OCULAR SENESCENCE

R. A. Weale

Age Concern Institute of Gerontology, King's College
London (University of London), Cornwall House Annex
Waterloo Rd., London SE1 8TX

1. Introduction

In gerontological analyses it is not unusual for data in some
specialist field to be reviewed, and then for an attempt to be made to
fit them into an existing theoretical frame-work. If the two are
consistent with each other, a given theory may receive a boost over
rival ones. This procedure is based on an assumption frequently implicit
in assessments of data on senescence, namely that most, if not all,
manifestations of human aging can be described largely by but a single
mechanism.

An example of such a view is the idea that senescence results
mainly from the accumulation of noxious molecules, such as free radicals
(Harman, 1984). Another is that the progressive reduction of
immunological responses exposes the individual to successful assaults by
a hostile environment, possibly leading ultimately to death (Meites &
al., 1987). There is a variety of other hypotheses, many of them
successful in the limited fields to which they are applied, but at risk
when they are generalised. This has been demonstrated in connection with
Orgel's catastrophe theory (1963, 1973). It postulates that senescent
proteins, cells, organs, and bodies, progressively accumulate such a
large number of unrepaired errors as to reach the point of no return,
when catastrophic, and irreversible damage occurs. Studies on enzymes
(Gershon & Gershon, 1976), and on newly synthesised proteins (Johnson &
McCaffrey, 1985), to quote two of several examples, failed to
substantiate the occurrence of the type of transcription error which
Orgel had postulated in his imaginative concept. However, Laughrea
(1982) believes that such errors can occur, but it is uncertain whether
they can affect the rate of senescence.

There is, however, an even more fundamental problem to be faced
whenever an attempt is made to understand the various phenomena of
senescence. This is, for example, the question of why free radicals
should accumulate to harmful levels, why immunological protection should
break down, why errors in transcription should occur and become noxious,
when nothing of the sort appears to happen when we are young. In other
words, the above [and several other] hypotheses in many ways describe
satisfactorily how the system of survival is undermined, but fail to
explain why this should happen at all.

The Changing Visual System, Edited by P. Bagnoli and
W. Hodos, Plenum Press, New York, 1991

More general approaches dealing with this basic question tend to follow one of two lines. One school believes that senescence is planned (Beutler, 1986). In modern parlance this may imply that it is a genetically determined process, perhaps one based on specific genes ensuring that one or more mechanisms promoting aging shall be put into operation. A view expressed in different ways holds that, if senescence (and death) did not exist, the world would become overpopulated. In other words, some supreme, economically minded intelligence decreed in the name of justice that life is to be rationed. This is an example of an adaptive theory.

Another group, protagonists of the non-adaptive type (cf. Kirkwood, 1984), postulate in effect that senescence occurs faute de mieux. It is not planned, but results from evolutionary pressure, as is thought to be true of all biological phenomena. One of the more characteristic theories in this group is the "disposable soma" theory (Holliday, 1988). This is based on the idea that a large investment is made in the ability of a species to procreate. There is a pay-off between longevity and procreational potential, the two being related inversely. A sequel of this hypothesis is concerned with bio-economic aspects, emphasising that evolution operates on a shoe-string (Weale, 1990).

The reason for this is not hard to see. If a departure from the norm is found to be beneficial to a species, then, in the first instance, the relevant mutation is likely to be marginal. It becomes established by repeated reinforcement, until a new norm, with its own variance, becomes set up, and can be identified by statistical means. As, by implication, the new characteristic is heritable, and everyone dies at some time or other, there arises the question of whether senescence is heritable.

This is for several reasons of concern to those who are interested in the time course of visual performance. For example, virtually the whole of mankind becomes presbyopic at the age of 40+-10y (Weale, 1982), some variations having been reported due to sex, and also geographical location.

This raises the interesting point of the extent to which the senescence of our visual system may be governed by genetic and environmental factors, if any. In connection with other somatic changes, this type of problem has led to the above-mentioned postulate of special genes for senescence, and in several laboratories the hunt is one for their discovery.

It has to be stated at this point that, on the basis of Occam's razor, namely that the number of hypotheses required to explain observed phenomena should be a minimum, it is hard to see the need for such genes. The reason is as follows. There is ample evidence for the existence of genetically controlled repair processes in our bodies. The coagulation of blood exposed to the air is one such example, the existence of the condition of haemophilia emphasising its control by genes. Corneal scarring provides an example of a result of a less adequate repair process; although repair processes following some relatively minor trauma may allow the cornea to heal, its function may be permanently impaired. A similar instance can be quoted in connection with the retina: exposing it to a very intense stimulus may cause a temporary scotoma or blind spot. Recovery from such an insult has been known to extend from a week or two to several months (Duke-Elder & MacFaul, 1972), and has also been known to be complete.

Given, therefore, that our bodies are protected from trauma and other insults also by a complicated immunological system, the postulate of genes for senescence seems to be superfluous. A limited investment in the maintenance of repair processes is all that is required. Biological maintenance costs biological money, and there is no evidence of any liberality on the Donor's part. Senescence can be achieved either by cutting off a particular system itself or the route of the metabolic supplies to its maintenance system. This can be achieved in more than one way.

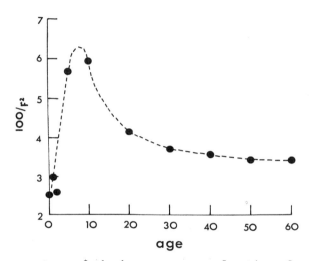

Fig.1. The aperture of the human eye as a function of age. (F=D/L, where D is the pupillary diameter in the light-adapted eye and L the effective focal length).

For example, there could be a limit on the maintenance capital; once this runs out, senescence begins. Ovulation and the menopause appear to illustrate such a device. The admission of light into the eye provides an example for the alternative. The aperture of the eye is maximal during early childhood (Fig.1).

This is a result of both the large size of the pupil, even under photopic or daylight conditions, and the relatively short ocular posterior nodal distance between the ages of 5 - 15y. The maximum pupillary diameter starts shrinking beginning with the early teens (cf. Weale, 1982). A variety of explanations has been advanced (Alexandridis, 1989) for age-related miosis, the statistically observed constriction of the light- and dark-adapted pupil. Histological evidence points to a more rapid age-related atrophy of the comparatively weak dilator muscle fibres than is true of the sphincter. Note that this offers an explanation of miosis, not one of the allegedly reduced contractility of the elderly iris. However, Meyer (priv. comm.) has recently shown by means of fluorescein angiography that the iridal vascular system tends to shrink with advancing years particularly in the region of the dilator fibres. It is undecided whether this is due to arteriolosclerosis or some local ocular events, but it serves to underline the view that functional changes associated with senescence may be consequences of more remote causes. It may therefore be conceptually simpler to envisage, and to look for, factors of limited duration in terms of life-span which are necessary for the performance of some specific function notably during the peak of our physical performance which coincides historically with the period of maximum fecundity than to search for genes for senescence the need for which may be hard to establish.

2. Peaks of achievement

The notion of bio-economics is well illustrated by the development, growth, and senescence of the visual system. Let us postulate that, speaking only from a biological point of view, the most important period of an individual's life is the period when he or she has produced offspring, and when they are being reared to an age when they, in turn, have matured biologically, and can continue the course of procreation.

This means that, if the period between birth and puberty is the period of development P, the acme of biological performance will fall approximately within the age interval lying between P and 2P; in other words, its duration will be of the order of P. The bio-economical hypothesis applied to this requirement would predict that any investment before and after this period should be minimal. Indeed, the investment during childhood, i.e. development, should be geared, on this view, merely to the optimisation of performance during the age span of P - 2P. If it is true, that, after the age of 2P, the individual's biological value drops to zero, then one has to try and find an explanation of why our visual faculties do not decay more rapidly than is, in fact, the case. It need hardly be mentioned that this question does not arise specifically just in connection with the visual system, but is of general interest.

The cost of maintenance of an individual varies with its duration. If it were constant throughout life the situation would be described by the horizontal line shown in Fig.2a. However, if the main thrust of evolutionary economics is to concentrate on the period of keeping a

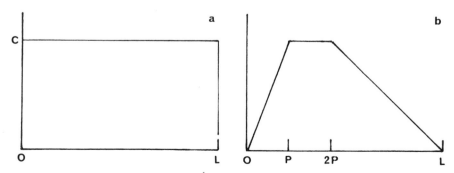

Fig.2. (a) Constant biological expenditure throughout life; (b) the situation when economies are achieved before and after the period of maximum fertility.

14

species going then the main expenditure is likely to occur within the period P – 2P. Obviously some type of economic investment is required during the period of development 0 – P, but, though large, it can be comparatively small in terms of energy expenditure per unit mass. It is therefore possible literally to cut corners as shown in Fig.2b.

Again, once the next generation is in a position to assume its biological role, investment in the parents can drop if not altogether stop, unless it can be shown that its continuation would serve a useful purpose. To a first approximation one may therefore cut the second corner (Fig.2b).

The shape of this hypothetical trapezium can be considered as follows. The ratio between the duration of the horizontal part P – 2P to the life-span 0 – L should be as large as possible; the downward period is evidently sheer waste but its length may result from earlier constraints. This is exemplified by the variation of the amplitude of ocular accommodation as a function of age, which is considered below. The rising period is needed to make P -> 2P as effective as possible. It therefore needs to be short in the interest of economy, but sufficiently long to ensure adequate returns from the horizontal portion.

In connection with the development of the visual system, the rising phase contains several unresolved puzzles. For example, the retina is sufficiently well developed in 5m old foetuses to enable such prematurely born individuals to attain useful vision. This seems to run counter the above ideas on biological economy. However, it suggests that term used to be much shorter during earlier stages of human evolution. A reflexion of this may be seen in the observation that an undernourished population has a much greater prevalence of premature births than is true of well-to-do industrialised countries. In India, for example, the rate is 45% of births as compared with the United Kingdom's 6%.

Another puzzle is why young children should be able to accommodate with powers paradoxically extending up to 15 or 16 dioptres. This corresponds to a distance of 6 or 7cm from the eyes, and there is no biological activity that would seem to demand that. They find nipples by touch or by smell, they guide their thumbs into their mouths probably haptically but certainly not visually, and there are enough distant, i.e. high-frequency, stimuli present in most environments for contrast sensitivity to develop if the ocular media are normal.

Bito & Miranda (1987) mention in connection with a review of work on the accommodative amplitude of rhesus monkeys that rhesus babies spend much of their early time close to the mother, and hypothesise that a sharp image of her ventral detail may stimulate visual development. It should be noted that the rhesus baby's accommodative amplitude is more than twice as powerful as is true of that of an infant. While this hypothesis is probably valid for the animals, human babies are not nurtured in a remotely similar fashion: if present-day aboriginal evidence is anything to go by, they are carried on the mother's back to enable her to work, and have every opportunity to look into the distance. If human visual development depended on the early existence of a powerful accommodative mechanism, the considerable prevalence of accommodative insufficiency (Daum, 1983) might well be correlated with amblyopia: no report on such a conclusion appears to have been published.

In an attempt to resolve the above paradox, Weale (1990) postulated that there is a need for accommodation to have a power of some 4

dioptres (D) up to the age of 30y on the assumption that,
prehistorically, this age was approximately equal to 2P (cf. Fig.2b).
However, if this was to be vouchsafed to virtually every human being,
then 4D could not be an average, for otherwise half of mankind would
have an accommodation smaller than this postulated minimum value. In
order to ensure the basic biological requirement of universality, some 5
standard deviations had to be added by evolutionary pressures to 4D,
bringing the average requirement to 8D. This ensured that only about 1
individual in 10**6 or 10**7 would fall short of what was needed. Since
the world population before the stone age has been estimated at ½10**6
(McEvedy & Jones, 1978), this would appear to be a plausible condition.

A second hypothesis concerned the biological cost of accommodation,
and that of its run-down when the faculty is no longer needed.
Essentially, two constants are required to describe a varying mechanism:
one determines an original value, the other the rate of change. A
negative exponential would meet the case, but it can be shown that it
would be too expensive in terms of Fig.2b. The most cost-effective
mechanism was found to obey the equation

$$A/A(c) + Y/2P = 2$$

where A(c) is the amplitude of accommodation at the age 2P. Fig.3 shows
experimental measurements due to (1) Donders (1864), (2) Duane (1912),
(3) Hamasaki & al. (1956), and (4) Brückner & al. (1987). The
regression calculated for the points does not differ significantly from
the above equation.

This example provides a tentative explanation of why useful
physiological functions can continue well beyond a biologically fruitful
period. Cutting them off quickly might require the evolution of ad hoc
devices which would be costly either in terms of biological space or in
maintenance. It also shows that the same principle of bio-economics may
help to elucidate apparently wasteful functions during some parts of the
life-span. It is possible that the length of the latter, too, is the
result of an evolutionary pressure for the minimisation of overall

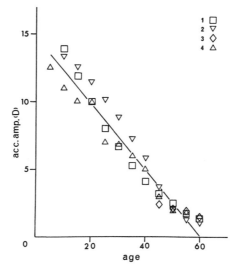

Fig.3. The variation of the amplitude of accommodation with age.
For refs. see text (Weale, 1990).

16

metabolic expenditure rather than that it should represent a part of a
hedonistic design. In fact, it can be shown that what appears to be long
for the human life-span (>100y), as compared with the period of human
fertility, is a consequence of the historic duration of P ($\frac{1}{4}$15y), the
number of years prehistorically intervening between successful
pregnancies, and the need for the maintenance of numbers of a species to
prevent its extinction.

3. The parabola of vision

The physical limit of the visual system as expressed by the
absolute visual threshold is set by the quantum nature of radiation.
Insofar as the visual pigments contained in the retinal photoreceptors
are present in early infancy (Fulton & Hansen, 1987), there is no reason
to doubt for the moment that we are born with the ability to be
stimulated by, though not necessarily to respond to, a small number of
quanta of radiation absorbed by the retina.

In practice there is, however, no need for low-threshold responses
in an infant's everyday life. It is also likely that ocular development
raises the threshold notwithstanding the age-related variation of ocular
aperture in early life, shown in Fig.1. In the first place, the amount
of light admitted into the eye is governed by the filtering properties
of the crystalline lens. These increase with age A(y) exponentially
according to the expression D = D(0).exp(βA), where D is the absorbance,
D(0) its value at birth, and β is an exponent, all three values varying
with the wavelength (cf. Fig.4, Weale, 1988). It follows that the amount
of radiation entering the eye and available for stimulating the retina
is progressively reduced, and this loss has to be allowed for in
threshold measurements.

The early accumulation of lipofuscin in the retinal pigment
epithelium (Wing & al., 1978; Feeney-Burns & al., 1984) may also
conceivably modify retinal performance. The reason is that lipofuscin
fluoresces when irradiated with relatively long-wavelength ultra-violet
radiation (UVA). The accumulation of this so-called "age-pigment" has
been linked tentatively to a photogenic effect of UVA, and the large
ocular aperture in early life (Fig.1) could be consistent with this

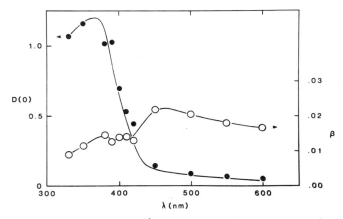

Fig.4. The values of D(0) and β, which enable one to estimate
      lenticular absorbance for large pupils. For pupils smaller
      than 4mm in diameter, these constants provide
      underestimates of the real situation for wavelengths <460nm
      (Weale, 1991). Courtesy: Editors, Journal of Physiology.

hypothesis. Weiter & al. (1986) have suggested that increasing lenticular yellowing may explain the slowing down of lipofuscin accumulation during the third decade of life, an idea that has recently been quantified (Weale, 1989, 1991). Lipofuscin fluorescence could generate a sort of haze in the retina, thereby interfering with some visual functions.

One of the most important of these is contrast vision. Several authors who have studied its threshold as a function of age (for summary, see Weale, 1982) have noted that it tends to decrease up to about the fourth decade of life and to rise thereafter. The optimal values obtained by McGrath & Morrison (1981) illustrate this (Fig.5a). This may be seen also in measurements of the visual acuity VA, usually expressed in terms of reciprocals of the least visual angle that can be resolved. If representative samples of VA (cf. Weale, 1982) are expressed in terms of their reciprocal (Fig.5b), the ensuing age-related variation echoes the plot for optimal contrast thresholds.

No reason for this parabolic variation does so far seem to have been advanced. But it can be seen on a qualitative basis that the hypothetical fluorescence of lipofuscin (and, indeed, of other retinal components) may play a role. Remember that though this fluorescence increases with age, the intensity of the radiation giving rise to it reaches the retina in ever decreasing quantities. However, even if there were no intrinsic senescence known to occur in the retina and its subsequent neural pathways, the progressive reduction in fluorescence could be counterbalanced by the increasing fluorescence of the crystalline lens (Lerman, 1988; Weale, 1985). This, too, can produce a haze, and potentially interfere with the perception of contrast.

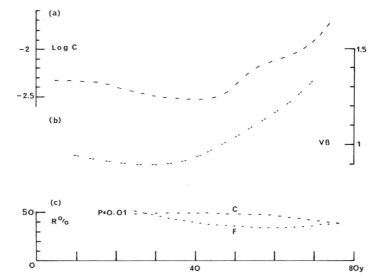

Fig.5. (a) The age-related variation of minimum values of [log]contrast thresholds (after McGrath & Morrison, 1981); (b) dtto for the smallest resolvable visual Snellen angle $'(from Weale, 1982); (c) dtto for percentage preferences of fluorescent tube illumination (C) with, and (F) without a UVA content (Weale, 1992). The P-value in (c) indicates that parabolas fit the experimental data much better than do linear regressions.

A recent study is relevant in this connection. Volunteers whose ages were divided into six decades (20-80y) were seated in a room illuminated with two white fluorescent tubes. One of these was covered with a filtered absorbing UVA radiation, the other was covered with a neutral filter to equate the luminances of the two when they were switched on in turn. The observers were given three tasks for each of which they had to say which of the two illuminants they preferred or whether they were indifferent to them. The tasks consisted of an assessment of coloured photographs, of reading fine print (4p), and also coarse print (22p). As there was no systematic significant difference as between the results for one task and another, the percentages of the responses were bulked, the "don't knows" having been negligibly small. Fig.5c shows that about 40% of those tested preferred the filtered light, which was a surprisingly large minority. Regression analysis for both groups showed that a parabolic regression function fitted the data better than did a linear one (Weale, 1992). This is consistent with the above hypothesis, namely that retinal fluorescence may hamper the young, while lenticular noise may tend to impede the vision of the elderly.

Other examples of age-related parabolic variations in vision are bound to occur to the reader. Reaction times and some aspects of colour vision spring to mind. It is noteworthy, however, that they manifest not at the retinal, but at more central levels: there is no such parabolic variation to be found in the number of photo-receptors or in the concentration of visual pigments. Yet, as we just noted, lenticular and retinal changes between them could possibly conspire to imprint onto the data-processing system of the eye the type of pattern shown in Fig.5, and so promote the kind of biological economy outlined earlier.

REFERENCES

Alexandridis, E. (1989). Iris und Pupillenreaktion im Alter. Ch.11. In: Handbuch der Gerontologie: Augenheilkunde (Platt, D. ed.) Gustav Fischer: New York.
Beutler, E. (1986). Planned obsolescence in humans and in other biosystems. Persp. Biol. Med. 29:175-179.
Bito, L. Z. & Miranda, O. C. (1987). Presbyopia: The need for a closer look. Ch.62. In: Presbyopia (Stark, L. & Obrecht, G. eds.). Fairchild Publications: New York.
Brückner, R., Batschelet, E. & Hugenschmidt, F. (1987). The Basel longitudinal study on aging (1955-1978). Docum. Ophthal. 64:235-310.
Daum, K. M. (1983). Accommodative dysfunction. Docum Ophthal. 55:177-198.
Donders, F. C. (1864). On the anomalies of accommodation at all ages. New Sydenham Society, London.
Duane, A. J. (1912). Normal values of the accommodation at all ages. Amer. Med. Assoc. 59:1010-1013.
Duke-Elder, Sir W. S. & MacFaul, P. (1972). A System of Ophthalmology. Vol. XIV. Henry Kimpton: London.
Feeney-Burns, L., Hildebrand, S. E. & Eldridge, S. (1984). Aging human RPE: Morphometric analysis of macular, equatorial and peripheral cells. Invest. Ophthal. Vis. Sci. 25:195-200.
Fulton, A. B. & Hansen, R. M. (1987). The relationship of retinal sensitivity and rhodopsin in human infants. Vision Res. 27:697-704.
Gershon, D. & Gershon, H. (1976). An evaluation of the "error catastrophe" theory of aging in the light of recent experimental results. Gerontology, 22:212-219.
Hamasaki, D., Ong, J. & Marg, E. (1956). The amplitude of accommodation in presbyopia. Amer. J. Optom. 33:3-14.

Harman, D. (1984). Free radical theory of aging: The "free radical" diseases. Age, 7:111-131.

Holliday, R. (1988). Toward a biological understanding of the ageing process. Persp. Biol. Med. 32:109-123.

Johnson, T. E. & McCaffrey, G. (1985). Programmed aging or error catastrophe? An examination by two-dimensional polyacrylamide gel electrophoresis. Mech. Ag. Dev. 30:285-297.

Kirkwood, T. B. L. (1984). Towards a unified theory of cellular ageing. Monogr. Devl. Biol. 17:9-20.

Laughrea, M. (1982). On the error theories of aging. Exp. Geront. 17:305-317.

Lerman, S. (1988). Human lens fluorescence aging index. Lens Res. 5:23-31.

McEvedy, C. & Jones, R. (1978). Atlas of World Population History. Allen Lane: London.

McGrath, C. & Morrison, G. D. (1981). The effects of age on spatial frequency perception in human subjects. Quart. J. Exp. Physiol. 66:253-261.

Meites, J., Goya, R. & Takehashi, S. (1987). Why the neuroendocrine system is important in aging processes. Exp. Gerontol. 22:1-15.

Orgel, L. E. (1963). The maintenance of the accuracy of protein synthesis and its relevance to aging. Proc. Nat. Acad. Sci. USA 49:517-521.

Orgel, L. E. (1973). Aging of clones of mammalian cells. Nature 243:441-445.

Weale, R. A. (1982). A Biography of the Eye - Development, Growth, Age. H. K. Lewis: London.

Weale, R. A. (1985). Human lenticular fluorescence and transmissivity, and their effects on vision. Exp. Eye Res. 41:457-473.

Weale, R. A. (1988). Age and the transmittance of the human crystalline lens. J. Physiol. (London) 395:577-587.

Weale, R. A. (1989). Do years or quanta age the retina? Photochem. Photobiol. 50:429-438.

Weale, R. A. (1990). Evolution, age and ocular focus. Mech. Ag. Dev. 53:85-89.

Weale, R. A. (1991). The lenticular nucleus, light, lens, and the retina. Exp. Eye Res. in press.

Weale, R. A. (1992). Personal preferences for fluorescent tubes with and without UVA. Lighting Research and Technology, in press.

Weiter, J. J., Delori, F. C., Wing, G. L. & Fitch, K. A. (1986). Retinal pigment epithelium lipofuscin and melanin and choroidal melanin in human eyes. Invest. Ophthal. Vis. Sci. 27:145-152.

Wing, G. L., Blanchard, G. C. & Weiter, J. J. (1978). The topography and age relationship of lipofuscin concentration in the retinal pigment epithelium. Invest. Ophthal. Vis. Sci. 17:601-607.

ANIMAL MODELS OF LIFE-SPAN DEVELOPMENT

William Hodos[*]

Age Concern Institute of Gerontology
Kings College London
London SE1 8TX, U.K.

At this NATO Advanced Study Institute we are concerned with the changes that occur in the visual system throughout life from the embryo through the juvenile phase, adulthood and senescence. The research that will be discussed at this meeting has been performed on a variety of species: various non-human mammalian species, birds, humans, fishes, etc. Since many of these animals differ in their life span and in their life expectancy, we must consider how to compare changes observed in one species with a short life span with comparable changes that occur in a species with relatively long longevity. This problem is of particular concern to those who would compare animal data with human data.

In this paper, I shall (1) discuss some of the reasons for studying aging in non-human animals; (2) make some recommendations as to which groups of animals are the most appropriate for various purposes; and (3) suggest a method for comparing animal species that differ in their life span.

Before I begin, let me define some of the terms that will be used in this paper. "Life span" is the maximum reported age for a given species or other group. "Mortality rate" is the cumulative percentage of a population that have died at a particular age. "Life expectancy" is the age at which the mortality rate is 50%. "Longitudinal studies" are those in which the same group of individuals is studied at several (or many) different ages or stages of development. "Cross-sectional studies" are those in which different groups of individuals are studied, each at a different age or stage of development.

WHY ANIMAL MODELS?

1. Most animals have shorter lives than humans, which means that life-span longitudinal studies can be carried out within a reasonable proportion of the experimenter's life.

---

[*]Present address: Department of Psychology, University of Maryland, College Park, MD 20742-4411, USA.

The Changing Visual System, Edited by P. Bagnoli and
W. Hodos, Plenum Press, New York, 1991

2. Many animals show age-related changes in one or more biological systems that are very similar to age-related changes in comparable systems in humans.

3. Some experiments cannot be done on humans for bioethical reasons.

4. Rapid feedback from the effects of experimental treatments on longevity is possible.

5. The relatively shorter animal life offers the possibility to separate "age-related" or "developmental" effects from mere "calendar" effects.

Developmental or age-related effects are those that are determined, at least in part, by intrinsic, genetically determined mechanisms that come into operation at a certain phase in the life span. Various theories have been proposed to account for changes that occur at the senescent end of the life span (Sacher, 1978; Merry, 1987). These include, the notions of specific genes that induce aging, failure of the organism to tolerate DNA damage, or an accumulation of errors of transcription and translation from DNA during protein synthesis. Kirkwood (1981, 1990) has proposed a natural-selection theory of aging, the disposable-soma theory, which states that organisms that inhabit high-risk environments improve the survival of their species if they invest their bodily resources heavily in reproduction and related activities, such as parental care, rather than in the maintenance of their own somatic cells. Such creatures will tend to have large numbers of offspring and relatively short life spans due to an accumulation of unrepaired somatic defects. Species in low-risk environments, however, can afford the luxury of investment in the repair of their somatic tissues and thereby will have greater longevity. These classes of theories are not necessarily mutually exclusive.

Changes that occur at a particular phase of the life span also may occur because the individual has been progressively exposed to certain environmental factors. Such causes may be termed "exposure" effects or "calendar" effects. For example, we can easily show that the seasonal darkening of Caucasian skin during the summer months is a calendar effect due to number of hours of exposure to ultraviolet light and not a genetically programmed annual event. An example closer to the subject of this conference has to do with the age-related yellowing of the human crystalline lens. The human lens becomes progressively more pigmented with increasing age to the extent that by the sixth decade, the effective light reaching the retina has been reduced to 40% of the intensity that reaches the retina in a 20-year old (Weale, 1982). A widely accepted theory is that a major contributory factor in the yellowing is caused by exposure to short-wavelength light (Weale, 1982, 1989). In contrast, the lenses of old pigeons and old quail are colorless. Is this difference due to the fact that pigeons and other birds are capable of detecting ultraviolet light (Remy and Emmerton, 1989) and therefore have evolved a mechanism to protect their lenses from yellowing with exposure? Or are we merely observing a calendar effect? In other words, if years of exposure are the culprit in lens yellowing, why would we expect a deeply yellow lens in a 17-year old (elderly) pigeon any more than we would in a 17-year old (young) human? An answer to this would be to compare pigeons with parrots, which have a life span that is more comparable to that of humans. Indeed, Christopher Murphy, a veterinary ophthalmologist at the University of Wisconsin, who specializes in birds, has informed me that there is no reported evidence of lens yellowing with age in any species of bird that has been studied, even elderly specimens of long-longevity species such as parrots. If cumulative ultraviolet exposure is the causative agent in lens darkening, then birds may have evolved a protective mechanism against this to protect their ability to detect and discriminate ultraviolet light.

Some cautions must be observed in extrapolating from animal studies to humans. Although they may appear to be similar to humans in their biological and psychological processes, the actual mechanisms of function in the animal model may be different; hence the causes of aging and the prevention and/or treatment of aging may differ in the animal model and in humans. For example, the avian eye is similar to the human eye in both the morphology and in the functions of its individual parts. But the intraocular muscles of birds are not smooth as they are in humans, but rather are striated muscles, which means that their pharmacology and some aspects of their physiology are quite different. Thus studies of both the causes and treatment of presbyopia in birds may have limited applicability to humans.

WHICH ANIMALS MAKE THE BEST MODELS?

If we are interested in studying life-span or senescent changes in a particular biological system, such as the visual system, rather than longevity of the animal, the choice of animal should be determined by the extent of development of the system of interest as well as rate of aging of that system. In addition, certain practical considerations should be taken into account:

1. The animals should be readily available.

2. They should be inexpensive to obtain and maintain.

3. They should have a fairly short life span so that life-span longitudinal studies are possible.

4. They should be sufficiently plentiful for cross-sectional studies, which often require larger sample sizes.

5. For purposes of extrapolation to human aging, the animals do not necessarily have to look like humans, so long as the particular biological system of interest is similar. Thus, non-human primates are not the only useful animal models of human aging. As we depart from close genetic affinity with humans, however, we must exercise caution in interpretation because other variables can affect our ability to apply the conclusions directly to humans.

Table 1. presents my assessment of the relative degree of appropriateness of various groups of animals for various purposes. The list certainly is not exhaustive, but it does present a number of important characteristics. The reader is hereby warned that the ratings given in the table are my subjective assessments based on my reading of the comparative anatomy and comparative behavior literatures. Other experts might make somewhat different assessments, but I suspect that their evaluations might not differ too greatly from mine. A final caveat: since the animal

TABLE 1. Survey of the Suitability of Various Vertebrate Groups as Animal Models

	NON-HUMAN PRIMATES	NON-PRIMATE MAMMALS	BIRDS	REPTILES	AMPHIBIANS	FISHES
LARGE BRAIN	+ + + +	+ + +	+ + +	+	+	+
BIPED	-	+	+ + + + +	-	-	-
EXCELLENT VISION	+ + + + +	+ +	+ + + + +	+ + + +	-	-
EXCELLENT HEARING	+ + + + +	+ + + +	+ + +	+ +	+ +	+
COMPLEX VOCAL REPERTOIRE	+ +	+ +	+ + + +	+	+	+
COMPLEX SOCIAL REPERTOIRE	+ + + + +	+ + + +	+ + + +	+	+	+ +
STRONG PAIR BOND	+ +	+ +	+ + + +	-	-	+
EXTENDED PARENTAL CARE	+ + + + +	+ + + + +	+ + + + +	+ +	+	+
INTELLIGENT	+ + + +	+ + +	+ + +	+	-	+

+ + + + + ALL OR NEARLY ALL   + + + + MOST   + + + MANY
+ + SOME   + A FEW   - NONE OR HARDLY ANY

subjects of my own research are birds, do not be surprised to find them scoring rather well in the table.

If a large brain relative to body size is important, many birds, whales and dolphins and most non-human primates may be considered. If bipedal locomotion is important then one must look to birds, kangaroos and other hopping mammals, but not to the non-human primates because their locomotion is not bipedal even though they can stand on their hind legs and walk bipedally for short distances. With regard to the subject matter of this conference, vision, researchers can turn to some reptiles, most birds, many mammals and the great majority of non-human primates. Similar choices could be made for hearing.

The table also contains recommendations for animal choices for the study of vocal communication (many birds, some mammals, some non-human primates), social organization (many birds, many mammals, many non-human primates), strong pair bond (many birds, some mammals, some non-human primates), extended parental care (some fishes, a few amphibians, a few reptiles, all birds, all mammals, including non-human primates) and intelligence (many birds, many mammals, nearly all non-human primates).

As you can see, birds have more characteristics in common with humans than do most mammals. Some mammals, however, and especially non-human primates may be adequate models for life-span development and aging of specific systems, such as the visual system, if the rest of the animal can safely be ignored. Two additional factors that are of great importance in the choice of any animal for life-span developmental studies are the life span and the relative rate of aging. These will be the focus of the remainder of this chapter.

BIOLOGICAL SYSTEMS AGE AT DIFFERENT RATES

Studies of aging typically deal in such actuarial statistics as life span or longevity and life expectancy or mortality rate (Sacher, 1978; Kirkwood, 1985; Finch, Pike and Witten, 1990). Such data are of great importance for evaluating the survivability of the species under various circumstances, but one must consider that these actuarial data include death from *all causes*. Thus an actuarial approach may be quite misleading for an individual system of the body that ages at a different rate from that indicated by the survivability curve for the whole animal. Some systems may age less rapidly than those that result in loss of life; other systems may age more rapidly yet their degeneration may not frequently lead to death. An example of the latter is the greying of hair in mammals, which commonly occurs with advanced years but invariably begins well before death. Greying of the hair, however, should not affect the rate of mortality unless it increased the risk of predation by making the animal more visible. On the other hand, if a major cause of death beyond a certain age is due to fragility of the skeletal system, this could drastically affect longevity, but may have little or no effect on the rate of aging of the visual system. Moreover, measures that increase longevity by reducing skeletal fragility may not necessarily affect the rate of senescence in the eye or central visual pathways.

Finch, Pike and Witten (1990) suggest that acceleration of the mortality rate, as represented by the time required for the mortality rate at puberty to double, is a useful way to make cross-species comparisons of relative rates of aging. This approach would appear to have merit in an actuarial context; i.e., it represents well how the effects of changes in or intervention in a particular biological system, such as the endocrine system, may affect the longevity of the animal as a whole. Unfortunately, this and other actuarial methods are not at all useful for studying the rate of aging with that system itself unless changes in that system are the cause of death.

RELATIVE RATES OF AGING

When considering the age of an animal model, one must take into account both absolute age and relative age. For calendar effects, absolute age, which could correspond to the absolute amount of exposure to the variable in question, may be a pertinent consideration irrespective of absolute age. But for developmental or aging studies of animals with life spans that are very different from those of humans, a more appropriate measure may be the relative age of the animal. In other words, if we are studying an animal such as a laboratory hamster with a life span of three years (Finch, Pike and Witten, 1990) to which human age would you compare such an animal when it was six months old? One could compare each species on the basis of age as a proportion of life span (i.e., absolute age divided by the life span) and compare the animal and the human on that basis. In this example, six months is 17% of the life span. If we estimate human life span to be 120, then a hamster at six months would correspond to a human 20 years old. Using the time required for the mortality rate to double (MRD) as Finch, Pike and Witten suggest, the hamster would have MRD = 0.5 and the human would have MRD = 8.0. Neither of these or other actuarial approaches, however, would be of help in determining relative rates of aging in individual body systems such as the endocrine system or the subject of our meeting, the visual system. My point here is that animal biological systems are a mosaic of autonomous or semi-autonomous mechanisms and almost certainly age at different rates. These differences are obscured by any actuarial approach to life span.

BIOMARKERS OF AGING

An approach that may be more suitable to the comparison of differing rates of development or aging of individual systems and in different species than the actuarial approach is based on the concept of "biomarkers" (Baker and Sprott, 1988). A biomarker is a biological or behavioral variable measured at a point in the life span

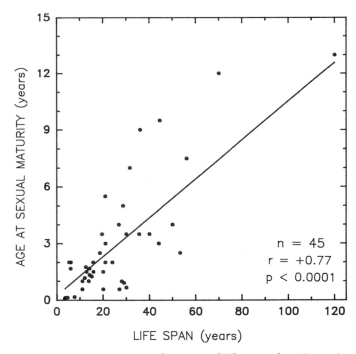

Fig. 1. Age at sexual maturity as a function of life span for 45 species of birds, reptiles, mammals and amphibians.

and that is capable of predicting the functional integrity of that biological system at a later age. The direction of change of the biomarker (whether it represents an increase or decrease of function) is of no importance; changes in either direction are of value. An important difference between the actuarial approach and the biomarker approach is that for actuarial data, the time course of changes in any given biological system is irrelevant; only the age of the animal at the time of death is critical. For the biomarker approach to life span, the time course of such changes is the basic datum. The biomarker approach recognizes that different biological systems age at different rates and these rates can only be determined by reference to events that occur during the life history of that system independently of when the animal may die from whatever cause. For our purposes here, our only concern with the death of the animal would be if it were caused by failing vision.

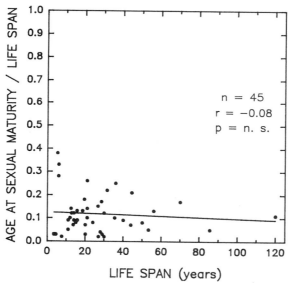

Fig. 2. Age at sexual maturity as a proportion of life span plotted as a function of life span for the same 45 species as in Fig. 1.

As an illustration of one way to use the biomarker approach, let us look at the relationship between the age of onset of reproduction as a function of age. Figure 1 presents a plot of the age of puberty as a function of life span for 45 species of mammals, reptiles, amphibians and birds. The data were taken from tables in the Biology Data Book (Altman and Dittman, 1974). Where several values were given, an average was taken. The figure shows a systematic relationship between the onset of puberty and life span, which would seem to be consistent with some of the notions implicit in Kirkwood's (1981, 1985, 1990) disposable-soma theory of aging. The coefficient of correlation between age at puberty and life span is $r = +0.77$, p <0.0001, which indicates that 59% of the variance in age at puberty is accounted for

Table 2. Relative Reproductive Aging

SPECIES	LIFE SPAN (years)	AGE OF ONSET OF PUBERTY (years)	RATIO OF AGE OF PUBERTY TO LIFE SPAN
human	120	13	0.11
quail	3.79	0.13	0.03
pig	27	0.58	0.02
cow	30	0.67	0.02
gorilla	36	9	0.25

by the variance in life span. How can we make a biomarker out of these data? One way is to transform age at sexual maturity to relative age at sexual maturity; i.e., age at puberty as a proportion of life span. When the relative age at puberty is plotted as function of life span the result is a virtual constant, except for the animals with very short life spans. The median proportion is 0.095, which means that for these 45 vertebrate species, the onset of reproduction occurs at approximately 10% of the life span. The coefficient of correlation is r = -0.08, which is not significant. Within these vertebrate classes, birds and non-primate mammals generally begin their reproductive behavior at about 3-8% of life span, primates tend to begin reproduction at about 12% of life span and amphibians and reptiles begin at about 13-16% of life span. The value of these data is that the constancy of the relative age at which reproduction begins offers us a way to compare rates of reproductive aging that is based on age-related events that occur in the neuroendocrine system relative to the life span rather than dealing only with age-specific death rates as in the actuarial approach. This particular way of using biomarkers could be termed an "inflection biomarker" because it takes advantage of a consistent inflection point in the biomarker curve rather than merely tracking the course of a biological event through the life span.

Let us now look at some specific examples shown in Table 2. Let us compare a human female with a life span of 120 years with an ovulating female quail with a life span of 3.8 years (Woodard and Abplanalp, 1971). The female quail reaches puberty in 4-5 weeks after hatching. Thus a female quail is sexually mature at 3% of her life span. In contrast, a human female who reached puberty at age 13 would have done so at 11% of her life span. These differences mean that a simple linear transformation of the animal model's age into human years based on life-span data alone may lead to very different conclusions about relative development or aging rates in specific biological systems than would a comparison based on significant events (biomarkers) within those systems themselves. The biomarker approach would suggest that the quail was developing more rapidly than the human because she reached sexual maturity at a relatively earlier point in her life span. A similar analysis could be performed for the age of menopause.

Some further examples: pigs have a life span of 27 years and an age of onset of reproduction of 0.58 years, which is 2% of life span. Cows have similar values: 30 years for life span and 0.67 years for reproductive onset. In contrast, gorillas, which have a similar life span of 36 years, have an age of puberty of 9 years, which is 25% of life span. Compared to humans, quail, cows and pigs show a more rapid development of reproduction because a smaller proportion of their life span is required for this event to occur.   Since gorillas do not begin reproduction until a quarter of their life span has passed, their reproductive systems develop at a much slower rate. Note also that even though ovulating female quail have a much shorter life span and a much earlier onset of ovulation (4.5 weeks = 0.13 years), this biomarker occurs at approximately the same proportion of the life span as in pigs and cows; therefore the three species have approximately the same rate of reproductive development even though their life spans and ages of onset differ greatly. If one accepts this line of reasoning, then it follows that although a short life span makes an animal species convenient for life-span longitudinal studies, a short life span by itself does not mean that every biological system of that species necessarily develops or ages faster than humans.

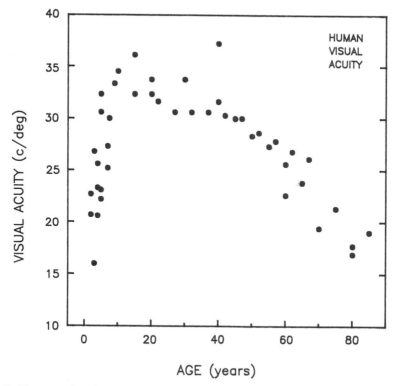

Fig. 3. Human visual acuity as a function of age. Adapted from Weale (1982).

DEVELOPMENT AND AGING OF THE VISUAL SYSTEM

A number of indicators of visual function have been described that could serve to quantify the rates of development and aging in the visual system. Such biomarkers also could be used to determine whether the entire visual system ages at the same rate or whether the individual components age separately? For example, does aging of the crystalline lens occur at the same rate as aging of the retina? Does the retina age at the same rate as the visual cortex? Do rods age as quickly as cones? Do all layers of the visual cortex age at the same rate?

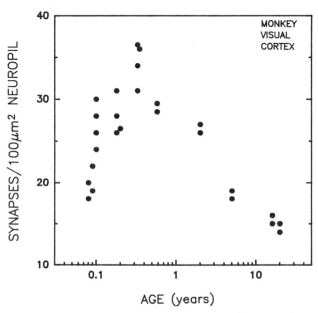

Fig. 4. Density of synaptic spines in the primary visual cortex of monkeys as a function of age. The data have been replotted from Rakic et al., (1986).

One visual biomarker is the time required to recover from the effects of glare (Reading, 1968). This duration remains roughly constant through the fourth decade in humans after which it shows a rapid acceleration upward when plotted against the life span. Other visual phenomena show a different pattern of change; i.e., an early improvement in performance, a peak in young adulthood or middle life followed by a later decline. For example, the ability to arrange a group of color samples in the correct spectral order rises to a peak at about age 20 and thereafter declines. This has been reported both in normal and color-defective humans (Verriest et al., 1962; Lakowski, 1974). Similar results have been reported for color matching (Lakowski, 1958). A temporal-resolution biomarker is the ability to discriminate the interval between two closely spaced flashes of light; performance on this task is optimal in the late teens (Amberson et al., 1959). Finally, visual acuity can serve as a useful biomarker. Figure 3 shows data adapted from data compiled by Weale (1982). This figure is a composite of the work of a number of scientists, some who studied the entire life span and others who investigated narrower ranges. The figure reveals that in humans acuity continues to improve from infancy until the middle twenties; thereafter it shows a progressive decline. An example of a morphological inflection biomarker for the visual system may be seen in the numbers of synaptic spines in monkey primary visual cortex (Rakic et al.,1986) and shown in Figure 4.

We have found an acuity peak in female quail that were studied in a longitudinal design (Hodos, et al., this volume) that appears similar to the human acuity peak. Ovulating female quail have their acuity peak at about 10 months, which is about 22% of their life span. The quail peak occurs at about the same relative portion of the life span as does the human peak, which occurs at about 21% of life span. Thus, even though female quail and humans have very different life-span durations, their visual systems are aging at about the same rate relative to their own life spans.

Some pitfalls of the inflection biomarker approach should be considered. First, we must be able to rule the possibility that the post-peak decline is actually a developmental process and not an exposure or calendar effect. Second, we must consider the possibility that the ascending limb of the inflection-biomarker curve may be due to one process and the descending limb due to another. The latter situation would not necessarily invalidate the biomarker, but it would make interpretation more complicated.

CONCLUSIONS

Non-human animal species can play a useful role in studies of development and aging. In general, animals with short life spans are the most practical for longitudinal studies because their life span is a relatively small proportion of the experimenter's life span. Although development and aging may be studied meaningfully within a single species, a problem arises when comparisons are to be made between species with very different life spans. Relative rates of aging of the entire organism, its individual biological systems or its behavioral processes can be assessed by the relative location of significant events (inflection biomarkers) within the life span of the species to be compared. Where the inflection biomarker occurs after a smaller proportion of the life span has elapsed, the rate of aging or development can be assumed to be higher than where the significant event has occurred relatively later in the life span. The inflection-biomarker approach indicates that although an animal may have a shorter life span than a human, it does not necessarily develop or age more rapidly.

ACKNOWLEDGEMENTS

This article was written while the author was a Visiting Professor at the Age Concern Institute of Gerontology, Kings College London. I am most grateful to the Director, Professor Anthea Tinker, for making the visit possible by generously providing space and administrative support in the stimulating environment of the Institute and to Professor Robert A. Weale for his encouragement and for sharing his insights in the course of many thought-provoking and instructive discussions about vision, aging and life-span development. Thanks also are due to Professor Weale and to Dr. T. B. L. Kirkwood for their valuable comments on an earlier draft of this paper.

This work was partially supported by grants from the US National Eye Institute through grants EY-00735 and EY-04742.

REFERENCES

Amberson, J. I., Atkeson, B. M., Oottack, R. H. and Malatesta, V. J., 1959, Age differences in dark-interval threshold across the life-span. Exper. Aging Res., 26:407-417.

Baker, G. T. III and Sprott, R. L., 1988, Biomarkers of Aging. Exp. Gerontol., 23:223-239.

Altman, P. L. and Dittman, D. S., 1974, "Biology Data Book," Federation of Societies of Experimental Biology, Bethesda, Maryland.

Finch, C. E., Pike, M. C. and Witten, M., 1990, Slow mortality rate accelerations during aging in some mammals and birds approximate that of humans. Science, 249:902-905.

Lakowski, R.,1958, Age and colour vision. Adv. Sci., 59:231-236.

Lakowski, R., 1974, Effects of age on the 100-hue scores of red-green deficient subjects. Mod. Problems Ophthalmol., 13:124-129.

Kirkwood, T. B. L., 1981, Repair and its evolution: survival versus reproduction, in "Physiological Ecology: An Evolutionary Approach to Resource Use," C. R. Townsend and P. Calow, (eds.), Blackwell, Oxford.

Kirkwood, T. B. L., 1985, Comparative and evolutionary aspects of longevity, in "Handbook of the Biology of Aging," C. E. Finch and E. L. Schneider, eds., van Nostrand Reinhold, New York.

Kirkwood, T. B. L., 1990, The disposable soma theory of aging, in "Genetic Effects on Aging II," D. E. Harrison, ed., Telford, Caldwell, NJ.

Merry, B. J., 1987, Biological mechanisms of ageing. Eye, 1:163-170.

Rakic, P., Bourgeois, J. -P., Eckenhoff, M, Zecevic, N. and Goldman-Rakic,P.S., 1986, Concurrent overproduction of synapses in diverse regions of primate cerebral cortex. Science, 232:232-235.

Reading, V. M., 1968, Disability glare and age. Vision Res., 8:207-214.

Remy, M. and Emmerton, J., 1989, Behavioral spectral sensitivities of different retinal areas in pigeons. Behav. Neurosci., 103:170-177.

Sacher, G. A., 1978, Evolution of longevity and survival characteristics in mammals, in "The Genetics of Aging," E. L. Schneider (ed.), Plenum, New York.

Verriest, G., Vandevyvere, R. and Vanderdonk, R., 1962, Nouvelles recherches se rapportant à l'influence du sexe et de l'âge sur la discrimination chromatique ainsi qu'à la signification practique des résultats du test 100 hue de Farnsworth-Munsell. Rev. d'Optique, 41:499-509.

Weale, R. A. 1982, "A Biography of the Eye: Development, Growth Age", Lewis, London.

Weale, R. A. 1989 Do years or quanta age the retina? Vision Res., 50:429-438.

Woodard, A. E. and Abplanalp, H., 1971, Longevity and reproduction in Japanese quail maintained under stimulatory lighting. Poultry Sci., 50:688-692.

ONTOGENETIC CLUES TO THE PHYLOGENY OF THE VISUAL SYSTEM

Bernd Fritzsch

Creighton University, Dept. Biomed. Sci.
Omaha, Nebraska 68178, USA

"To suppose that the eye with all its inimitable contrivancies for adjusting the focus to different distances, for admitting different amounts of light, and for the correction of spherical and chromatic aberration, could have been formed by natural selection, seems, I freely confess, absurd in the highest possible degrees. "

C. Darwin (1859)

INTRODUCTION

The visual system of vertebrates has long presented a puzzle for evolutionary biology: Darwin himself pointed out the difficulties of understanding how such a perfect dioptric apparatus with extra- as well as intraocular muscles, motoneurons, and connections for neuronal analysis could have evolved through stages where this entire system was at best functioning rather differently. Fossil vertebrates have been of very limited help because they either had no eyes or fully developed lateral eyes. Moreover, the relationship of fossil jawless vertebrates to living vertebrates, in particular to hagfish, is largely obscure (Carroll, 1988). The gap in our knowledge of vertebrate lateral eye evolution was addressed in a number of pertinent papers at the turn of the century. The hope at that time was that studies of the organization of the visual system of primitive craniate vertebrates, like hagfish, might provide clues to the ancestral condition of jawed vertebrates. Retzius (1893) was the first to conclude that the eye of hagfish is regressed rather than primitive. Older and more recent suggestions along this line (Franz, 1934; Walls, 1942; Duke-Elder, 1958; Holmberg, 1978; Wicht and Northcutt, 1990) were rooted in the belief that hagfish are modern descendents of fossil jawless vertebrates known to have had large eyes and were supported by the apparent similarities between the hagfish eye and the regressed eyes of some amphibians (Franz, 1934; Wake, 1985) and fish (Franz, 1934; Peters and Peters, 1984). Unfortunately, the

The Changing Visual System, Edited by P. Bagnoli and
W. Hodos, Plenum Press, New York, 1991

differences between the retinae of jawless (Holmberg, 1978) and jawed vertebrates have not been put into an evolutionary context. Consequently, the substantial evidence for evolutionary changes at least in the neural retina as presented here went unrecognized for almost a century.

In the absence of any obvious way to solve the problem of eye evolution through analysis of existing visual systems, ontogenetic data (as a model of phylogenetic recapitulation) in conjunction with hypotheses about the evolution of the visual system were used to bridge that gap in our knowledge (Franz, 1934; Sarnat and Netsky, 1974). Common to all these models is that at any stage of eye formation the existing structure must have served some function, otherwise it would not have provided any adaptive advantage that helps to propagate the bearer of this change more efficiently than its contemporaries.

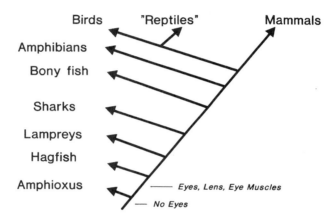

Fig. 1. This simplified cladogram shows the contemporary view of the evolution of the vertebrate eyes as expressed in many textbooks. The eye has apparently evolved without leaving any detectable tract of its evolution and was already fully differentiated more or less in its present form in fossil jawless vertebrates.

One of these models was proposed first by Balfour (1885), independently by Franz (1934), and was later modified by Sarnat and Netsky (1974), among others. This model takes as a starting point the fact that there is a general light sensitivity around the ventricle of the forebrain and suggests that these forebrain neurons were transformed in the course of evolution into an assemblage of neurons capable of analyzing strictly visual information rather than any other information carried to this area by other input neurons. The processed visual information was transferred through relay neurons (the future ganglion cells) to the contralateral part of the brain. In subsequent generations, this primordial retina evaginated and eventually transformed into the lateral eyes of extant vertebrates.

Appealing as these hypotheses may be, they largely focus on the morphogenetic process of eye formation rather than on the transformation of an area of the forebrain into the neural retina. Consequently the following problems have not been discussed:

1) During ontogeny, the vertebrate eye does not recapitulate this proposed evolutionary scenario and, instead, first develops through morphogenetic movements of the forebrain before any differentiation of the retina takes place (Gilbert, 1988). Furthermore, recent experimental evidence shows that morphogenesis and differentiation of the retina are two independent developmental processes which may have evolved independently and were rearranged in their timing during evolution.

2) Given that the retina apparently represents a transformed part of the forebrain which has acquired a distinct neuronal organization, one may ask how this transformation occurred. Data on the different distributions of ganglion cells in the retina of jawed and jawless vertebrates will be presented below and compared to the organization of the forebrain of vertebrates and to the derived pattern of retinal organization of jawed vertebrates.

3) The different distributions of ganglion cells in jawless and jawed vertebrates may be parallelled by different patterns of retinal projections. Evidence will be provided that indicates that a bilateral rather than a completely crossed, contralateral projection may have been primitive for craniate vertebrates.

4) Prior to the transformation of a part of the forebrain into the retina, this forebrain area must have had an input from other parts of the brain and performed a rather different function. Presumably, this input was later modified and eventually substituted by the input generated by illumination. Quantitative data suggest that there is a higher proportion of retinopetal neurons in jawless vertebrates and it will be argued that this reflects the above suggested modification/substitution which is not fully realized in jawless vertebrates.

5) The last part will introduce the different patterns of extra- and intraocular muscles in vertebrates and will speculate on possible reasons for the observed differences.

Together these changes strongly suggest that major aspects of the evolution of the neural retina and the motor systems of the eye can be studied in living vertebrates.

1) EVIDENCE THAT MORPHOGENESIS OF THE EYE AND DIFFERENTIATION OF THE RETINA ARE UNRELATED PROCESSES

During ontogenetic development the eye forms through a complex interaction between neuroectoderm, mesoderm and endoderm. First, the eye field is induced by pharyngeal endoderm and head mesoderm in the neural plate. Second, the eye anlage evaginates and then invaginates to form the outer and inner layers of the optic cup. Subsequently, the inner part of the eyecup differentiates into the neural retina and the outer part into the pigment epithelium. Finally, when the optic cup reaches the overlying epidermis it will induce the formation of the lens placode at that specific location (Jacobson and Sater, 1988; Gilbert, 1988).

Clearly, this ontogenetic scenario is not a recapitulation of the above proposed phylogenetic scenario. If interpreted in a strict sense of Haeckelian recapitulation, it rather suggests that the evagination of the eyecup took place before any differentiation of the retina occurred. However, heterochronic changes, i.e. changes of the relative timing of appearance, are among the best characterized evolutionary events (Arnold et al., 1989). Thus, it can not be ruled out that the ontogeny of the vertebrate eye reflects a heterochronic transformation of evolutionary events rather than the original temporal pattern. This suggestion implies that the morphogenesis of the eye and the differentiation of the neural retina are two independent events whose temporal sequence can be freely rearranged. We have recently tested this suggestion experimentally by employing the vitamin A metabolite retinoic acid (RA).

RA showes features of a vertebrate morphogen and alters the normal development of the forebrain (Durston et al., 1989, Sive et al., 1990). We have tested the effect of RA on the morphogenesis and differentiation of the **Xenopus** retina (Manns and Fritzsch, 1991). Complete blockade of eye formation was achieved with 10^{-5} M RA applied for 20 minutes at **Xenopus** stages 9-11. Eye features developed more normally as RA-concentrations were applied at increasingly later stages. At stage 12 there was a concentration dependent effect of RA which often resulted in the complete blockade of eye morphogenesis without noticeable effects on the differentiation of the retina. In the most severe cases, the eye developed as an apparently functional area within the forebrain. The dorsal part of the forebrain contained the pigment epithelium whereas the adjacent ventral part of the forebrain differentiated into a retina. In these cases, the outer segments of the receptor cells protruded into the third ventricle and were nowhere close to the pigmented epithelium (Manns and Fritzsch, 1991).

These data clearly show that RA affects the two apparently independent developmental processes differently: morphogenesis and differentiation of the eye. This experimental separation of the two processes is therefore

compatible with the suggestion that the development of the
vertebrate eye is a uniquely derived heterochronic
rearrangement of two processes and that ontogeny does not
necessarily reflect the evolutionary sequence in which both
changes were introduced. In other words, the observed
sequence of normal developmental events of the eye does not
recapitulate evolution but rather reflects a temporal
ontogenetic rearrangement.

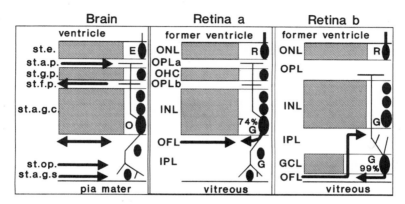

Figure 2. The distribution of cells (hatched areas), areas of neuropil, input regions
(arrows toward the right), and output regions (arrows toward the left) of the lamprey
optic tectum (brain), the lamprey retina (retina a) and jawed vertebrate retina (retina
b) are shown. The cell layering and the fiber organization are very similar in the
lamprey retina and tectum. Both are different from retina b. Thin lines connected to
output (O) and ganglion cells (G) are dendrites. Numbers indicate the proportion of
ganglion cells (G) in this layer. E, ependymal cells; G, ganglion cells; GCL, ganglion cell
layer; INL, inner nuclear layer; IPL, inner plexiform layer; O, major output neurons; OFL,
optic fiber layer; OHC, outer horizontal cells; ONL, outer nuclear layer; OPL (a,b), outer
plexiform layer (a,b); R, receptor cells; st.a.g.c., stratum album et griseum centrale;
st.a.g.s., stratum album et griseum superficiale; st.a.p., stratum album periventriculare;
st.e, stratum ependymale; st.f.p., stratum fibrosum profundum; st.g.p., stratum griseum
periventriculare; st.op., stratum opticum. Modified after Nieuwenhuys (1977) and
Fritzsch and Collin (1990).

2) ORGANIZATION OF THE VERTEBRATE RETINA

     Having shown that the transformation of the forebrain
into the neural retina is a problem in its own right, it is
obviously relevant to compare the organization of the retina
in different vertebrates to find evidence for evolutionary
changes. Although a detailed description of all cells and
their synaptic interactions is beyond the scope of this

paper, it is worthwhile to comment on the different organization of the ganglion cell and fiber layers among vertebrates.

In lampreys, most ganglion cells are in a layer where only a few, ectopic ganglion cells are found in jawed vertebrates. Moreover, in lampreys the ganglion cell axons course between the inner plexiform and inner nuclear layers and not along the vitreal layer as in jawed vertebrates (Tretjakov, 1916; Fritzsch and Collin, 1990). Outgroup comparisons show a somewhat similar organization of the hagfish retina (Holmberg, 1978), although the details are less clear than in lampreys. Comparison of the lamprey retina with the adjacent parts of the brain (i.e. the preoptic, tectal and hypothalamic regions) reveal striking similarities in the distribution of cells and fibers (Fig. 2). In contrast, the retina of jawed vertebrates shows a very different distribution of ganglion cells and their fibers when compared either to brain organization or the lamprey retina. The ganglion cells are separated only by the optic fiber layer from the vitreous (Fig. 2). This difference is particularly noteworthy given that there is not a single area in the brain of any vertebrate in which virtually all output neurons are segregated below the meninges and furthermore are separated by an area of neuropil from the vast majority of interneurons, as it is the case with the ganglion cells in the jawed vertebrate retina.

Comparing the organization of the eyes of hagfish and lampreys with areas of the brain adjacent to the optic chiasm in lampreys indicates remarkable similarities in the distribution of cells and fibers. Thus the retina of both lamprey and hagfish may represent the primitive pattern of craniate vertebrates. In contrast, the pattern of distribution of ganglion cells and their fibers in jawed vertebrates likely represents a derived pattern. Consistent with this hypothesis, recent data on the organization of amacrine cells shows some differences between lampreys and jawed vertebrates (Versaux-Botteri et al., 1991).

It is not clear how, why or when the reorganization of the presumably primitive lamprey (and hagfish) retina into the jawed vertebrate retina occurred. The virtual absence of physiological data on the function of the lamprey retina (Rovainen, 1982; Vesselkin et al., 1989) is particularly disappointing given the vast amount of data we have about the functional neuroanatomy of many aspects of the jawed vertebrate retina. Owing to this absence of data there is no way to speculate about the advantages and disadvantages of either type of retina. Nevertheless, it is noteworthy that the reorganization of the retina coincides with a number of changes including the reorganization of eye muscles (see below) and the formation of myelin.

3) IS THERE AN EVOLUTIONARY CHANGE OF THE RETINAL PROJECTION PATTERN?

The data presented above clearly show that the lamprey retina is different from jawed vertebrates with respect to

fiber course and distribution of the ganglion cells.
Therefore it appears reasonable to ask whether these
differences are reflected in the pattern of retinal
projections. Three major retinal fiber tracts are present in
virtually all vertebrates: 1) the basal optic tract; 2) the
axial (or medial) optic tract, and 3) the marginal optic
tract. The presence or absence of any of these tracts may
provide clues to the evolution of the retinal projection.

Among at least some vertebrates a unique class of
ganglion cells, the displaced ganglion cells project
selectively through the basal optic root to the basal optic
nucleus (Reiner, 1981; Fite, 1985). These displaced ganglion
cells comprise less than 1% of all ganglion cells in jawed
vertebrates but about 74% in lampreys (Fritzsch and Collin,
1990). Neither published data (Kosareva, 1980; Rubinson,
1990) nor our own preliminary data indicate any large scale
projection through the basal optic root in lamprey. To the
contrary, our data indicate that, if all the unfasciculated
fibers lateral to the marginal optic tract are considered to
be basal optic root fibers, it is a very disorganized
pathway. The basal optic root and nucleus do not exist in
hagfish (Wicht and Northcutt, 1990). This can either be a
primitive or a derived feature of hagfish which may be
related to the absence of the oculomotor nucleus.
Interestingly, some amphibians with reduced vision have only
a few ganglion cell fibers that comprise a small basal optic
root and also have a reduced number of oculomotor neurons
(Fritzsch et al., 1985).

A second major retinal tract present in virtually all
jawed vertebrates is the axial (or medial) optic tract
(Fritzsch et al., 1985, for review). Lampreys clearly have
an axial optic tract, but it consists of retinopetal or
efferent fibers rather than retinofugal fibers (Kosareva,
1980; Rubinson, 1990; Fritzsch and Northcutt, in prep.).
Distinct marginal and axial optic tracts do not exist in
hagfish. Rather, it appears that all retinofugal and
retinopetal fibers run within the same tract which may be
homologous to the axial optic tract of other vertebrates
(Wicht and Northcutt, 1990).

The proportion of crossed and uncrossed fibers that run
in the marginal or the axial optic tract varies among
jawless and jawed vertebrates. The marginal optic tract of
lampreys and most jawed vertebrates contains the majority of
ganglion cell axons. This tract is predominantly crossed in
jawed vertebrates but in lampreys it is partially uncrossed
(Rubinson, 1990). Prominent bilateral projections are found
in most jawed vertebrates where they run in the axial optic
tract (Fritzsch et al, 1985). Similarly, in the hagfish 15%
of the fibers in the axial optic tract are uncrossed (Wicht
and Northcutt, 1990). The bilateral projection of the axial
optic tract appears to represent a feature associated with
regressed vision in both hagfish and jawed vertebrates
(Fritzsch et al., 1985). Alternatively, it may be the
ancestral condition of craniate vertebrates which has been
retained in hagfish. In any case, the bilateral projection
of the ganglion cells running in the marginal optic tract of
lampreys appears to be a derived feature of lampreys shared
only by some mammals (Wilm and Fritzsch, 1990).

In summary, the differences in ganglion cell distribution of jawed and jawless vertebrates are not reflected in major reorganizations of the optic projections. Both hagfish and lampreys have a large uncrossed projection which was probably a primitive feature of craniate vertebrates. However, the presence of uncrossed fibers in the marginal optic tract (in lampreys) rather than in the axial optic tract (as in hagfish and many jawed vertebrates) appears to be a derived feature (Fritzsch et al., 1985; Wicht and Northcutt, 1990). The appearance of an axial optic tract, comprised exclusively of retinopetal fibers, is a uniquely derived feature of lampreys. Reduction of retinopetal fibers in the axial optic tract of jawed vertebrates is now proposed to be a derived feature (see below). The ancestral condition may be a single optic tract that contained all retinofugal and retinopetal fibers, similar to the organization seen in hagfish. Segregation and differential loss of retinal fibers may have resulted in the derived conditions seen in extant vertebrates.

4) WHAT ARE THE EVOLUTIONARY CHANGES IN THE RETINOPETAL OR EFFERENT SYSTEM

Every area of the brain receives at least one major input and projects to at least one other area of the brain. The retinae of many jawed vertebrates clearly violate this rule and have few, if any, cells projecting to them (Uchiyama, 1989; Reperant et al., 1989). This reduction or absence of efferents may be a derived feature that reflects the evolution of the retina towards the exclusive processing of visual information rather than the processing of information carried into the retina by the efferent fibers. Lampreys and hagfish are supposed to have presumably homologous populations of efferent cells (Wicht and Northcutt, 1990). Given that the retinae of lampreys and hagfish appear to represent the ancestral condition, these retinal efferents may likewise represent the ancestral condition.

This suggestion is corroborated by the proportionally large number of efferents which amounts to about 2% of all optic nerve fibers in lampreys as compared to 0.5% and less in most jawed vertebrates (Vesselkin et al., 1989; Fritzsch and Collin, 1990; Uchiyama, 1989). Preliminary quantitative data on Pacific hagfish suggests an even higher proportion of about 5% of efferent fibers (unpublished observations). The presence of efferents to the eye is particularly relevant for the interpretation of the visual system of the hagfish as being primitively undeveloped vs. derived: no other vertebrate yet studied with a secondarily reduced eye has any efferents at all. This fact strongly suggests to me that the visual system of hagfish reflects, at least with respect to the organization of the efferent system, the primitive vertebrate pattern. I suggest that the reduced presence of efferents in most vertebrates is a derived condition which may be related to the differences in the organization of the retina (Fig. 2).

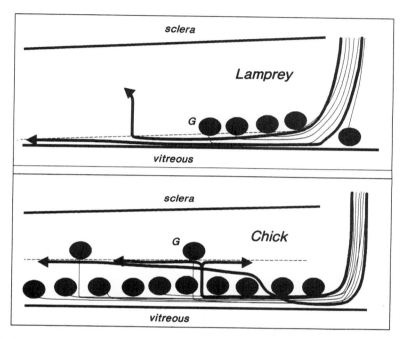

Figure 3. This scheme outlines some of the differences in the development of efferent innervation in the lamprey and chicken retinae. In lamprey efferent fibers (arrows) extend from the optic nerve head along the inner limiting membrane beyond the area of differentiated ganglion cells (G) and may be the first fibers present in the developing inner plexiform layer . In contrast, many ganglion cells in the chicken retina have differentiated and an inner plexiform layer has formed by the time the efferent fibers will arrive. Consequently after these efferent fibers leave the optic fiber layer they must navigate through the inner plexiform layer to reach their target. Dashed lines indicate the inner nuclear/inner plexiform boundary.

The limited data on the development of the retina of lampreys (Rubinson, 1990; Fritzsch and Northcutt, 1990; De Miguel et al., 1989; 1990) are not yet sufficient to propose a detailed scheme to explain the evolution of lamprey and jawed vertebrate retinae. However, some clues are provided by the very different routes taken by the efferent fibers within the retina and the differences in timing of efferent and ganglion cell development (Figs. 2,3). In chickens and in cichlid fish the current evidence argues that ganglion cell axons project into the brain before the efferent fibers reach the optic nerve head (Clarke et al., 1976; Crapon de Caprona and Fritzsch, 1983; Fritzsch et al., 1990b).

Lampreys show a noteworthy difference in the timing of development as compared to both birds and fish. In the latter two the efferent fibers reach the retina **after** afferents have reached the brain whereas the efferents of lampreys project throughout the retina several years **before** this part of the retina develops any neurons (Fritzsch and Northcutt, 1990; De Miguel et al., 1990). The early presence of efferents throughout the undifferentiated retina of lampreys suggests that efferents may actually guide the afferents within the retina. Clearly this is not possible in fish or birds where the efferents arrive after the ganglion cells have reached the brain with their axons (Fritzsch et al., 1990b). Early ablation of the efferent nucleus in lampreys is needed to provide more evidence for this assumption.

An important point here is that the efferents will be right next to their target cells, amacrine and displaced ganglion cells (Uchiyama, 1989; Reperant et al., 1989), at the inner plexiform/inner nuclear layer boundary in lampreys but the entering efferent fibers will have to pass through the partly developed inner plexiform layer in jawed vertebrates (Fig. 3). Owing to the changed spatiotemporal pattern of development of afferent and efferent cells and their fibers only those efferent cells will reach their target which have evolved the appropriate mechanisms to navigate through the ganglion cell layer and inner plexiform layer. This hypothesis implies that the reorganization of the jawed vertebrate retina, either alone or in conjunction with a change in timing of efferent fiber arrival, is responsible for the large reduction of efferents in most jawed vertebrates. Obviously, the efferent fibers can reach their target only when they know where to leave the fiber layer and grow into the inner plexiform layer, a behavior that is not at all understood at present (Fritzsch et al., 1990b). It is equally unknown how the increased problems in target finding may have affected such well known developmental mechanisms as cell death (Catsicas et al., 1987). It is conceivable that only after the mechanisms for proper pathfinding were evolved there could be a secondarily increase in the proportion of efferents as in some bony fish and in birds (Uchiyama, 1989). Whether these efferent cells represent a re-evolution of contacts to the area of the brain that were once present before this area was transformed into the retina, or are newly formed connections will likely remain obscure.

5) THE EVOLUTION OF THE VESTIBULO-OCULAR MOTORSYSTEM

Having listed some differences in adult organization and development of the lamprey and jawed vertebrate retinae, it will come as no surprise that the extra- and intraocular muscles of lampreys and jawed vertebrates are also different. We have recently shown that the old suggestion for a different pattern of eye muscle organization of lampreys extends to the oculomotor connectivities as well (Fritzsch et al., 1990a). Lampreys appear to have a primitive pattern of oculomotor innervation (Fritzsch et al., 1990a) from which two, equally derived patterns in jawed vertebrates may have evolved (Graf and Brunken, 1984). Moreover, lampreys and hagfish have no internal eye muscles, no ciliary ganglion, and no Edinger-Westphal nucleus. This suggests that the dioptric apparatus of the eye of jawed vertebrates may have continued to evolve beyond the condition in jawless vertebrates. Consequently, clues to these evolutionary changes can be studied in extant vertebrates.

As noted before there is no relationship between the evolution of the retinal organization and the evolution of the dioptric apparatus of the eye. Likewise, it is difficult to understand how the reorganization of the ocular muscles could have been related to the reorganization of the retina and the dioptric system. A more likely explanation is that the reorganization of the extraocular muscles is related to changes in the organization of the inner ear as proposed by Graf and Brunken (1984) and Fritzsch et al. (1990a). This hypothesis is based on the observations that (1) lampreys and hagfish lack a horizontal canal and (2) that lampreys have a very different pattern of eye muscles and eye muscle innervation than jawed vertebrates. How the vestibulo-ocular pattern of innervation is assembled differently in lampreys and jawed vertebrate development is not known. However, there are several significant differences in the central wiring of the vestibular system onto the ocular motoneurons in lampreys and jawed vertebrates. First, the vestibular system appears to project directly onto the dorsal dendrites of the trochlear motoneurons (Fritzsch and Sonntag, 1988). Second, following the evolution of a horizontal canal, its connections must be implemented into the existing wiring (Fig. 4). This requires some rewiring of existing connections and this rewiring may have occurred independently and differently in elasmobranchs and in the ancestral lineage leading to all other jawed vertebrates (Graf and Brunken, 1984).

The driving forces for all of these rearrangements remains obscure. However, the reorganization of the cranial neural crest to form the jaws in jawed vertebrates is likely linked to the formation of the neural crest derived ciliary ganglion, presumably primitively absent in all jawless vertebrates. Whether this reorganization of the neural crest between jawless and jawed vertebrates had also influenced other reorganizations, like the eye muscles, formation of a horizontal canal, or changes in the retinal layers is not clear.

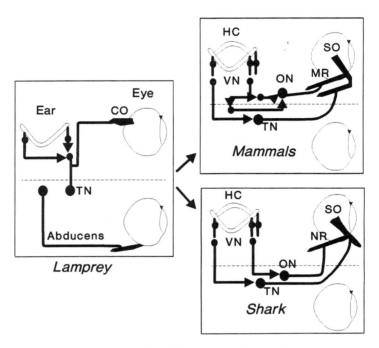

Fig. 4. This scheme shows some of the differences in the oculomotor connections among vertebrates. In lampreys afferents from the vestibular ganglion project directly onto the motoneurons of the trochlear nucleus (TN). Lampreys have no horizontal canal and have not one but two (out of six) eye muscles innervated by the abducens and only three by the oculomotor nucleus (fewer muscles are shown to simplify the diagram). All jawed vertebrates, represented here by a mammal and a shark, have four eye muscles innervated by the oculomotor nucleus. The additional muscle (MR in mammal, NR in shark) is innervated by an uncrossed projection of oculomotor motoneurons (OC) in jawed vertebrates except elasmobranchs where it receives a crossed projection. As would be expected, the connections of the horizontal canal (HC) via the vestibular nuclei (VN) onto these neurons is different in sharks and mammals: direct and indirectly, respectively . CO, caudal oblique; HC, horizontal canal; MR, medial rectus; NR, nasal rectus; ON, oculmotor nucleus; SO, superior oblique; TN, trochlear nucleus; Vn, vestibular nuclei. Dashed line indicates the midline, Modified after Graf and Brunken (1984) and Fritzsch and Sonntag (1988).

SUMMARY

The evolution of the retina, the retinofugal and
retinopetal projections and the ocular muscles is reviewed.
Experimental evidence shows that the morphogenesis of the
eye and differentiation of the retina are two independent
developmental events. It is concluded that their
evolutionary sequence of appearance has been
heterochronically shifted to achieve the spatiotemporal
pattern observed in vertebrate development.

The retina can be grouped into two recognizable
patterns of organization: the lamprey and the jawed
vertebrate pattern. Comparing the organization of the
lamprey and hagfish retinae and with that of the lamprey
forebrain indicates that the retinal organization in
lampreys likely reflects the primitive vertebrate pattern,
whereas that in jawed vertebrates is derived.

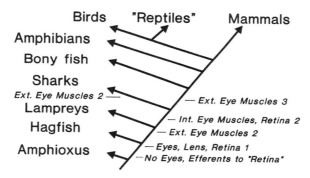

Fig. 5. This cladogram shows a modified view of the reorganization of the neural
components of the eye. A "neural retina" including "efferents" was presumably present
before the morphogenesis of the lateral eye, i.e. in ancestral vertebrates, but not in
Amphioxus. Morphogenesis dislocated the neural retina and further reorganization
formed a sclera and a lens. At this stage the retina presumably was not too different
from the one present in lampreys. The lens and distinct layering were lost in modern
adult hagfish as a secondary reduction, but the large proportion of efferents was
retained. External eye muscles evolved in the common ancestors of lampreys and jawed
vertebrates. Internal eye muscles and the reorganization of the retina and the external
eye muscles occurred in the ancestors of jawed vertebrates. Finally, the external eye
muscles were reorganized into two different patterns of eye muscles in jawed
vertebrates.

The differences in the organization within the retina
are not reflected in obvious changes in the retinal
projection. Hagfish may reflect a primitive pattern with
afferents and efferents running together in a single axial
tract. Lampreys differ from jawed vertebrates in that the
axial tract contains all efferent fibers and no ganglion
cell axons. Further, a bilateral projection may be primitive
for craniate vertebrates, but the detailed organization
differs in hagfish, lampreys and jawed vertebrates.

The efferent system is proportionally large. This pattern is suggested to represent the primitive organization. In contrast, most jawed vertebrates show reduced proportions of efferents. The differences in retinal organization are hypothesized to be related to evolutionary changes in the timing of arrival of efferents in the retina.

Finally, the organization of ocular muscles in lampreys is different from that of jawed vertebrates. These differences may be causally related to the reorganization of the vestibular system. After the horizontal canal was introduced in ancestral jawed vertebrates, there was the addition of the neural crest derived ciliary ganglion and the internal eye muscles. It is unclear how these changes were related to each other and what the driving force was.

In conclusion then, the evolutionary changes of the visual system of vertebrates are more pronounced then most textbooks make us believe. Moreover, provided proper physiological data would be at hand, we may be able to create a more detailed scenario of changes including the adaptivity of each retinal and eye muscle organization.

ACKNOWLEDGEMENTS

This work has been supported by the German Science Foundation. I wish to express my sincere thanks to Drs. L.L. Bruce, S.P. Collin, T. J. Neary and R.G. Northcutt for the invaluable discussions on numerous aspects of the visual system presented here. I am particularly gratefull to Drs. L.L. Bruce and T.J. Neary for their help in converting my ideas into readable English.

REFERENCE CITATIONS

Arnold, S.J. (rapporteur) et al. , 1989, How do complex organisms evolve? In: D.B. Wake and G. Roth (eds.) Complex Organismal Functions: Integration and Evolution in Vertebrates. Dahlem Conference, Wiley and Sons, Chichester, p. 403-433.

Balfour, F.M. 1885, A treatise on comparative embryology. Macmillan, London, pp 483-511.

Carroll, R.L., 1988, Vertebrate paleontology and evolution. W.H.Freeman, New York.

Catsicas, S., Thanos, S. and Clarke, P.G.H., 1987, Major role for neuronal death during brain development: refinement of topographical connections. Proc. Natl. Acad. Sci., USA, 84: 8165-8168.

Clarke, P.G.H., Rogers, L.A., and Cowan, W.M., 1976, The time of origin and the pattern of survival of neurons in the isthmo-optic nucleus of the chick. J. Comp. Neurol., 167: 125-142.

Crapon de Caprona, M.-D. and Fritzsch, B., 1983, The development of the retinopetal nucleus olfacto-retinalis of two cichlid fish as revealed by horseradish peroxidase. Develop. Brain Res., 11:281-301.

Darwin, C., 1859, On the origin of species by means of natural selection or the preservation of favoured races in the struggle for life. London, Murray.

De Miguel, E., Rodicio, M.C. and Anadon, R., 1989, Ganglion cells and retinopetal fibers of the larval lamprey retina: an HRP ultrastructural study. Neurosci. Lett., 106:1-6.

De Miguel, E., Rodicio, M.C. and Anadon, R., 1990, Organization of the visual system in larval lampreys: An HRP study. J. Comp. Neurol., 302:1-14.

Duke-Elder, S. 1958, System of ophthalomology. 1. The eye in evolution. Mosby, St. Louis.

Durston, A. J., Timmermanns, J.P.M., Hage, W.M., Hendriks, A.F.J., De Vries, N.J. and Nieuwkoop, P.D., 1989, Retinoic acid causes an antero-posterior transformation in the developing central nervous system. Nature, 340: 140-144.

Fite, K.V., 1985, Pretectal and accessory-optic visual nuclei of fish, amphibia and reptiles: theme and variations. Brain, Behav., Evol., 26: 71-90.

Franz, V., 1934, Vergleichende Anatomie des Wirbeltierauges. In: L. Bolk, E. Goeppert, E. Kallius and W. Lubosch (eds.) Handbuch der Vergleichenden Anatomie der Wirbeltiere, Urban und Schwarzenberg, Wien, pp. 989-1292.

Fritzsch, B., Himstedt, W. and Crapon de Caprona, M.-D., 1985, The visual projections of larval Ichthyophis kohtaoensis (Amphibia: Gymnophiona). Develop. Brain Res., 23: 201-210.

Fritzsch, B. and Sonntag, R., 1988, The trochlear motoneurons of lampreys: location, morphology and numbers as revealed with horseradish peroxidase. Cell Tissue Res., 252: 223-229.

Fritzsch, B. and Collin, S.P., 1990, The dendritic organization of two populations of ganglion cells and the retinopetal fibers in the retina of the silver lamprey, Ichthyomyzon unicuspis. Visual Neurosci., 4: 533-545.

Fritzsch, B., Crapon de Caprona, M.-D., and Clarke, P.G.H., 1990b, The development of two fiber types projecting to the retina of chicken as revealed with DiI. Journal of Comparative Neurology, 300: 405-421.

Fritzsch, B. and Northcutt, R.G., 1990, Retinopetal and retinofugal projections in larval and adult lamprey: an in vitro study with HRP and fluorescent dextran-amines. Soc. Neurosci. Abstr. 16: 127.

Fritzsch, B., Sonntag, R., Dubuc, R., Ohta, H. and Grillner, S., 1990a, Organization of the six motor nuclei innervating the ocular muscles in lamprey. Journal of Comparative Neurology, 294: 491-506.

Gilbert, S.F., 1989, Developmental Biology, Sinauer, Sunderland.

Graf, W., and Brunken, W.J., 1984, Elasmobranch oculomotor organization: Anatomical and theoretical aspects of the phylogenetic development of vestibulo-oculomotor connectivity. J. Comp. Neurol., 227: 569-581.

Holmberg, K., 1978, The cyclostome retina. In: F. Crescitelli (ed.) Handbook of Sensory Physiology, Vol. VII/5, The visual system in vertebrates. Springer, Berlin, pp. 47-94.

Jacobson, A.G. and Sater, A.K., 1988, Features of embryonic
    induction. Development, 104: 341-359.
Kosareva, A.A., 1980, Retinal projections in lamprey
    (Lampetra fluviatilis). J. Hirnforsch., 21: 243-256.
Manns, M. and Fritzsch, B., 1991, The eye in the brain:
    Retinoic acid effects morphogenesis of the eye and
    pathway selection of axons but not the differentiation
    of the retina. Neurosci. Lett., 127:150-154.
Nieuwenhuys, R., 1977, The brain of the lamprey in a
    comparative perspective. Ann. N.Y. Acad. Sci., 299:
    970-145.
Peters, N. and Peters, G., 1984, On the ontogenesis of
    rudiments. Fortschr. Zool. Syst. Evol. 3: 36-55.
Reiner, A., 1981, A projection of displaced ganglion cells
    and giant ganglion cells to the accessory optic nuclei
    in turtle. Brain Res., 204:403-409.
Reperant, J., Miceli, D., Vesselkin, N.P., and
    Molotchnikoff, S., 1989, The centrifugal visual system
    of vertebrates: a century-old search reviewed. Int.
    Rev. Cytol., 118: 115-171.
Retzius, G., 1893, Das Gehirn und das Auge von Myxine.
    Bilogische Untersuchungen, 5: 55-68.
Rovainen, C.M., 1982, Neurophysiology. In: M.W. Hardisty and
    I.C. Potter (eds.) The biology of lampreys. Academic
    Press, London, pp. 1-136.
Rubinson, K., 1990, The developing visual system and
    metamorphosis in the lamprey. J. Neurobiol., 21: 1123-
    1135.
Sarnat, H.B. and Netsky, M.G., 1974, Evolution of the
    nervous system. Oxford Univ. Press, London.
Sive, H.L., Draper, B.W., Harland, R.M., and Weintraub, H.,
    1990, Identification of a retinoic acid-sensitive
    period during primary axis formation in Xenopus laevis.
    Genes and Develop. 4: 932-942.
Tretjakoff, D.K., 1916, The sense organs of the lamprey
    (Lampetra fluviatilis). University of Novorossijsk,
    Odessa, German in Morphol., Jb. 64 (1926).
Uchiyama, H., 1989, Centrifugal pathways to the retina:
    influence of the optic tectum. Vis. Neurosci., 3:183-
    206.
Versaux-Botteri, C., Dalil, N., Kenigfest, N., Reperant, J.,
    Vesselkin, N. and Nguyen-Legros, J., 1991,
    Immunohistochemical localization of retinal serotonin
    cells in the lamprey (Lampetra fluviatilis). Vis.
    Neuroscie., in press.
Vesselkin, N.P., Reperant, J., Kenigfest, N.B., Rio., J.P.,
    Miceli, D., and Shupliakov, O.V., 1989, Centrifugal
    innervation of the lamprey retina. Light- and electron
    microscopic and electrophysiological investigations.
    Brain Res. 493: 51-65.
Wake, M.H., 1985, The comparative morphology and evolution
    of the eyes of caecilians (Amphibia, Gymnophiona).
    Zoomorphology, 105: 277-295.
Walls, G.L., 1942, The vertebrate eye and its adaptive
    radiation. Cranbrook Inst. of Science, Bloomfield
    Hills.
Wicht, H., and Northcutt, R.G., 1990, Retinofugal and
    retinopetal projections in the Pacific hagfish,
    Eptatretus stouti (Myxinoidea). Brain Behav. Evol., 36:
    315-328.

Wilm, C. and Fritzsch, B., 1990, The ipsilateral retinofugal
    projection in a percomorph fish: Its induction,
    accuracy and maintenance. Brain, Behavior and
    Evolution, 36: 271-300.

ARE VISUAL HIERARCHIES IN THE BRAINS OF THE BEHOLDERS?

CONSTANCY AND VARIABILITY IN THE VISUAL SYSTEM

OF BIRDS AND MAMMALS

Harvey J. Karten[1] and Toru Shimizu[2]

[1]Department of Neurosciences
University of California, San Diego
La Jolla, California 92093

[2]Department of Psychology
University of South Florida
Tampa, Florida 33620

INTRODUCTION

Contemporary concepts of the organization of the visual system began to emerge in the mid to late 19th century. It had long been appreciated that penetrating wounds of the occipital region of the brain resulted in blindness. Lesions of more lateral portions of the hemisphere often resulted in varying degrees of visual agnosias, though it was not until the middle third of the twentieth century that the contribution of such cortical areas to visual performance became an object of interest.

The prevalent view of the organization of the cortical visual pathways is that they are organized in a largely hierarchical manner. That is to say, the major input to the mammalian cortical visual regions is derived from a sequence of projections from the lateral geniculate nucleus (LGN) upon the striate cortex, and from the striate cortex, via a series of direct and indirect connections, upon a vast region of the temporal and parietal cortices. An anatomical analysis from such a view was elegantly summarized in Felleman and Van Essen's scholarly work (1991; see Figure 1).

Many electrophysiological data appear to be consistent with hierarchical models derived from such connectivity. Thus, the striate cortex (i.e., V1 or area 17) contains units that respond to rather simple properties of the visual stimuli, such as "line" elements. On the other hand, units in the temporal and parietal cortices, i.e., extrastriate cortices (e.g., V2, V3, V4, or MT) respond to more "complex" features, such as "motion" or "objects". Thus, in keeping with hierarchical models, visual input first arrives at the striate cortex, where it undergoes an initial stage of processing, and is then passed on to other visual cortical areas for further analysis.

However, the extrastriate cortex is also known to receive a direct and distinct projection from thalamic nuclei. This pathway to the extrastriate cortex does not include the LGN or the striate cortex, but includes the extrageniculate thalamic nuclei which in turn receive input from the superior colliculus (optic tectum). The extrastriate system, as well as the striate system, is one of the structures providing additional visual input mediating parallel processing of visual information. Indeed, the extrastriate system is the major visual ascending pathway in the majority of nonmammalian vertebrates.

The Changing Visual System, Edited by P. Bagnoli and
W. Hodos, Plenum Press, New York, 1991

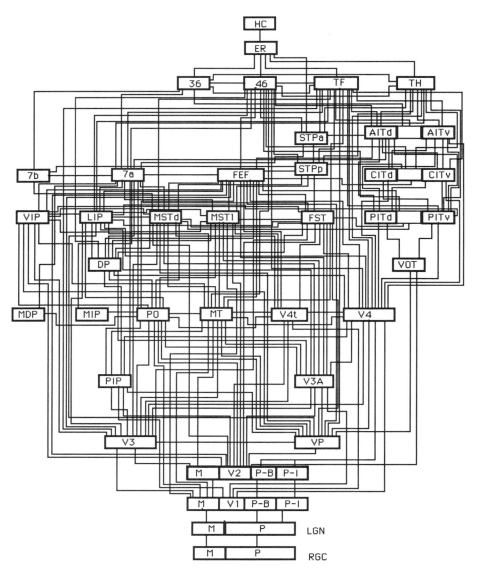

Figure 1. Hierarchy of primate visual areas. (From Felleman and Van Essen, 1991).

Our suggestion is that the functional relationship between the striate and extrastriate systems is not a simple hierarchical one; rather they are equally significant for parallel processing, and complementary rather than dependent. In the present paper, the geniculo-striate pathway is referred to as the *thalamofugal* pathway and the colliculo-thalamo-cortical pathway is referred to as the *tectofugal* pathway.

ASSUMPTIONS FOR HIERARCHICAL MODELS

The notion that visual processing is hierarchically ordered relies directly or indirectly upon several assumptions. However, these assumptions are often questionable from a point of view based on comparative analysis of brains of various animals. For instance, one of the most commonly held current notions about the evolution of the mammalian visual system is that the striate cortex is the first cortical visual region to have elaborated in evolution. Other visual cortical regions are postulated to have emerged from the original striate cortical region. Such a point of view is most explicitly stated in the writings of Allman (e.g., 1977). Our interpretation regarding the evolution of the cortex has been discussed elsewhere (Karten and Shimizu, 1989). In contrast to the argument for hierarchical models, we suggest that the *tectofugal* pathway was elaborated earlier than the *thalamofugal* pathway as a major visual pathway to the telencephalon. The telencephalic visual pathways in amniotic vertebrates have not evolved in a linear fashion. There is no simple relationship between the antiquity of various components of the visual system and their functional roles in visual discrimination.

In the present paper, we will question two more assumptions that are often associated with hierarchical models. Using data from comparative analyses, we then shall attempt to argue against the dominance of the striate cortex. These assumptions are:

Assumption 1 - The extrastriate cortex should be inoperative in the absence of the striate cortex (assuming that the lateral geniculate nucleus outputs are limited to the striate cortex - a condition that may only obtain in the brains of some species of primates);

Assumption 2 - The development of the striate cortex, i.e., its connectivity and the onset of function, should precede that of the extrastriate cortices.

TWO VISUAL PATHWAYS

The existence of two separate visual pathways to the telencephalon, the thalamofugal pathway (including the striate cortex) and the tectofugal pathway (including various extrastriate cortices), appears to be a phylogenetically conservative plan. The two visual cortical or telencephalic areas are identifiable in many vertebrates, including nonmammals.

Functional segregation of visual functions have been suggested by several authors. For instance, Schneider (1969) proposed that two major components of visual function operate through two different structures: "where is it" is mediated by the tectofugal pathway and "what is it" is mediated by the thalamofugal pathway. However, Schneider did not include the cortical components of the tectofugal pathway in his formulation.

Amongst nonmammals, the visual system of birds provides a particularly useful model, as they have extremely well-developed visual systems, and possess superb color vision and a high degree of visual acuity. In birds, the *visual wulst* in the telencephalon, receives afferent connections from retino-recipient dorsal thalamic nuclei (the thalamofugal pathway). As in the striate cortex of mammals, the visual wulst has efferent projections to the visual nuclei of the brainstem (e.g., the retino-recipient dorsal thalamic nuclei and optic tectum).

The target of the tectofugal pathway in birds is located in the area called the dorsal ventricular ridge (DVR) in the lateral telencephalon. A characteristic feature of the DVR is its nonlaminated (cluster) organization, in contrast to the laminar organization of homologous neuronal populations seen in mammalian cortex. The general similarities of the two visual pathways between mammals and birds are shown schematically in Figure 2.

In a previous paper (Karten and Shimizu, 1989), we suggested that both birds and mammals have similar microcircuitry that mediates the visual processing in the telencephalon, despite this laminar versus cluster organization. Thus, neurons within individual laminae of the mammalian cortex may correspond to those in discrete nuclear groups within the DVR in birds.

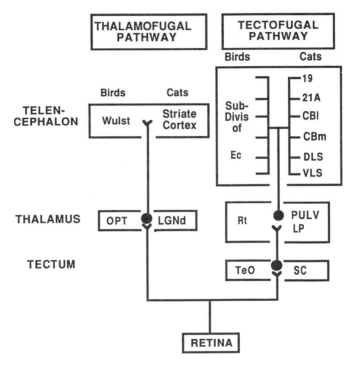

Figure 2. Schematic representation of the major visual pathways to the telencephalon in birds (chicks, pigeons and owls) and in cats. Note the extensive similarity in the organization of major pathways, despite the overall absence of lamination in the telencephalic component of the tectofugal pathways in birds.

Our hypothesis suggests that one major consequence of the organizational pattern in mammals is that these nuclear groupings are stretched out horizontally in apposition to each other, with greater interlaminar interactions. This proposed microcircuitry is shown in Figure 2. We further suggest that the evolution of the basic microcircuitry preceded that of lamination. Thus, we postulate that lamination is an independent evolutionary event involving modification of more ancient neuronal constituents into the laminae characteristic of mammalian neocortex (Karten and Shimizu, 1989).

A. Circuitry in Mammalian Cortex

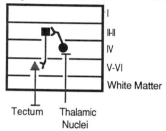

B. Equivalent Circuitry in Avian DVR

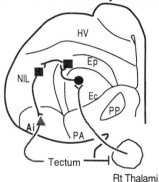

Figure 3. A. Schematic representation of a general pattern of cortical organization characteristic of many sensory cortical areas. B. Schematic representation of organization of a major visual sensory pathway in birds comparable to an extrastriate visual pathway in mammals. Individual nuclei within the DVR of birds and reptiles correspond to cells within individual laminae of the neocortex.

EFFECTS AFTER LESIONS IN THE VISUAL WULST OF BIRDS

In the most extreme formulation of hierarchical models, the operations of the extrastriate cortex are completely and exclusively dependent on processed information exported from the striate cortex. Thus, lesions in the striate cortex should interrupt functions of the extrastriate cortex. However, many behavioral and electrophysiological studies in both mammals and nonmammals have indicated that the extrastriate cortex is still functional and active even after lesions of structures in the striate system.

Birds, pigeons in particular, seem to show little or no changes after damage to the thalamofugal pathway. Pattern or intensity discrimination was disrupted only slightly after lesions of the dorsal thalamic nuclei or the wulst (Hodos et al., 1973). Almost no effect was observed on intensity-difference and visual acuity thresholds following the destruction of the thalamofugal pathway (the dorsal thalamic nuclei: Hodos and Bonbright, 1974; Macko and Hodos, 1984; wulst: Pasternak and Hodos, 1977; Hodos et al., 1984).

In pigeons, the tectofugal pathway appears to be more significant for visual behavior than the thalamofugal pathway. Studies of the after-effects of lesions in the tectofugal pathway reveal severe deterioration of visual behavior in birds (Hodos, 1976; Kertzman, 1988). Lesions in any structures in the pathway of pigeons disrupted performance on pattern and intensity discriminations. The effects can be permanent, or, even if partial recovery occurs, birds require prolonged retraining to return preoperative performance levels (optic tectum: Hodos and Karten, 1974; Jarvis, 1974; the thalamic nucleus: Hodos and Karten; 1966; DVR: Hodos and Karten, 1970). When psychophysical methods were used to study changes in thresholds after surgery, intensity-difference and visual acuity thresholds were found to be substantially decreased (the thalamic nucleus: Hodos and Bonbright, 1974; Macko and Hodos, 1984; DVR: Hodos et al., 1984).

Thus, although the function of the wulst and the thalamofugal pathway is still unknown, the DVR of the tectofugal pathway seems to analyze and process most of the visual input. Therefore, in pigeons, the analysis within the wulst cannot be regarded as a sensory-filter mechanism that proceeds analysis within DVR. The analysis in DVR is, rather, independent of the wulst. This flow of information processing is opposite to that implied in the prevailing assumption that visual information is conveyed from the striate to extrastriate cortex to achieve visual perception in mammals.

EFFECTS AFTER LESIONS IN THE STRIATE CORTEX OF MAMMALS

The functional significance of the tectofugal pathway has been shown not only in birds, but also in mammals. The effects of striate lesions appear to be more severe in primates than non-primates. However, recent findings in studies of the primate visual system have indicated the existence of significant residual ability after such lesions.

In humans, patients with striate lesions are, at least at their conscious level, blind in the affected regions of their visual fields. It is now known, however, that these patients retain significant residual visual ability after striate lesions, and that these residual functions may be attributed to the tectofugal pathway. Interestingly, these people do not have conscious awareness of their "sight". Such residual functions, including coarse pattern and motion discriminations, are called "blindsight", and are described in detail in a series of studies by Weiskrantz and his co-workers (see a review by Weiskrantz, 1986).

In monkeys, the effects of lesions in the striate cortex are profound although they are less severe than those in humans, and often reversible. Since many extended reviews of studies using monkeys are available, we present only one example here.

The extrastriate cortex of the macaque monkey contains a region called the middle temporal area (MT). Single units within MT were found to respond selectively to direction of motion in the visual field. MT has attracted the attention of many researchers studying the mechanism of motion detection (e.g., Movshon et al., 1985; Ullman, 1986). The striate cortex and V2 (which is completely dependent on striate cortex for visual responsiveness) send projections to MT. Thus, at the computational and physiological levels, MT has been regarded as a structure that analyzes the visual information derived from the striate cortex. However, a study done by Rodman et al. (1989) provides a new perspective on the relationship between the striate cortex and MT. In their study, Rodman and co-workers collected unit-recordings of MT after striate lesions in order to examine the dependency of MT on striate input. Despite massive striate lesions, the majority of MT neurons were still found to respond to visual stimuli in the absence of any input from the striate cortex. Although the residual activity was weaker than before the striate lesions, the neurons of MT maintained direction selectivity and binocularity to visual stimuli. This study apparently indicates that the visual responsiveness of units in MT is not dependent exclusively on the striate input. The authors suggested that this residual ability is attributable to the other MT afferents deriving from the lateral and inferior portions of the pulvinar. The inferior pulvinar receives an input from the superior colliculus. The optic tectum is known to contain cells with directional selectivity. The thalamic nucleus in the tectofugal pathway (i.e., nucleus rotundus in birds and inferior pulvinar in mammals) is known to receive bilateral inputs from tectum/superior colliculus. Thus, the tectofugal pathway appears to be important for motion analysis in MT. Similar motion detection units are also found in avian tectum (Frost, 1982) and mammalian superior colliculus (reviewed in Chalupa, 1984). These observations pose a serious challenge to the assumption that the hierarchical processing involving the striate cortex is essential in order for cells in the extrastriate cortex to exhibit directional selectivity.

In cats, several workers (e.g., Sprague et al., 1981; Antonini et al., 1985) have described the effects of destruction of various regions of the visual cortex on visual ability, and showed functional segregation of the striate and extrastriate cortex. Cats show almost perfect performance in pattern discrimination when lesions are limited to areas 17 and 18 whereas visual acuity after the same lesions deteriorated significantly. In contrast, lesions in the extrastriate cortex (i.e., the suprasylvian gyrus) produced severe deficits in pattern discrimination, but no changes in visual acuity. Their suggestion was that the striate system is critical for analysis of local details of visual stimuli, whereas perception of pattern, based on the general configuration of such stimuli, may require the extrastriate system.

RELATIVE TEMPORAL ONTOGENY OF VISUAL TELENCEPHALIC AREAS

Using tritiated thymidine, Tsai et al., (1981) reported that, in birds, neurons within DVR develop earlier than neurons in the wulst. According to this study, neurons of the visual centers in DVR develop about day 4 to 5 of embryogenesis which is several days earlier than development of neurons in the wulst. Our unpublished observations, based on a *Phaseolus vulgaris* tract-tracing study, also indicate that the thalamofugal pathway appears to be functional much later (perhaps after hatching) than the tectofugal pathway. Furthermore, using $[^{14}C]$2-deoxyglucose, Rogers and Bell (1989) found age-dependent changes in neuronal metabolic activity in the two visual pathways. Thus, in 2-day-old chicks, high levels of metabolic activity occurred in the tectofugal pathway whereas very low-levels activity were observed in the thalamofugal pathway. However, in 23-day-old chicks, high levels of activity occurred in the both visual pathways (Rogers and Bell, 1989).

In regards to the relative temporal ontogeny of the two visual telencephalic areas in mammals, we are desperately short of information, particularly concerning the development of the extrastriate cortices. Nevertheless, some studies suggest that the lateral region of the mammalian neocortex appears to develop earlier than the dorsal region (e.g., Fernandez and Bravo, 1974; Smart and Smart, 1977). Further analyses are essential since dorsal and lateral regions of the neocortex may not necessarily directly correspond to the striate cortex and extrastriate cortex.

The consistent observation in birds and many mammals that the extrastriate and tectofugal pathways develop before the striate system raises the possibility that a given cortical region may perform different functions at different stages of development. Indeed, the role of the striate and extrastriate cortices may change over a period of several years, as in the development of the visual system in humans. Some linear models of development of the visual system have assumed that all cortical visual regions are relatively synchronized in their time course of maturation. Certainly the notion that all cortical areas rely upon input from the striate cortex would imply that maturation of the striate cortex is the rate limiting factor in the functional development of cortical visual systems. If, however, the extrastriate cortical regions attain operational capabilities prior to the maturation of striate cortex, the extrastriate regions may be dominant in visual function at earlier stages of life. Thus, we would suggest that there may be a shift in regional dominance during development. Different cortical areas may play more significant roles in visual performance at different stages of development.

CONCLUSION

In the central nervous system of vertebrates, there are multiple cortical areas mediating each sensory modality. The visual system is only one of them, and we suspect that similar processing mechanisms may operate in other sensory systems. Furthermore, we suggest that this basic mechanism may be common to motor systems and may play a role in higher cognitive functions.

Attributing an hierarchical order to each of these cortical regions has provided a useful model for and prompted a large body of inspired and interesting research on the visual system. However, the current hierarchical model is not easily reconciled with the less extensive, though still growing body of information on the evolution, comparative anatomy, development, and behavioral functions of the different components of the telencephalic visual regions. We do not deny the significance of hierarchical processing from the striate cortex to the extrastriate cortex. Rather, our suggestion complements and extends such hierarchical models in that hierarchical processing may be only one aspect of visual information processing by the forebrain.

ACKNOWLEDGEMENTS

The authors are grateful to Dr. Daniel J. Felleman for permission to use material from his publication and Dr. Kent T. Keyser for reading the manuscript. We also thank Ms. E. B. Watelet for secretarial assistance. This work was supported to NEI grant EY-06890, NINDS grant NS24560, and ONR contract N00014-88-K-0504.

REFERENCES

Allman, J., 1977, Evolution of the visual system in the early primates, in: "Progress in Psychobiology and Physiological Psychology. Vol. 7," J. M. Sprague, and A. M. Epstein, eds., Academic Press, New York.

Antonini, A., Berlucchi, G. and Sprague, J. M., 1985, Cortical systems for visual pattern discrimination in the cat as analyzed with the lesion method, in: "Pattern recognition mechanisms," C. Chagas, R. Gattass, and C. Gross, eds., Springer-Verlag, New York.

Chalupa, L.M., 1984, Visual physiology of the mammalian superior colliculus, in: "Comparative neurology of the optic tectum," H. Vanegas, ed., Plenum Press: New York.

Felleman, D. J. and Van Essen, D. C., 1991, Distributed hierarchical processing in the primate cerebral cortex, Cerebral Cortex, 1: 1.

Fernandez, V. and Bravo, H., 1974, Autoradiographic study of development of the cerebral cortex in the rabbit, Brain Behav Evol., 9: 317.

Frost, B. J., 1982, Mechanisms for discriminating object motion from the self-induced motion in the pigeon, in: "Analysis of visual behavior," D. J. Ingle, M. A. Goodale, and R. J. W. Mansfield, eds., MIT Press, Cambridge, MA.

Hodos, W., 1976, Vision and the visual system: A bird's eye-view, in: "Progress in Psychobiology and Physiological Psychology. Vol. 6," J. M. Sprague, and A. M. Epstein, eds., Academic Press, New York.

Hodos, W., Bonbright, J. C., Jr. and Karten, H. J., 1973, Visual intensity and pattern discrimination deficits after lesions of the thalamofugal visual pathway in pigeons, J. Comp. Physiol. Psych., 148: 447.

Hodos, W. and Bonbright, J. C., Jr., 1974, Intensity difference thresholds in pigeons after the tectofugal and thalamofugal visual pathways, J. Comp. Physiol. Psych., 87: 1013.

Hodos, W. and Karten, H. J., 1966, Brightness and pattern discrimination deficits in the pigeon after lesions of nucleus rotundus, Exp. Brain Res., 2: 151.

Hodos, W. and Karten, H. J., 1970, Visual intensity and pattern discrimination deficits after lesions of ectostriatum in pigeons, J. Comp. Neurol., 140: 53.

Hodos, W. and Karten, H. J., 1974, Visual intensity and pattern discrimination deficits after lesions of the optic lobe in pigeons, Brain Behav. Evol., 9: 165.

Hodos, W., Macko, K. A. and Bessette, B. B., 1984, Near-field visual acuity changes after visual system lesions in pigeons. II. Telencephalon, Behav. Brain Res., 13: 15.

Jarvis, C. D., 1974, Visual discrimination and spatial localization deficits after lesions of the tectofugal pathway in pigeons, Brain Behav. Evol., 9: 195.

Karten, H. J. and Shimizu, T., 1989, The origins of neocortex: connections and lamination as distinct events in evolution, J. Cog. Neurosci., 1: 291.

Kertzman, C. and Hodos, W. (1988). Size-difference thresholds after lesions of thalamic visual nuclei in pigeons, Visual Neurosci., 1: 83.

Macko, K. A. and Hodos, W., 1984, Near-field visual acuity changes after visual system lesions in pigeons. I. Thalamus, Behav. Brain Res., 13: 1.

Movshon, J. A., Adelson, E. H., Gizzi, M. S. and Newsome, W. T., 1985, The analysis of moving visual patterns, in: "Pattern recognition mechanisms," C. Chagas, R. Gattass, and C. Gross, eds., Springer-Verlag, New York.

Rodman, H. R., Gross, C. G. and Albright, T. D., 1989, Afferent basis of visual response properties in area MT of the macaque: Effects of striate cortex removal, J. Neurosci., 9: 2033.

Rogers, L. J. and Bell, G. A., 1989, Different rates of functional development in the two visual systems of the chicken revealed by [^{14}C]2-deoxyglucose, Dev. Brain Res., 49: 161.

Schneider, G. E., 1969, Two visual systems, Science, 163: 895.

Smart, I. H. M. and Smart, M., 1977, The location of nuclei of different labelling intensities in autoradiographs of the anterior forebrain of postnatal mice injected with [^{3}H] thymidine on the eleventh and twelfth days post-conception. J. Anat., 116: 515.

Sprague, J. M., Hughes, H. C. and Berlucchi, G., 1981, Cortical mechanisms in pattern and form perception, in: "Brain mechanisms and perceptual awareness," 0. Pompeiano, and C. A. Marsan, eds., Raven press, New York.

Tsai, H. M. Garber, B. B. and Larramendi, L. M. H., 1981, ^{3}H-thymidine autoradiographic analysis of telencephalic histogenesis in the chick embryo: I. Neuronal birthdates of telencephalic compartments in situ. J. Comp. Neurol., 198: 275.

Ullman, S., 1986, Artificial intelligence and the brain: Computational studies of the visual system, Ann. Rev. Neurosci., 9: 1.

Weiskrantz, L., 1986, "Blindsight: A case study and implications," Clarendon Press: Oxford.

THE CENTRIFUGAL VISUAL SYSTEM: WHAT CAN COMPARATIVE STUDIES TELL US ABOUT ITS EVOLUTION AND POSSIBLE FUNCTION?

Roger Ward [1,2], Jacques Repérant[1,3] and Dom Miceli[2]

[1]Laboratoire d'Anatomie Comparée
Muséum National d'Histoire Naturelle
55 rue Buffon
75005 Paris, France

[2]Laboratoire de Neuropsychologie
Université du Québec à Trois-Rivières
C.P. 500, Trois-Rivières QC
Canada G9A 5H7

[3]INSERM U-106
Hôpital de la Salpêtrière
75013 Paris, France

A wide variety of techniques has been used during the last century to investigate the possibility that some nerve fibers arise from neurons within the central nervous system and terminate in the retina. These techniques vary from the classical silver impregnation of what appear to be free nerve endings, the demonstration of differential rates of degeneration of axons in the proximal and distal stumps of the transected optic nerve, through the retrograde labelling of cell bodies after intraocular injection of a variety of tracers, to the immunohistochemical identification of cell bodies and fibers characterized by a particular neurotransmitter or neuropeptide.

Each technique in isolation has a number of disadvantages; the impregnation of free nerve endings runs the risk of giving rise to the "Martian canal" effect, the factors influencing the rates of degeneration of transected axons are not well understood (Repérant et al. 1991a), cell bodies may be labelled by transsynaptic leakage rather than retrograde transport(Weidner et al. 1983; Schnyder & Künzle 1984), and immunohistochemical techniques may be so sensitive that they reveal the presence of small quantities of the target antigen which do not necessarily have any physiological effect(Hökfelt et al. 1984). While a single study may therefore be open to criticism on a number of technical grounds, the mass of anatomical evidence that has accumulated since Cajal's initial study (1888) of the avian retina cannot be simply set aside.

The anatomical data, which have been recently reviewed by Repérant et al. 1989 and by Uchiyama 1989, may be summarised as follows.

(1) The location of retrogradely or immunochemically labelled intracerebral neurons varies widely from species to species. Such cells have been described in the

Mesencephalon
Tegmentum;
    Cyclostomes;Myxinoids - *Epatretus* (Wicht & Northcutt 1990) and
        Petromyzontiforms - *Lampetra* (Repérant et al. 1980;Vesselkin et
        al. 1980), *Ichthyomyzon* (Fritzsch & Collin 1990)
    Brachiopterygians; *Polypterus* (Meyer et al. 1983)
    Teleosts; *Esox* (Schilling &Northcutt 1987)

Some reptiles - Crocodiles; *Caiman* (Ferguson et al. 1978), Turtles;
   Pseudemys (Weiler 1985), Lizards; *Gerrhonotus* (Halpern et al.
   1986), *Varanus* (Hoogland &Welker 1981) and*Ophisaurus*
   (Kenigfest et al. 1986)
Birds; the isthmo-optic nucleus (ION)(Cowan & Powell 1963) and cells
   "ectopic" to the ION (Hayes & Webster 1981)
Tectum;
   Elasmobranchs; *Ginglymostoma* (Luiten 1981)
   Some teleosts; (references in Repérant et al. 1989 and Uchiyama 1989;
      Ebbesson & Meyer 1989)
   Superior colliculus of gerbils (Larsen & Møller 1985)
Oculomotor nuclei;
   Rats (Hoogland et al. 1985)
Peri-aqueductal gray matter
   Rats (Itaya & Itaya 1985)
Dorsal raphe nucleus
   Rats (Villar et al. 1987)

Diencephalon
Meso-diencephalic junction;
   Teleosts in general (references in Repérant et al. 1989 and Uchiyama 1989)
   Urodeles (Fritzsch & Himstedt 1981)
   Rats (Itaya 1980; Itaya & Itaya 1985; Villar et al. 1987)
Ventrolateral thalamus;
   Coenophidian snakes; *Crotalus* (Schroeder 1981), *Thamnophis* (Halpern et
      al. 1976), *Vipera* (Repérant et al. 1981)
   Lizards; *Cordylus* (Halpern et al. 1976)
Dorsal thalamus (GL pars dorsalis)
   Gerbils (Larsen & Møller 1985)
Hypothalamus
   Some teleosts (Gerwertzhagen et al. 1982; Uchiyama & Ito 1984; Matsutani et
      al. 1986)
   Dogs (Terubayashi et al. 1983);   *Microcebus* (Bons & Petter 1986)

Telencephalon
N.olfactoretinalis
   Teleosts in general (references in Repérant et al. 1989 and Uchiyama 1989)
Septal area
   Anurans (Wirsig-Wiechmann & Basinger 1988; Uchiyama et al. 1988)
Basal telencephalon
   Hoenophidian snakes; *Python* (Hoogland & Welker 1981)

Repérant et al. 1989 point out that in both amphibians and mammals attempts to visualize the cells of origin of the centrifugal visual fibers by conventional retrograde labelling have produced both inconsistent and highly controversial results, but that such techniques appear to give consistent results in other vertebrates. While some of the theoretical issues underlying labelling by retrograde transport are discussed in Cowan & Cuénod 1975, it is not clear why this is the case.

The logical difficulties that exist with these data are that (1) it is possible that some neurons are labelled by trans-synaptic leakage of tracer (e.g. Schnyder & Künzle 1984), (2) extraretinal leakage of injected tracer may label structures that are attached to, for example intraocularor extraocular (e.g. Weidner et al. 1983) muscles, or (3) the tracer may enter retinal blood vessels, to be distributed systemically and to leak back through the blood-brain barrier being eventually taken up by neurons (Peyrichoux et al. 1977).   As Repérant et al. 1989 point out, not all published studies present adequate control data that alow these possibilities to be ruled out.

The number of neurons involved in these systems is generally small compared to the numbers of retinal ganglion cells, between 1 - 5% in teleosts, about 1 - 2% in lampreys and *Vipera*, about 0.5% in birds, and considerably less in amphibians, turtles, and mammals,

(2)   These groups of neurons can be divided into two major groups on the basis of their afferent connections, where this has been demonstrated. Uchiyama 1989 has pointed out

that in one of these groups, typified by the avian isthmo-optic nucleus and which he terms the "ION-type" system, the centrifugal visual neurons form part of a retino-retinal feedback loop which passes by way of the tectum, while in the second "nonION-like" system, exemplified by the teleostean *n. olfactoretinalis*, the afferent supply to the centrifugal visual neurons is nonvisual in origin.

In cyclostomes, the two populations of tegmental centrifugal visual neurons form parts of two feedback loops. The nucleus M5 in the lamprey is innervated by optic fibers which terminate in the tegmental mesencephalic optic area (MOA) and thus forms part of the loop retina - MOA - M5 - retina (Repérant et al. 1988); the cells of the reticular mesencephalic area of the lamprey, on the other hand, are supplied by fibers from the superficial layers of the tectum (Repérant et al. 1988) and thus form part of the loop retina - tectum - RMA - retina. Wicht & Northcutt 1990 describe a similar state of affairs in the hagfish *Epatretus*, and claim that the two groups of cells that they describe are the myxinoid homologues of the cells described in M5 and the MRA of the lamprey.

In fish other than teleosts the data are extremely scanty and await confirmation by additional studies. Meyer 1983 describes centrifugal visual neurons in the tegmentum of the brachyopterygian *Polypterus*, and Luiten 1981 describes retrogradely labelled neurons in the *z. externum* of the *s. cellulare externum* of the tectum in the shark *Ginglymostoma*, but the afferent supplies of these cells remain to be demonstrated.

As both Repérant et al. 1989 and Uchiyama 1989 point out, the data concerning teleosts are simultaneously extensive, somewhat contradictory, and show a considerable degree of interspecific variation. Depending on the species, between one and five structures have been shown to contain retrogradely labelled neurons, while in other species no such cells have been demonstrated. As a general principle, however, it appears that the modern acanthopterygian teleosts contain two structures that project to the retina, the diencephalic preoptic retinopetal nucleus (PRN) and the telencephalic *n. olfactoretinalis*. The former receives an afferent supply from the tectum, primarily from cells located in the deeper *ss. periventriculare* or *album centrale* (Uchiyama et al. 1986), which have their dendritic arborizations horizontally distributed within small (0.01 mm^2) areas of the superficial *ss. opticum* and *griseum et fibrosum superficiale*. Furthermore, quantitative studies by the same authors show that the number of tectal neurons, retrogradely labelled by HRP injected into the PRN, is about the same as the number of neurons in the PRN.

The neurons of the teleostean *n. olfactoretinalis*, on the other hand, fall into two cytological classes, a minority of large (25 μm) multipolar neurons and a majority of smaller (12-15 μm) pear-shaped neurons. The dendritic processes of the latter penetrate the olfactory bulb and appear to make contact with mitral cells of the olfactory glomeruli (Matsutani et al. 1986). Three categories of axon appear to leave the nucleus (von Bartheld & Meyer 1986b); the first type crosses the midline twice, in the anterior commissure and the chiasm, to terminate in the ipsilateral retina, those of the second type cross in the chiasm to terminate in the contralateral retina, while those of the third type have extensive collateral branches which pass both to the contralateral retina and to central structures in the telencephalon, diencephalon or mesencephalon. Some cells of the *n. olfactoretinalis* have also been shown to project bilaterally to both retinae (Stell et al. 1984).

In amphibians, the afferent connections of the centrifugal visual neurons that have been demonstrated, either by retrograde labelling in the pretectum of urodeles (Fritzsch & Himstedt 1981) or immunohistochemically or by HRP in the septal area of anurans (Uchiyama et al. 1988), remain to be elaborated.

The available reptilian data are scanty. In the turtle *Pseudemys*, the centrifugal visual neurons are located in a poorly defined region of the caudal reticular formation of the mesencephalon (Schnyder & Künzle 1983; Weiler 1985) and are extremely few in number, 4-12 neurons projecting contralaterally and 1-3 projecting ipsilaterally. Their afferent supplies have not apparently been demonstrated.

In the coenophidian snakes *Crotalus* (Schroeder 1981), *Thamnophis* (Halpern et al. 1976) and *Vipera* (Repérant et al. 1981), retrogradely labelled cells are located in a ventrolateral thalamic nucleus described as the nucleus of the ventral commissure (Halpern et al. 1976; Schroeder 1981) or the centrifugal thalamic optic nucleus (Repérant et al. 1981), a structure which is known to receive tectal afferents (Wang & Halpern 1977) and thus forms part of an ION-like feedback loop.

In the hoenophidian snake *Python*, retinopetal fibers arise from neurons in the basal telencephalon (Hoogland & Welker 1981) which are scattered throughout a region rostral to the anterior thalamus, equal numbers of cells projecting ipsilaterally and contralaterally; after injection of different fluorochromes into the two eyes, Hoogland and Welker 1981 did not observe any doubly labelled cells.

In the lizards *Gerrhonotus* (Halpern et al. 1976), *Varanus* (Hoogland & Welker 1981), *Ophisaurus* (Kenigfest et al. 1986), retrogradely labelled cells have been observed in the caudal tegmentum, and in *Cordylus* (Halpern et al. 1976) in the ventral thalamus. Unfortunately, as is the case for *Python*, the sources of the afferent supply to these cells remains to be demonstrated.

In the crocodile *Caiman*, the centrifugal visual cells are located in the tegmentum and have an afferent supply from the tectum (Ferguson et al. 1978).

In birds, an extensive series of investigations by a number of workers (reviewed by Repérant et al. 1989 and Uchiyama 1989) have shown that the majority of cells projecting to the retina are located in the isthmo-optic nucleus (ION), lying caudally in the dorsal tegmentum.. This nucleus, while of variable size depending on the species, is described in classical neuroanatomical studies of all avian species that have been studied except the kiwi, the ibis and the ostrich.

By far the greater portion of the experimental studies of the ION have, however, been carried out in pigeons, chickens and quails. The cells of the ION receive afferent connections from neurons located in the *s. griseum et fibrosum superficiale* of the tectum (Crossland & Hughes 1978; Uchiyama & Watanabe 1985) as well as from other structures (Angaut & Repérant 1978). Virtually all neurons of the ION ($8 - 11 \times 10^3$ in pigeons and chickens) project to the contralateral retina; ipsilateral centrifugal projections from this structure are rare (O'Leary & Cowan 1982; Weidner et al. 1987).

A second, smaller population of centrifugal visual neurons (between 15 and 30% of the number of neurons on the ION), lying outside the IONand initially described as "ectopic" to this structure (Cowan and Clarke 1976), has been described in a number of avian species. The "ectopic" centrifugal neurons are larger than those of the ION (18 μm versus 15 μm in Golgi preparations), and receive afferent fibers from the tectum by way of the tectoisthmic tract (O'Leary & Cowan 1982). A moderate proportion of these cells project to the ipsilateral retina, the greater part projecting contralaterally.

Recent investigations (Catsicas et al. 1987; Fritzsch et al. 1990) have shown that the patterns of terminal arborizations of the axons arising from neurons of the ION and from "ectopic" neurons are different. The former are restricted to small areas of the retina, while the latter ramify over larger areas.

While numerous attempts have been made to label centrifugal visual neurons in mammals (see Repérant et al. 1989 for review) their outcomes are extremely controversial (e.g. Schnyder & Künzle 1984). The largest number of retrogradely labelled cells in mammals appears to exist in the hypothalamus of the dog (Terubayashi et al. 1983), but it is unkown whether these receive visual afferents. An additional, fairly consistent finding is the presenxce of a small number of retrogradely labelled neurons in the medial pretectal area (Itaya 1980; Itaya & Itaya 1985; Bunt et al. 1983; Villar et al. 1987). Villar et al. also describe a small population of labelled neurons in the dorsal raphe, destruction of which leads to a marked decrease in retinal serotonin. Their suggestion that these cells are thus serotoninergic has recently been confirmed by an investigation in which intraocular injection of [^{3}H]-serotonin was combined with immunochemical demonstration of serotoninergic neurons (Araneda et al., unpublished).

In addition, in hagfishes (Wicht & Northcutt 1990), anurans (Toth & Straznicky 1989), chicken embryos (McLoon & Lund 1982), developing rats (Bunt & Lund 1981; Bunt et al. 1983) and adult rats and rabbits (Müller & Holländer 1988), injection of tracer into one eye can lead to the retrograde labelling of ganglion cells in the contralateral eye.

(3) Prior to the adoption of retrograde labelling techniques, a number of older studies presented evidence either that axons survived in the central stump of the optic nerve after

transection or degenerated more rapidly in the peripheral stump (see Repérant et al. 1989 for a review of these studies).

While in the viper, the number of surviving axons seen 4 months after retinal ablation (Repérant et al. 1981) is comparable to the 600 or so cells that are retrogradely labelled after intraocular injection of tracer(Repérant et al. 1980), there exist two difficulties of interpretation of these results.   In nonmammalian species, particularly reptiles, the rate of degeneration of optic fibers is extremely variable (Repérant et al. 1991b), and thus the early degeneration of fibers in the distal stump together with the long-term survival of fibers in the proximal stump may not necessarily reflect the presence of a population of centrifugal fibers.   In addition, many of the mammalian results have not been repeated by other investigators.

(4)   Free nerve endings in the retina have been described by a number of investigators, using either classical Golgi (Cajal 1888) or reduced silver impregnation techniques (e.g. Repérant & Gallego 1976), anterogradely transported HRP (e.g. Vesselkin et al. 1988, 1989), immunochemical labelling (e.g. Schütte & Weiler 1988) or antibodies directed against neurofilaments (e.g. Dräger et al. 1984). In snakes, crocodiles, birds and mammals the centrifugal fibers are generally large and myelinated, while in the majority of species they are small and unmyelinated (Repérant et al. 1989).   Except in birds, in which the terminal areas of the fibers are small and nonoverlapping (Hayes & Holden 1983), the fibers generally ramify to cover wide areas of the peripheral retina.

The logical difficulty in interpreting these findings is that in some cases (notably the mammalian data) evidence as to the location of the cells of origin of these endings is lacking.   It is thus possible that the fibers may be recurrent collaterals of retinofugal fibers that branch postchiasmatically, or may be misrouted fibers arising from the contralateral retina (e.g. Frizsch et al. 1990).

(5)   The termination of centrifugal fibers within the retina appears to be considerably more consistent than the location of their cells of origin.

In cyclostomes, the thin (0.2-0.3 μm) unmyelinated centrifugal fibers, labelled with HRP, terminate within the external zone of the inner plexiform layer, and make symmetrical Type I synaptic contacts with either unlabelled cell bodies, unlabelled profiles containing synaptic vesicles, or more rarely with labelled dendrites of retinal ganglion cells (Vesselkin et al. 1988, 1989).

In teleosts, the fibers reaching the retina from the n. olfactoretinalis terminate either on amacrine cells (Carassius; Stell et al. 1988) or on dopaminergic interplexiform cells (Perca; Zucker & Dowling 1987).

The peptidergic centrifugal fibers of amphibians course through the inner plexiform layer, branching frequently, and appear to terminate at the proximal boundary of the amacrine cell layer (Wirsig-Weichmann & Basinger 1988).

In the turtle retina, the small number of peptidergic (Weiler 1985) or serotoninergic (Schütte & Weiler 1988) centrifugal fibers arborize extensively within the inner plexiform layer.

In birds, Dogiel 1895 was the first to observe two different patterns of terminal arborizations of centrifugal fibers, a "widespread" type in which tangential arborizations cover an area of several hundred microns in the inner plexiform layer close to the inner nuclear layer, and a "restricted" type in which the terminal arborizations form a basket around a single amacrine cell.   A more recent study (Fritzsch et al. 1990) has confirmed this observation. Fibers giving rise to restricted endings are relatively thick and devoid of varicosities, and run for a short distance in the scleral level of the inner plexiform layer after leaving the optic fiber layer.   The fibers giving rise to widespread endings are thinner and varicose, and ramify extensively within the inner plexiform layer.

Several investigators have described centrifugal fibers in the mammalian retina, using either Golgi, reduced silver impregnation (references in Repérant et al. 1989) or immunochemical techniques (Dräger et al. 1984).   These fibers are generally large and myelinated, few in number (less than 10 in human retinae; Repérant & Gallego 1976) and branch extensively in the inner plexiform layer, where they appear to terminate.

(6)   A number of possible neurotransmitters and neuropeptides have been identified in centrifugal visual neurons or in their retinal arborizations;

Serotonin (*Pseudemys* - Schutte & Weiler 1988; rats - Villar et al. 1987)
GABA (cyclostomes - Repérant et al. 1988)
Substance P (teleosts - Zucker & Dowling 1987; amphibians - Uchiyama et
    al. 1988; Wirsig-Weichmann & Basinger 1988)
GnRH (teleosts - Stell et al. 1988)
LHRH (teleosts - Zucker & Dowling 1987)
FMRF amide (teleosts - Zucker & Dowling 1987; amphibians - Uchiyama et
    al. 1988; Wirsig-Weichmann & Basinger 1988)
Met-enkephalin (*Pseudemys* - Weiler 1985)
Acetylcholine (birds - Hayes 1982; mammals - references in Repérant et al. 1989).

In some cases two or more of neuropeptides may coexist within the same terminals (Stell et al. 1984; Zucker & Dowling 1987)

(7)   Developmental studies of the centrifugal visual system are fewer in number than those in adult vertebrates.

In the marine lamprey *Petromyzon*, the two populations of retinopetal neurons that exist in M5 and MRA of adults can be demonstrated by HRP in young (<70 mm) larvae, before retinal differentiation is complete (de Miguel et al. 1987, 1990; Rubinson 1990). Some of the theoretical implications of this finding are discussed below.

In teleosts, the number of neurons in the *n. olfactoretinalis* increases throughout the life of the fish (Crapon de Caprona & Fritzsch 1983), a state of affairs which is reminiscent of the continuous generation of retinal ganglion cells in teleosts (Meyer 1978; Johns 1981), and the retinopetal fibers appear early in development, those arising from the *n. olfactoretinalis* slightly earlier than those from the diencephalon (Rusoff & Hapner 1990).

In chicken embryos, the cells of the ION are generated between the fifth and seventh day on incubation, within the caudal mesencephalic alar plate, and migrate ventrolaterally to aggregate as the anlage of the nucleus. Centrifugal fibers penetrate the retina by the ninth day of incubation in the chick, and the number of cells projecting to the retina decreases by about 50 - 60% between days 13 and 17, stabilising thereafter. The "ectopic" neurons and the neurons of the ION differentiate at the same time, but it is not altogether clear whether the "ectopic" cells are simply misdirected during migration from the neuroepithelium or represent a different neuronal population (Repérant et al. 1989). This latter possibility is strengthened by the cytological differences between the two populations of cells, referred to in (2), and the finding that cells of the ION and "ectopic" cells have different patterns of termination within the retina (Catsicas et al. 1987; Fritzsch et al. 1990).

Both in birds and in teleosts, an association appears to exist between the importance of the centrifugal system and the mode of life of the species. Uchiyama 1989 points out that, in teleosts, the largest number of diencephalic retinopetal neurons is found in the balistid filefish *Navodon* and accounts for about 1% of the optic nerve fibers (Ito & Murakami 1984), and in birds the number of neurons in the ION is considerably greater in Galliforms and Columbiforms than in raptors (Weidner et al. 1987). Even so, the 10×10^4 cells of the ION of the pigeon (Weidner et al. 1987) only account for about 0.4% of the 2.5 x 10^6 fibers of the optic nerve (Bingelli & Paule 1969), this proportion being even smaller (about 0.04%) in raptors (Repérant et al. 1989).

Balistid fish are slow-moving, highly manoeuvrable inhabitants of coral reefs that are specialised to feed on sessile food rather than free-swimming prey (Lorenz 1962), and Galliform and Columbiform birds feed by pecking at objects - generally small seeds - on the ground.   Both groups perform frequent eye-head movements (Goodale 1983; Lanchester & Mark 1975), and during feeding behavior the target is located at a short viewing distance.   The centrifugal systems of these species may thus, as both Uchiyama 1989 and Repérant et al. 1989 have suggested, be involved in the modulation of retinal sensitivity either to supress blurring of the retinal image during eye movements or to facilitate detection of a target.   On the other hand, both ground-feeding birds and filefish are likely to be the objects of attention of predators, and the function of the centrifugal system may be more directly related to the early detection of a distant, oncoming and menacing object (Rogers & Miles 1972; Uchiyama 1989; Holden 1990).

Functional investigations

Physiological studies of the avian centrifugal visual system are extensive, and began with the investigations by Miles 1971and Galifret et al. 1971 of the isthmo-optic nucleus. In an extensive series of investigations in decerebrate chickens, Miles 1972a-d showed that the effects of manipulations of the ION on the physiological properties of retinal ganglion cells could be summarised as follows. Stimulation of the ION facilitates the visual responses of retinal ganglion cells, and cooling of the structure produces a decrease in the magnitude of the response of ganglion cells to visual stimulation. In both cases, however, the type of stimulus producing a maximal response of the ganglion cell - which Repérant et al. 1989 call the "trigger feature" - is unchanged. Cells within the ION that are responsive to visual stimulation have large receptive fields, up to five times the size of the receptive fields of retinal ganglion cells, habituate rapidly to repetitive stimulation, and appear to be most responsive to anteroposterior movement of dark edges.

Since the centrifugal visual fibers terminate on amacrine cells in the avian retina (Dowling & Cowan 1966), Miles 1972b,c suggested that the facilitatory influence of these fibers is due to their inhibition of inhibitory effects of amacrine cells on retinal ganglion cells. It is unfortunately not clear whether these effects are limited to a particular category of retinal ganglion cell or not. Uchiyama 1989 points out that while the morphological features and physiological features of ganglion cells projecting to the avian tectum, thalamus, pretectum, hypothalamus and tegmentum are different (Bravo & Pettigrew 1981; Burkhalter et al. 1979), and that centrifugal influences can only be demonstrated in 70-80% of avian retinal ganglion cells (Miles 1972b; Pearlman & Hughes 1976) it remains to be shown whether centrifugal influences apply equally to all categories of ganglion cell. If ganglion cells are categorised by their response properties rather than morphology, the data are contradictory. Nondirectional ganglion cells with on-off responses, nondirectional cells with on-responses and directionally sensitive cells with on-off responses account together for over 90% of the population in birds (Holden 1982); Miles 1972b found no major difference of the degree of centrifugal effects among these three types, while Pearlman & Hughes 1976 reported a higher proportion of directionally sensitive or motion-sensitive cells responding to centrifugal influences.

In a study of the ION in chronically prepared, unanesthetized pigeons, Marin et al. 1990 present findings which generally support Miles 1972b but with some quantitative differences; the receptive fields of cells in the ION were smaller than those reported by Miles 1972b, and the degree of habituation to repetitive stimulation was neither as strong nor as frequent as in the decerebrate chick. The question whether these differences are due to decerebration or represent an interspecific difference remains open. The major finding of Marin et al. 1990 was that the tonic activity of cells in the ION decreased or disappeared altogether during saccades and the fast recovery phase of optokinetic nystagmus.

Physiological investigations in nonavian species other than mammals are less extensive. Vesselkin et al. 1989 present electrophysiological evidence to support the notion that centrifugal fibers in the lamprey terminate on amacrine cells and sometimes on ganglion cells, in support of morphological data to the same effect. In balistid teleosts, stimulation of the centrifugal fibers produces a facilitatory effect on retinal ganglion cells (Sandeman & Rosenthal 1974) similar to that found in birds, and application of the neuropeptides contained in the olfactoretinal terminals (FRMF amide and LHRH) increases the spontaneous activity of the isolated goldfish retina (Stell et al. 1984). Murakami & Shimoda 1977 found excitatory post-synaptic potentials (EPSPs) in some amacrine cells of the carp retina.

In frogs, EPSPs contingent on optic nerve stimulation have been described in amacrine cells by Byzov & Utina 1971 and by Matsumoto 1975.

Marchiafava 1976 observed EPSPs in amacrine cells of the turtle retina, produced by stimulation of the optic nerve. Also in turtles, Cervetto et al. 1976 found that when the retinal ganglion cell was subjected simultaneously to photic stimulation and to centrifugal influences, the distribution of excitatability over the receptive field of the ganglion cell changed, the center becoming more excitable at the expense of the periphery.

It is somewhat surprising that in spite of the highly controversial anatomical data concerning the retinopetal system in mammals, a fairly extensive physiological literature exists (cf Repérant et al. 1989) in which central affects on mammalian retinal function have been demonstrated.

Both Dodt 1956 and Ogden & Brown 1964 found evidence of electrophysiological events following the antidromic action potential evoked in ganglion cells by stimulation of the optic nerve. In rats, cryogenic blockade of the visual cortex or pretectum (Molotchnikoff & Tremblay 1983, 1986) modifies the response properties of retinal ganglion cells, in particular those that show off-responses. Spinelli & Weingarten 1966 reported that, for about 10% of the optic nerve fibers that they studied, responses could be elicited by auditory or somesthetic stimili, and that the association of nonvisual stimuli with flashes of light led to a decrease in the latency of the response to visual stimulation.

A number of studies in which section of the mammalian optic nerve led to increases in the amplitude of the electroretinogram (references in Repérant et al. 1989) have not been replicated by other workers (e.g. Brindley & Hamasaki 1962). The claim that the human ERG can be manipulated by the selective attention of the observer (Eason et al. 1983) has similarly not been confirmed (Mangun et al. 1986).

Behavioral studies of the effects of manipulations of the centrifugal visual system are extremely few in number. Somewhat surprisingly, in view of the wealth of anatomical data concerning the avian centrifugal visual system and the widespread use of pigeons in operant conditioning and psychophysical studies (see Wright 1979 for a brief review), only four behavioral studies appear to have been carried out. Intensity and pattern discriminations in pigeons are unimpaired by bilateral lesions of the ION (Hodos & Karten 1974). Pecking behaviour in pigeons, directed towards grain scattered on the floor, is either diminished (Shortess & Klose 1977) or unaffected (Knipling 1978) by such lesions.

The most extensive study appears to be that by Rogers & Miles 1972. Young (1-2 week old) chicks were either subjected to complete bilateral lesions of the ION, incomplete bilateral lesions, or a sham-operative procedure in which all surgical procedures except the creation of anodal electrolytic lesions were carried out, and were compared to intact control birds. The behavioral variables examined were the efficiency of picking up grain scattered on a uniform clear floor, the ability to discriminate between grain and pebbles of the same size, shape and color scattered over a black-and-white checkerboard, and the response of the chicks while feeding from a food hopper to a novel object approaching from the rear. The results indicate that lesioned chicks need to make more pecks than controls in order to pick up a given number of grains, that their ability to discriminate between grain and pebbles in dark squares (but not in light squares) of a checkerboard is reduced, and that their reactivity to an approaching novel object is reduced. In addition, Rogers & Miles 1972 mention that lesioned birds showed two abnormalities; they frequently made pecking movements with the beak closed, and pecked at non-food objects such as specks of dirt on the walls of the testing chamber. It is extremely unfortunate that these authors did not incorporate an additional control group of chicks, with lesions of comparable size in a structure other than the ION.

Conclusions

The extensive morphological and biochemical variation of the centrifugal system leads to considerable difficulties in trying to analyse its possible evolution. Uchiyama 1989 makes a start at the question by considering the "ION-like" retino-retinal feedback loop separately from the "nonION-like" system. The ION-like system can in turn be divided into at least two subgroups, one with retinopetal neurons in the tegmentum, the second with the cell bodies in the ventral thalamus or pretectum.

The situation is complicated by the fact that for some vertebrate groups (notably urodeles and lizards) retinopetal cells are found in the same area as the ION-like neurons of other groups, but their afferent connections remain to be demonstrated, and the system thus awaits classification as ION-like or nonION-like.

However, the anatomical evidence indicates that ION-like systems, characterised by the involvement of the tectum, exist in cyclostomes, teleosts, some reptiles, and birds, while nonION-like systems in which the tectum is not involved exist in teleosts, other reptilian species and possibly in mammals. While the neurochemical data are somewhat fragmentary, the presence of neuromodulatory peptides in teleosts (in which an important centrifugal influence on the retina is the nonION-like olfactoretinal projection)and anurans (in which the retinopetal cell bodies are in the septal area and thus probably nonION-like) and of chemically simpler neurotransmitters in the ION-like systems of cyclostomes and birds together with the absence of neuropeptides in the avian ION (de Lanerolle et al. 1981; Woodson et al. 1989) suggests that the ION-like and nonION-like systems may possibly be distinguished on the basis of the neuroactive substances involved (Uchiyama 1989). It is obvious, as both Repérant et al. 1989 and Uchiyama 1989 point out, that further neurochemical investigations are called for.

An additional difference between the two centrifugal influences on the retina is that the fibers of ION-like neurons project to small, discrete areas of the retina, while the nonION-like fibers ramify extensively. This state of affairs suggests that the functions of the two systems may be different.

At this point any discussion of the phylogeny of the two systems runs into a number of difficulties. Two populations of retinopetal neurons exist in cyclostomes (Vesselkin et al. 1980, 1984; Repérant et al. 1980; Frizsch & Collin 1990; Wicht & Northcutt 1990). Since the Petromyzontiforms are considered the sister group of jawed vertebrates (Janvier 1981), we may enquire whether these groups of cells are the common origin of the ION-like and non-ION-like centrifugal systems of more modern vertebrates.

Sufficient evidence exists to make this possibility highly unlikely. The homologue of the teleostean *n. olfactoretinalis* (the ganglion of the *n. terminalis*) appears to exist in all vertebrate classes (Kuhlenbeck 1977; von Bartheld et al. 1987). Neither in larval (de Miguel et al. 1990; Rubinson 1990) nor adult cyclostomes (Vesselkin et al. 1980, 1984) are neurons in this structure labelled by intraocular tracer, neither can such neurons be demonstrated in *Polypterus* (von Bartheld & Meyer 1986a) nor in selacians (Luiten 1981), and we are thus forced to accept that the retinopetal neurons of the teleostean *n. olfactoretinalis* have an origin independent of that of the retinopetal neurons of cyclostomes.

An alternative type of scenario has been proposed by Ebbesson 1980 and Ebbesson & Meyer 1981. It may be the case that the evolution of the nervous system proceeds by the progressive elimination of more and more connections from an initially diffuse network. This "parcellation" theory requires us to suppose that, in the more primitive vertebrates, retinopetal projections arose from a diversity of central structures, more and more of which were eliminated with each divergence from the ancestral stock. Together with the reader we are thus required to suppose that the sources of retinopetal axons are more widespread in ancient vertebrates or in embryonic forms, and less extensive but more diverse in modern adult forms. The developmental data are not as extensive as they might be; they do, however, indicate that in larval cyclostomes (Rubinson 1990; de Miguel et al. 1990) the same two cell groups are found as in adults, one in M5 and one in the mesencephalic reticular area, a finding which rules out the possibility that some additional groups of retinopetal neurons might exist in larval cyclostomes but disappear during development.

In teleosts, the number of neurons in the *n. olfactoretinalis* increases during development (Crapon de Caprona & Frizsch 1983), a state of affairs reminiscent of the continuous growth of the retina and tectum in teleosts (Meyer 1978; Johns 1981) and in marked contrast to the reduction that takes place in the developing avian ION (Cowan & Clarke 1976). As in cyclostomes, no transient groups of retinopetal neurons that disappear during development have been reported (Crapon de Caprona & Fritzsch 1983; Rusoff & Hapner 1990).

In addition, none of the developmental studies reviewed by Repérant et al. 1989 refer to the existence of populations of retinopetal neurons other than those of the ION and the "ectopic" neurons in avian ambryos. In adult forms, the parcellation theory runs into the difficulty that the number of structures containing retinopetal neurons is more extensive in some teleosts than in cyclostomes, in contradiction to expectation.

Both Repérant et al. 1989 and Uchiyama 1989 have suggested that the centrifugal visual systems of different vertebrate groups may be polyphyletic in origin and have arisen independently on a number of occasions. Northcutt 1984, using cladistic analysis, has pointed out that separate, independent origins of homoplastic (Lankester 1970) characters in the central nervous system are commoner than one might expect; as examples he cites the ascending spinothalamic pathways in elasmobranchs and amniotes, the descending palliospinal pathways in birds and mammals, and the electroreceptive systems of teleosts and other anamniotes.

The available data are unfortunately too fragmentary to enable us to pursue the question of homologous or analogous origins of the different populations of centrifugal cells in detail, but the notion that a number of these populations have indepenent origins does give a reasonable account of some of the data.

Centrifugal visual neurons exist in the tegmentum of a large number of vertebrates {see (1)}.   In birds and the closely related crocodiles these cells may possibly be homologous (although this remains to be shown), but the absence of such cells in elasmobranchs, most teleosts, and amphibians clearly rules out the possibility that the "crocodilio-avian" group of tegmental centrifugal neurons is homologous with those of cyclostomes.

Centrifugal neurons have also been described in the tectum of a number of species of teleost.   If we accept (Ebbesson & Meyer 1989) that these are not due to methodological errors in spite of the contradictory nature of the data, the presence of these cells in some families but not others (Repérant et al. 1989; Uchiyama 1989) or in some species of the same family but not others (Ebbesson & Meyer 1989) also suggests strongly that these populations of cells may be homoplasous rather than homologous.

The presence of two arrangements of the retinopetal neurons in lizards, either in the mesencephalon or in the thalamus, is reminiscent of the attempt to distinguish between Type I lacertomorph and Type II dracomorph lizards (Northcutt 1972, 1978; Platel 1975) on the basis of neuroanatomical differences. However, both the dracomorph *Varanus* and the lacertomorph *Gerrhonotus* have mesencephalic retinopetal neurons, and the lacertomorph *Cordylus* has thalamic centrifugal visual neurons.   Thus, as for the ipsilateral retinofugal projections in lizards (Repérant et al. 1991b), interspecific differences in the arrangement of the lacertilian retinopetal system do not correspond to the distinction between Type I and Type II lizards.

An additional, intriguing possibility is indirectly suggested by Wicht & Northcutt 1990. These authors, in discussing the primary visual system of the myxinoid *Epatretus*, point out that hagfishes are benthic, and active at night.   The eyes lack a lens, iris and extraocular muscles.   The behavioral studies to which they refer indicate that the only known visually guided behavior of these creatures is negative phototaxis, which is not abolished by destruction of the eyes.   The authors contrast these findings with the elaborate retinofugal and retinopetal connections that they demonstrate, and enquire why these exist.   They suggest, among other possibilities, that the visual system of hagfishes may be nonfunctional, and that its components are under no direct selection pressure but persist because of selection for some other, unidentified, character. It is thus conceivable that the same may be true of the centrifugal visual neurons in some vertebrate groups.

It may also be the case (particularly for the direct retino-retinal projections that have been demonstrated in some species) that some retinopetal neurons may be the result of developmental accidents.

Discussions of the possible function of the centrifugal system (Repérant et al. 1989; Uchiyama 1989; Holden 1990) point out that central modulation of sensory input can be demonstrated in a number of other modalities.   The efferent fibers to the lateral line organs of fish and amphibians are activated during self-induced movement (Russel & Roberts 1974) and inhibit the afferent volleys that would otherwise be generated, and centrifugal fibers to the vestibular system of squirrel monkeys appear to be involved in extending the dynamic range of the system during head movements (Goldberg & Fernandez 1980).

A number of possible roles of the avian centrifugal visual system have been suggested.   The physiological data, showing that the centrifugal fibers supress inhibitory effects in the retina (Miles 1972b,c) and that they decrease in activity during eye movements (Marin et al. 1990) indicate that this system may be involved in a decrease in visual sensitivity during saccadic eye movements similar to that which has been demonstrated psychophysically in human observers (Stevenson et al. 1986). The effect of such a decrease in sensitivity may well be to supress the blurring of the retinal image that would otherwise take place. The physiological data are also consistent with the notion that the centrifugal visual system may be involved in the distinction between movement of the retinal image brought about by the animal's own movement (in particular, eye movements) and by movement of an external object with respect to the animal's retina (Repérant et al. 1989)

Alternatively, Uchiyama 1989 and Holden 1990 have suggested that the system may be involved in attentional processes; the two authors differ, however, as to the nature of these processes. Uchiyama 1989 points out the similarities in feeding behavior between ground-feeding birds and balisitid teleosts, two groups in which the ION-like system is pronounced, and suggests, with Weidner et al. 1987, that the system may be involved in the attentional processes associated with the discrimination of edible targets. On the other hand Holden 1990 points out that the receptive fields of neurons in the pigeon ION are principally located in the upper retina (on which the image of the nearby terrain falls during feeding), while the terminals of the centrifugal fibers are mainly located in the lower retina (which views the horizon and the upper visual field), suggesting that the system may be more involved in the attentional processes associated with predator detection.

One major difficulty with Holden's hypothesis is that the detection of a distant predator involves the detection of high spatial frequencies; a raptor with a wingspan of 50 cm, at a distance of 1 km, subtends a visual angle of about 1 min. arc, or 30 cycles/degree. The detection of such an object thus requires a fairly high degree of selectivity (Morgan & Ward 1985), yet the electrophysiological evidence indicates that the disinhibitory influence of the ION on retinal ganglion cells is to decrease selectivity.

While the possible role of the nonION-like centrifugal system is even less evident, the fairly consistent pattern of termination of termination of centrifugal fibers in the retina suggests that the nonION-like fibers may also influence the activity of amacrine cells. Uchiyama 1989 points out that a general feature of nonION-like retinopetal fibers is their extremely wide ramification within the retina; the single serotoninergic fiber described by Schütte & Weiler 1988 in *Pseudemys* arborizes within about one-third of the total retinal area, and the fibers described by Repérant & Gallego 1976 in the human retina may arborize within an entire retinal quadrant. It is thus highly unlikely that such fibers are involved in a process which selectively modifies the function of a restricted region of the retina, in contrast to the attentional processes which have been suggested for the ION-like system. Demski & Northcutt 1983 suggested that the centrifugal neurons of the n. *olfactoretinalis* of teleosts might be involved in an overall modulation of retinal sensitivity in response to olfactory cues such as pheromones, a hypothesis which appears to be invalidated by the subsequent finding that these neurons do not respond to olfactory stimulation (Fujita et al. unpublished, cited by Uchiyama 1989). Repérant et al. 1989 point out that the modification of retinal sensitivity brought about by dark adaptation is slow, yet in the majority of cases the amount of light that strikes the retina varies amost instantaneously as the environment is viewed; they suggest that a more rapid modulation of overall retinal sensitivity may be brought about by a small number of centrifugal fibers which ramify over wide areas of the retina.

References

Angaut, P. & J. Repérant (1978) A light- and electron-microscopic study of the nucleus isthmo-opticus in the pigeon. *Archives d'Anatomie Microscopique et de Morphologie Expérimentale* **67**:63-78

von Bartheld, C.S. & D.L. Meyer (1986a) Central projections of the nervus terminalis in the bichir, *Polypterus palmas. Cell and Tissue Research* **244**:181-186

von Bartheld, C.S. & D.L. Meyer (1986b) Retinofugal and retinopetal projections in the teleost (*Channa micropeltes*) (Channiformes). *Cell and Tissue Research* **251**:653-663

von Bartheld, C.S., H.W. Lindörfer & D.L. Meyer (1987) The nervus terminalis also exists in cyclostomes and birds. *Cell and Tissue Research* **250**:431-434

Bingelli, R.L. & W.J. Paule (1969) The pigeon retina: quantitative aspects of the optic nerve and ganglion cell layer. *Journal of Comparative Neurology* **137**:1-18

Bons, N. & A. Petter (1986) Afférences rétiniennes d'origine hypothalamique chez un primate prosimien: *Microcebus murinus*. Etude à l'aide de traceurs fluorescents rétrogrades. *Comptes Rendus de l'Académie des Sciences (Paris)* **303**:719-722

Bravo, H. & J.D. Pettigrew (1981) The distribution of neurons projecting from the retina and visual cortex to the thalamus and tectum opticum of the barn owl (*Tyto alba*) and the burrowing owl (*Speotyto cunicularia*). *Journal of Comparative Neurology* **199**:419-441

Brindley, G.S. & D.I. Hamasaki (1962) Histological evidence against the view that the cat's optic nerve contains centrifugal fibres. *Journal of Physiology* **184**:444-449

Bunt, S.M. & R.D. Lund (1981) Development of a transient retino-retinal pathway in hooded and albino rats. *Brain Research* **211**:399-404

Bunt, S.M., R.D. Lund & P.W. Land (1983) Prenatal development of the optic projection in albino and hooded rats. *Developmental Brain Research* **6**:149-168

Byzov, A.L. & I.A. Utina (1971) Centrifugal influence on amacrine cells in frog retina. (in Russian) *Neurofiziologia* **3**:293-300

Burkhalter, A., S.J. Wang & P. Streit (1979) Thalamic projection of retinal ganglion cells: distribution and classification. *Neuroscience Letters* (Supplement) **3**: S285

Cajal, S.R. (1888) Estructura de la retina de las aves. *Revista Trimestral de Histologia Normal y Patologia* **1**, August 1888. Reprinted 1924 in *Trabajos Escogidos* **1**:355-371 Madrid, Jimenez y Mollari

Catsicas, S., S. Thanos & P.G.H. Clarke (1987) Major role for neuronal death during brain development: refinement of topographical connections. *Proceedings of the National Academy of Sciences of the USA* **84**:8165-8168

Cervetto , L., P.L. Marchiafava & E. Pasina (1976) Influence of efferent retinal fibres on responsiveness of ganglion cells to light. *Nature* **260**:56-57

Cowan, W.M. & M. Cuénod (1975) *The use of axonal transport for studies of neuronal connectivity*. Amsterdam, Elsevier

Cowan, W.M. & P.G.H. Clarke (1976) The development of the isthmo-optic nucleus. *Brain, Behavior and Evolution* **13**:345-375

Cowan, W.M. & T.P.S. Powell (1963) Centrifugal fibres in the avian visual system. *Proceedings of the Royal Society B* **158**:232-252

Crapon de Caprona, M.-D. & B. Fritzsch (1983) The development of the retinopetal nucleus olfacto-retinalis of two cichlid fish as revealed by horseradish peroxidase. *Developmental Brain Research* **11**:281-301

Crossland, W.J. & C.P. Hughes (1978) Observations on the afferent and efferent connections of the avian isthmo-optic nucleus. *Brain Research* **145**:239-256

Demski, L.S. & R.G. Northcutt (1983) The terminal nerve: a new chemosensory system in vertebrates? *Science* **220**:43437

Dodt, E. (1956) Centrifuigal impulses in rabbit's retina. *Journal of Neurophysiology* **19**:301-307

Dogiel, A.S. (1895) Die Retina der Vögel. *Archiv für Mikroskopische Anatomie* **44**:622-648

Dowling, J.E. & W.M. Cowan (1966) An electron-microscope study of normal and degenerating centrifugal fibre terminals in the pigeon retina. *Zeitschrift für Zellforschung und Mikroskopische Anatomie* **71**:14-28

Dräger, U.C., D.L. Edwards & C.J. Barnstable (1984) Antibodies against filamentous components in discrete cell types of the mouse retina. *Journal of Neuroscience* **4**:2025-2042

Eason, R.G., M. Oakley & L. Flowers (1983) Central neural influences on the human retina during selective attention. *Physiological Psychology* **11**:18-28

Ebbesson, S.O.E. (1980) The parcellation theory and its relation to interspecific variability in brain organization, evolutionary and ontogenetic development, and neuronal plasticity. *Cell and Tissue Research* **213**:179-212

Ebbesson, S.O.E. & D.L. Meyer (1981) Efferents to the retina have multiple sopurces in teleost fish. *Science* **214**:924-926

Ebbesson, S.O.E. & D.L. Meyer (1989) Retinopetal cells exist in the optic tectum of steelhead trout. *Neuroscience Letters* **106**:95-98

Ferguson, J.L., P.J. Mulvanny & S.E. Brauth (1978) Distribution of neurons projecting to the retina of *Caiman crocodilus*. *Brain, Behavior and Evolution* **15**:294-306

Fritzsch, B. & W. Himstedt (1981) Pretectal neurons project to the salamander retina. *Neuroscience Letters* **24**:13-17

Fritzsch, B. & S.P. Collin (1990) Dendritic distribution of two populations of ganglion cells and the retinopetal fibers in the retina of the silver lamprey (*Ichthyomyzon unicuspis*). *Visual Neuroscience* **4**:533-545

Fritzsch, B., M.-D. Crapon de Caprona & P.G.H. Clarke (1990) Development of two morphological types of retinopetal fibers in chick embryos, as shown by the diffusion along axons of a carbocyanine dye in the fixed retina. *Journal of Comparative Neurology* **300**:405-421

Galifret, Y., F. Condé-Courtine, J. Repérant & J. Servière (1971) Centrifugal control in the visual system of the pigeon. *Vision Research* (Supplement) **3**:185-200

Gewurtzhagen, K., M.J. Rickmann, D.L. Meyer & S.O.E. Ebbesson (1982) Optic tract cells projecting to the retina in the teleost (*Pantodon buchholzi*). *Cell and Tissue Research* **225**:23-28

Goldberg, J.M. & C. Fernandez (1980) Efferent vestibular system in the squirrel monkey: anatomical location and influence on afferent activity. *Journal of Neurophysiology* **43**:986-1025

Goodale, M.A. (1983) Visually guided pecking in the pigeon (*Columba livia*). *Brain, Behavior and Evolution* **22**:22-41

Halpern, M., R.T. Wang & D.R. Coleman (1976) Centrifgal fibers to the eye in a nonavian vertebrate: source revealed by horseradish peroxidase studies. *Science* **194**:1185-1188

Hayes, B.P. (1982) The structural organization of the pigeon retina. *Progress in Retinal Research* **1**:197-226

Hayes, B.P. & A.L. Holden (1983) The distribution of centrifugal terminals in the pigeon retina. *Experimental Brain Research* **49**:189-197

Hayes, B.P. & K.E. Webster (1981) Neurons situated outside the isthmo-optic nucleus and projecting to the eye in adult birds. *Neuroscience Letters* **26**:107-112

Hodos, W. & H.J. Karten (1974) Visual intensity and pattern discrimination deficits after esions of ectostriatum in pigeon. *Journal of Comparative Neurology* **140**:53-68

Hökfelt, T., O. Johanson & M. Goldstein (1984) Chemical anatomy of the brain. *Science* **225**:1326-1334

Holden, A.L. (1982) Electrophysiology of the avian retina. *Progress in Retinal Research* **1**:179-196

Holden, A.L. (1990) Centrifugal pathways to the retina: which way does the "searchlight" point? *Visual Neuroscience* **4**:493-495

Hoogland, P.V. & E. Welker (1981) Telencephalic projections to the eye in *Python reticulatus*. *Brain Research* **213**:173-176

Hoogland, P.V., A. Vanderkrans, F. Koole & H.J. Groenewegen (1985) A direct projection from the nucleus oculomotorius to the retina in rats. *Neuroscience Letters* **56**:323-328

Itaya, S.K. (1980) Retinal efferents from the pretectal area in the rat. *Brain Research* **201**:436-441

Itaya, S.K. & P.W. Itaya (1985) Centrifugal fibers to the rat retina from the medial pretectal area and the periaqueductal grey matter. *Brain Research* **326**:362-365

Ito, H. & T. Murakami (1984) Retinal ganglion cells in two teleost species, *Sebasticus marmoratus* and *Navodon modestus*. *Journal of Comparative Neurology* **229**:80-96

Janvier, P. (1981) The phylogeny of the Craniata with particular reference to the significance of fossil "agnathans". *Journal of Vertebrate Palaeontology* **1**:121-159

Johns, P.R. (1981) Growth of fish retinas. *American Zoologist* **21**:447-458

Kenigfest, N.B., J. Repérant & N.P. Vesselkin (1986) Retinal projections in the lizard *Ophisaurus apodus* revealed by autoradiographic and peroxidase methods. (in Russian) *Journal of Evolutionary and Biochemical Physiology* **22**:181-187

Knipling, R.R. (1978) No deficit in near-field visual acuity of pigeons after transection of the isthmo-optic tract. *Physiology and Behavior* **21**:813-816

Kuhlenbeck, H. (1977) *The central nervous system of vertebrates*, vol. 5, I. *Derivatives of the prosencephalon: diencephalon and telencephalon*. Basel, Karger

Lanchester, B.S. & R.F. Mark (1975) Pursuit and prediction in the tracing of moving food by a teleost fish (*Acanthaluteres spilomelanurus*). *Journal of Experimental Biology* **63**:627-645

Lankester, E.R. (1870) On the use of the term homology in modern zoology, and the distinction between homogenetic and homoplastic agreements. *Annual Magazine of Natural History* **4**:34-43

Larsen, J.N.B. & M. Møller (1985) Evidence for efferent projections from the brain to the retina of the Mongolian gerbil (*Meriones unguiculatus*). A horseradish peroxidase tracing study. *Acta Ophthalmologica* (Supplement) **63**:11-14

Lazar, G. (1969) Distribution of optic terminals in the different optic centers of the frog. *Brain Research* **16**:1-14

Lorenz, K. (1962) The function of colour in coral reef fishes. *Proceedings of the Royal Institute of Great Britain* **39**:282-296

Luiten, P.G.M. (1981) Two visual pathways to the telencephalon in the nurse shark (*Ginglymostoma cirratum*). I. Retinal projections. *Journal of Comparative Neurology* **196**: 531-538

Mangun, G.R., J.C. Hansen & S.A. Hillyard (1986) Electroretinograms reveal no evidence for centrifugal modulation of retinal inputs during selective attention in man. *Psychophysiology* **23**:156-165

Marchiafava, P.L. (1976) Centrifugal actions on amacrine and ganglion cells in the retina of the turtle. *Journal of Physiology* **255**:137-155

Marin, G., J.C. Letelier & J. Wallman (1990) Saccade-related responses of centrifugal neurons projecting to the chicken retina. *Experimental Brain Research* **82**:263-270

Matsumoto, N. (1975) Responses of the amacrine cells to optic nerve stimulation in the frog retina. *Vision Research* **15**:509-514

Matsutani, S., H. Uchiyama & H. Ito (1986) Cytoarchitecture, synaptic organization, and fiber connections of the nucleus olfactoretinalis in a teleost (*Navodon modestus*). *Brain Research* **373**:126-138

Maturana, H.R. & S. Frenk (1965) Synaptic connections of the centrifugal fibers of the pigeon retina. *Science* **150**:359-362

McLoon, S.C. & R.D. Lund (1982)Transient retinofugal pathways in the developing chick. *Experimental Brain Research* **45**:277-284

de Miguel, E., M.C. Rodicio & R. Anadon (1987) HRP study of retinofugal and retinopetal projections in larval lampreys (*Petromyzon marinus*). *Acta Anatomica* **130**:23

de Miguel, E., M.C. Rodicio & R. Anadon (1990) Organization of the visual system in larval lampreys: an HRP study. *Journal of Comparative Neurology* **302**:529-542

Miles, F.A. (1971) Centrifugal effects in the avian retina. *Science* **170**:992-995

Miles, F.A. (1972a) Centrifugal control of the avian retina. I. Receptive field properties of retinal ganglion cells. *Brain Research* **48**:65-92

Miles, F.A. (1972b) Centrifugal control of the avian retina. II. Receptive field properties of cells in the isthmo-optic nucleus. *Brain Research* **48**:93-113

Miles, F.A. (1972c) Centrifugal control of the avian retina. III. Effects of electrical stimulationof the isthmo-optic tract on the receptive field properties of retinal ganglion cells. *Brain Research* **48**:115-129

Miles, F.A. (1972d) Centrifugal control of the avian retina. IV. Effects of reversible cold block of the isthmo-optic tract on thereceptive field properties of cells in theretina and isthmo-optic nucleus. *Brain Research* **48**:131-145

Meyer, R.L. (1978) Evidence from thymidine labelling for continuing growth of retina and tectum in juvenile goldfish. *Experimental Neurology* **59**:99-111

Meyer, D.L., K. Gerwerzhagen, E. Fiebig, F. Ahlswede & S.O.E. Ebbesson (1983) An isthmo-optic system in a bony fish. *Cell and Tissue Research* **231**:129-133

Morgan, M.J. & R. Ward (1985) Spatial and spatial-interval primitives in spatial-interval estimation. *Journal of the Optical Society of America* **2**:1205-1210

Molotchnikoff, S. & F. Tremblay (1983) Influence of the visual cortex on responses of retinal ganglion cells in the rat. *Journal of Neuroscience Research* **10**:397-409

Molotchnikoff, S. & F. Tremblay (1986) Visual cortex controls retinal output in the rat. *Brain Research Bulletin* **17**:21-32

Müller, M. & H. Holländer (1988) A small population of retinal ganglion cells projecting to the retina of the other eye. An experimental study in the rat and the rabbit. *Experimental Brain Research* **71**:611-617

Murakami, M. & Y. Shimoda (1977) Identification of amacrine and ganglion cells in the carp retina. *Journal of Physiology* **264**:801-818

Northcutt, R.G. (1972) The Teiid prosencephalon and its bearing on squamate systematics. *Abstracts of the 52nd Annual Meeting of the American Society for Ichthyology and Herpetology*, pp. 75-79

Northcutt, R.G. (1978) Forebrain and midbrain organization in lizards and its phylogenetic significance. *In* N. Greenberg & P.D. Maclean (ed.) *Behavior and Neurobiology of Lizards.* Rockville MD, DHEW Publication #77-491

Northcutt, R.G. (1984) Evolution of the vertebrate central nervous system: patterns and processes. *American Zoologist* **24**:701-716

Ogden, T.E. & K.T. Brown (1964) Intraretinal responses of the cynomologous monkey to electrical stimulation of the optic nerve and retina. *Journal of Neurophysiology* **27**:682-705

O'Leary, D.D.M. & W.M. Cowan (1982) Further studies on the development of the isthmo-optic nucleus with special reference to the occurrence and fate of ectopic and ipsilaterally projecting neurons. *Journal of Comparative Neurology* **212**:399-416

Pearlman, A.L. & C.P. Hughes (1976) Functional role of efferents to the avian retina. II. Effects of reversible cooling of the isthmo-optic nucleus. *Journal of Comparative Neurology* **166**:123-132

Peyrichoux, J., C. Weidner, J. Repérant & D. Miceli (1977) An experimental study of the visual system of cyprinid fish using the HRP methods. *Brain Research* **130**:531-537

Platel, R. (1975) Nouvelles données sur l'encéphalisation des Reptiles Squamates. *Zeitschrift für Zoologische Systematik und Evolutionsforschung* **13**:65-87

Repérant, J. & A. Gallego (1976) Fibres centrifuges dans la rétine humaine. *Archives d'Anatomie Microscopique et de Morphologie Expérimentale* **65**:103-120

Repérant, J., N.P. Vesselkin, T.V. Ermakova, N.B. Kenigfest & A.A. Kosareva (1980) Radio-autographic evidence for both orthograde and retrograde axonal transport of label compounds after intraocular injection of [^{3}H]-proline in the lamprey (*Lampetra fluviatilis*). *Brain Research* **200**:179-183

Repérant, J., N.P. Vesselkin, J.-P. Rio, T. Ermakova, D. Miceli, J. Peyrichoux & C. Weidner (1981) La voie visuelle centrifuge n'exist-t-elle que chez les oiseaux? *Revue Canadienne de Biologie Expérimentale* **40**:29-46

Repérant, J., N.P. Vesselkin, D. Miceli & J.-P. Rio (1988) Anatolical organization of the centrifugal visual system in the lamprey. *Abstracts of the 8th European Winter Conference on Brain Research* p. 96

Repérant, J., D. Miceli, N.P. Vesselkin & S. Molotchnikoff (1989) The centrifugal visual system of vertebrates: a century-old search reviewed. *International Review of Cytology* **118**:115-171

Repérant, J., J.-P. Rio, R. Ward, D. Miceli, N.P. Vesselkin & S. Hergueta (1991a) Sequential events of degeneration and synaptic remodelling in the viper optic tectum following retinal ablation. A degeneration, radioautographic and immunocytochemical study. *Journal of Chemical Neuroanatomy*, in press

Repérant, J., J.-P. Rio, R. Ward, S. Hergueta, D. Miceli & M. Lemire. (1991b) Comparative analysis of the primary visual system in reptiles. *In* C. Gans & P.S. Ulinski (ed.) *Biology of the Reptilia*, vol. 17, Neurology C. Chicago, University of Chicago Press, in press

Rogers, L.J. & F.A. Miles (1972) Centrifugal control of the avian retina. V. Effects of lesions of the isthmo-optic nucleus on visual behaviour. *Brain Research* **48**:147-156

Rusoff, A.C. & S.J. Hapner (1990) Development of retinopetal projections in the cichlid fish, *Herotilapia multispinosa*. *Journal of Comparative Neurology* **294**:431-442

Russel, I.J. & B.L. Roberts (1974) Active reduction of lateral-line sensitivity in swimming dogfish. *Journal of Comparative Physiology* **94**:7-15

Sandeman, D.C & N.P. Rosenthal (1974) Efferent axons in fish optic nerve and their effect on the retinal ganglion cell. *Brain Research* **68**:41-54

Schilling, T.F & R.G. Northcutt (1987) Amniotes and anamniotes may posess homoplastic retinopetal projectiuons from the isthmic tegmentum. *Society for Neuroscience Abstracts* **13**:130

Schnyder, H. & H. Künzle (1983) The retinopetal system in the turtle (*Pseudemys scripta elegans*). *Cell and Tissue Research* **234**:219-224

Schnyder, H. & H. Künzle (1984) Is there a retinopetal system in the rat? *Experimental Brain Research* **56**:502-508

Schroeder, D.M. (1981) Retinal afferents and efferents of an infrared sensitive snake, *Crotalus viridis*. *Journal of Morphology* **170**:29-42

Schütte, M. & R. Weiler (1988) Mesencephalic innervation of the turtle retina by a single serotonin-containing neuron. *Neuroscience Letters* **91**:289-294

Shortess, G.K. & E.F. Klose (1977) Effects of lesions involving efferent fibers to the retina in pigeons (*Columba livia*). *Physiology and Behavior* **18**:409-414

Spinelli, D.N. & M. Weingarten (1966) Afferent and efferent activity in single units of the cat's optic nerve. *Experimental Neurology* **15**:347-362

Stell, W.K., S.E. Walker, K.S. Chohan & A.K. Ball (1984) The goldfish nervus terminalis: a luteinizing hormone-releasing hormone and molluscan cardioexcitatory peptide immunoreactive olfactoretinal pathway. *Proceedings of the National Academy of Sciences of the USA* **81**:940-944

Stell, W.K., S.E. Walker & A.K. Ball (1988) Functional - anatomical studies on the terminal nerve projection to the retina of bony fishes. *Annals of the New York Academy of Science* **519**:80-96

Toth, P. & C. Straznicky (1989) Retino-retinal projections in three anuran species. *Neuroscience Letters* **104**:43-47

Terubayashi, H., H. Fujisawa, M. Itoi & Y. Ibata (1983) Hypothalamo-retinal centrifugal projection in the dog. *Neuroscience Letters* **40**:1-6

Uchiyama, H. (1989) Centrifugal pathways to the retina: influence of the optic tectum. *Visual Neuroscience* **3**:183-206

Uchiyama, H. & H. Ito (1984) Fiber connections and synaptic organization of the preoptic retinopetal nucleus in the filefish (Balistidae, Teleostei). *Brain Research* **298**:11-24

Uchiyama, H. & M. Watanabe (1985) Tectal neurons projecting to the isthmo-optic nucleus in the Japanses quail. *Neuroscience Letters* **58**:381-385

Uchiyama, H., S. Matsutani & H. Ito (1986) Tectal projections to the retinopetal nucleus in the filefish. *Brain Research* **369**:260-266

Uchiyama, H., T.A. Reh & W.K. Stell (1988) Immunocytchemical and morphological evidence for a retinopetal projection in anuran amphibians. *Journal of Comparative Neurology* **274**:48-59

Villar, M., M.L. Vitale & M.N. Parisi (1987) Dorsal raphe serotoninergic projection to the retina. A combined peroxidase tracing - neurochemical/high performance liquid chromatography study in the rat. *Neuroscience* **22**:681-686

Vesselkin, N.P., T.V. Ermakova, J. Repérant, A.A. Kosareva & N.B. Kenigfest (1980) The retinofugal and retinopetal systems in *Lampetra fluviatilis*. An experimental study using radioautographic and HRP methods. *Brain Research* **195**:453-460

Vesselkin, N.P., J. Repérant, N.B. Kenigfest, D. Miceli, T.V. Ermakova & J.-P. Rio (1984) An anatomical and electrophysiological study of the centrifugal visual system in the lamprey (*Lampetra fluviatilis*). *Brain Research* **292**:41-56

Vesselkin, N.P., J. Repérant, N.B. Kenigfest, J.-P. Rio, D. Miceli & O.V. Shuplyakov (1989) Centrifugal innervation of the lamprey retina. Light- and electron microscopic and electrophysiological investigations. *Brain Research* **493**:51-65

Wakakura, M. & S. Ishikawa (1982) Ultrastructural study on centrifugal fibers in trhe feline retina. *Japanese Journal of Ophthalmology* **26**:63-70

Wang, R. & M. Halpern (1977) Afferent and efferent connections of thalamic nuclei of the visual system of garter snake. *The Anatomical Record* **187**:741-742

Weidner, C., D. Miceli & J. Repérant (1983) Orthograde axonal and transcellular transport of different fluorescent tracers in the primary visual system of the rat. *Brain Research* **272**:129-136

Weidner, C., J. Repérant, A.-M. Desroches, D. Miceli & N.P. Vesselkin (1987) Nuclear origin of the centrifugal visual pathway in birds of prey. *Brain Research* **436**:153-160

Weiler, R. (1985) Mesencephalic pathway to the retina exhibits enkephalin-like immunoreactivity. *Neuroscience Letters* **55**:11-16

Wicht, H. & R.G. Northcutt (1990) Retinofugal and retinopetal projections in the Pacific hagfish, *Epatretus stouti* (Myxinoidea). *Brain, Behavior and Evolution* **36**:315-328

Witkovsky, P. (1971) Synapses made by myelinated fibers running to teleost and elasmobranch retinas. *Journal of Comparative Neurology* **142**:205-221

Wirsig-Weichmann, C.R. & S.F. Basinger (1988) FMRFamide-immunoreactive retinopetal fibers in the frog (*Rana pipiens*): demonstration by lesion and immunocytochemical techniques. *Brain Research* **449**:116-126

Woodson, W., T. Shimizu & H.J. Karten (1989) Transmitter and peptide content of the isthmo-optic nucleus in the pigeon (*Columba livia*): a study of non-tectal afferents. *Society for Neuroscience Abstracts* **15**:459

Wright, A.A. (1979) Color-vision psychophysics: a comparison of pigeon and human. In A.M. Granda & J.H. Maxwell (ed.) *Neural mechanisms of behavior in the pigeon*. New York, Plenum Press, pp. 89-128

Zucker, C.L. & J.E. Dowling (1987) Centrifugal fibres synapse on dopaminergic interplexiform cells in the teleost retina. *Nature* **330**:166-168

BLOCKADE OF PROTEOLYTIC ACTIVITY RETARDS RETROGRADE DEGENERATION OF AXOTOMIZED RETINAL GANGLION CELLS AND ENHANCES AXONAL REGENERATION IN ORGAN CULTURES

Solon Thanos

Res. Laboratory, Dept. of Ophthalmology, University of
Tübingen, School of Medicine, Schleichstr. 12, 7400
Tübingen, FRG

INTRODUCTION

Observations concerning the consequences of injury to the central nervous system, to the spinal cord and to the retina of higher vertebrates can be traced back to the early decades of the century (Cajal, 1928; James, 1933; Eayrs, 1952). In accord with these observations, which have been confirmed later, the course of retrograde adult retinal ganglion cell degeneration commences a few days after intraorbital transection of the optic nerve and progresses during the weeks and months following the axotomy, finally resulting in depletion of the retinal ganglion cell layer (GCL) (Richardson et al. 1982; Barron et al. 1986; Thanos, 1988; Villegas-Perez et al. 1988; Carmignoto et al. 1989). The failure of lesioned ganglion cells to regrow their axons within the distal portion of the optic nerve is assumed to be caused by the presence of differentiated oligodendrocytes whose myelin exerts inhibiting influences both on embryonic (Schwab and Caroni, 1988) and on adult ganglion cell axons (Vanselow et al. 1990). In addition to the inhibiting environment, insufficient growth-supporting agents within the optic nerve (Cajal, 1928) have been assumed to determine the fate of lesioned neurons, namely the progressive degeneration. External neurotrophic influences introduced by the apposition of peripheral nerve segments at the time of severing the optic nerve could rescue some ganglion cells, which then can regenerate into growth-permitting peripheral nerve transplants (Vidal-Sanz et al. 1987; Villegas-Perez et al. 1988). Factors released from peripheral nerves also support regrowth of axons in cultured retinal explants (Thanos et al. 1989). The responsiveness of lesioned ganglion cells to external administration of nerve growth factor (NGF) during the first weeks after lesion (Carmignoto et al., 1989) is in line with all previous observations that epigenetic influences can regulate the quantities of neurons which survive axotomy.

Further exploration and intervention into the responses of ganglion cells and of their glial environment to external violence may result in persistent increase of the numbers of neurons which can be then recruited to regrow and reconnect their axons. Since ganglion cell lesion and subsequent death cause a local inflamation within the ganglion cell and inner plexiform layers, local or generalized mechanisms of recognition and removal of cell debris are probably essential in order to protect the surrounding tissue from further lytic destruction. The investigation of the entire local response within the retina is therefore of crucial importance for understanding the mechanisms of lesion-induced cell death, and perhaps to preventing it. Besides neurons and the macroglia (astrocytes and the Müller's glia), microglia are the third major population of cells within the retina of mammals (del Rio-Hortega, 1932; Gammermeyer, 1970). Microglia are also localized in various areas of the developing, adult and lesioned CNS (Gammermeyer, 1965; Ling, 1982; Streit and Kreutzberg, 1987; Perry and Gordon, 1988; Schnitzer, 1989; Schnitzer and Scherer, 1990). The function of brain and retinal microglia in the repair process at the sites of injuries is not well defined, although several lines of evidence support the view that these cells are responsible for the immune response and phagocytosis (see Perry and Gordon, 1988, and Guilain, 1990 for reviews). Observations based on the temporal relation of the microglia to neuronal cell death in the lesioned adult rabbit retina (Schnitzer and Scherer, 1990) have assigned to the microglia a relationship to the dying cells.

The present work was based on the anticipation that retinal proteases which are probably produced by microglia are directly involved in the cascade of regressive events initiated by optic nerve transection. It basically monitored whether blockade of the proteolytic activities can rescue the lesioned neurons from degeneration. If so, the model predicts that axotomized and functionally altered ganglion cells are recognized by immunocompetent microglial cells (Streit et al. 1990), which respond to the alteration with onset of enzymatic neuron degradation and subsequent andocytosis. This possibility, called neurophagy, implies that microglia represent a local immune system devoted to the protection of the functional and structural retinal integrity. Consequently, such a mechanism also presumes that microglial cells use proteases (Guilain, 1990) to degrade severed ganglion cells. Administration of protease inhibitors would therefore influence ganglion cell degradation. To confirm this, the optic nerves of adult rats were transected beyond the eye cup and the retinal ganglion cells whose axons form the optic nerve were retrogradely labelled with the fluorescent dye 4Di-10ASP which accompanies the membrane particles after cell degradation and phagocytosis (Thanos et al. submitted). Usual protease inhibitors (Table 1) were injected into the vitreous body during the surgical optic nerve interruption. It is shown here that substantial numbers of vital ganglion cells can be rescued and express regenerative capacities in organ cultures, whereas in the same retinae, significant delay in the specific, phagocytosis-dependent transcellular labelling of microglia, indicates that the protease inhibitors may interact and inactivate microglial neurophagic activities.

EXPERIMENTAL PROCEDURES

Surgery at the Optic Nerve and Staining Procedures

Adult female rats (24) weighing 200 to 230 g from the Sprague-Dawley strain were used for the present study. In intraperitoneal chloral-hydrate anesthesia (0.42 mg/Kg body weight), the left optic nerve was intraorbitally exposed and after longitudinal incision of its meningeal sheath the nerve was completely transected. Care was taken to avoid damage of the retinal blood supply. In 20 rats, solid crystals (0.2 to 0.4 μm in diameter) of the fluorescent styryl dye [D291, N-4-(4-didecylaminostyryl)-N-methylpyridinium iodide, (4-di-10-ASP), Molecular Probes, Oregon] were deposited immediately after transection at the ocular stump of the optic nerve as reported for DiI (Thanos, 1988), in order to label the retinal ganglion cells retrogradely before they undergo degeneration. In 10 of these rats, 5 μl of a freshly prepared protease inhibitor solution (Table 1) were injected into the vitreous body of the axotomized eye with a 10 μl Hamilton syringe. The remaining 10 control rats which received optic nerve transection and 4Di-10ASP but not inhibitors, were either used to determine the normal course of retrograde ganglion cell degeneration and microglial labelling (8 rats), or they received intravitreal injection of 5 μl phosphate buffer (2 rats). In 6 further control rats (3 with optic nerve cut and protease inhibitor injection, and 3 with nerve cut but without injection), the dye was deposited at the optic nerve stump during a second surgical intervention, 2 days prior to the animal's death, in order to label only the population of ganglion cells which survived the primary axotomy.

Following survival times of 2, 8, 14, 30, 50 and 90 days, the rats were deeply anesthetized with 7% chloralhydrate. After intracardial perfusion with phosphate buffered saline, the animals were killed and fixed with 200 ml aquous 4% paraformaldehyde and their retinae were dissected, incised into four quadrants and flat-mounted on filters with the nerve fiber layer upwards.

Explantation of Retinal Stripes

Under chloralhydrate anesthesia, the left optic nerve of 20 rats was surgically exposed and crushed within its intraorbital segment with a jeweller's forceps, in order to produce a conditioning lesion, which has beneficial effects on the regenerative response of ganglion cells (Thanos et al. 1989). In 8 rats, 5 μl of the protease inhibitor solution was injected into the vitreous body. The remaining 12 rats were used as controls without any injection during the procedure of crush. One week after severing the optic nerve, the retinae of animals with protease inhibitor injection and these of the controls were dissected under sterile conditions and were used to produce organ cultures in a chemically defined medium devoid of serum and growth factors according to the technique of Thanos et al. (1989). Each retina was divided into 8 optic nerve head centered pieces, which were then explanted on petriperm dishes (Heraeus) coated with polylysine (MW 375,000 to 410,000 Da, Boehringer; 200 μg/ml, overnight at 37^{0}C) and with laminin (BRL, 20 μg/ml, 1h at 37^{0}C) with the ganglion cell layer facing the substrate. For examining the effects of protease inhibitors injected *in situ*, the 64 explants obtained from pretreated retinae were not supplemented with neurotrophic factors. Control explants were substituted with each of the following neurotrophic factors: (1) 20 explants with basic fibroblast growth factor (bFGF, 5 μg/ml). (2) 30 explants received purified brain-derived neurotrophic factor (Barde et al. 1982) at biologically active dilutions identical to these described by Thanos et al.(1989). (3) In an additional 32 explants derived from protease inhibitor-treated retinae *in situ*, BDNF was added to the organ cultures, in order to examine additive effects on axonal growth. (4) Further controls consisted of cultures of 32 retinal explants with *in situ* conditioned sciatic nerve exudate collected into implanted teflon tubes during nerve regeneration (Thanos et al. 1989) and dissociated cells from sciatic nerves which were precrushed 1 week prior to explantation.

TABLE 1. INTRAVITREALLY INJECTED SUBSTANCES WHICH RESCUED GANGLION CELLS FROM DEGRADATION.

Substance (Stability)	Biological Activity	Effective Concentr. [µg/ml]	Concentration used [µg/ml]	Total ammount injected [µg]
PEPSTATIN (moderate)	pepsin renin cathepsin	0.01 0.005 4.5	35-105	0.01-0.03
LEUPEPTIN (low)	plasmin trypsin chymotryps. kallikrein papain lysosomal cathepsin A B D	70 2 >500 >500 0.5 1680 0.4 109	60-180	0.01-0.05
APROTININ (high)	trypsin kallikrein plasmin chymotrypsin	17	17-51	0.005-0.015
N-NEURAMINIDASE-INHIBITOR (high)		14-20	14-20	0.870-2.610
E-64 (high)	calpain and other cysteine proteases	1-3 µM		0.01-0-003

LEGEND TO TABLE 1: Protease inhibitors were freshly prepared from frozen stock solutions (-20° C) containing 1.4 mg/ml pepstatin, 2.4 mg/ml Leupeptin, 1.7 mg/ml aprotinin and 2.9 mg/ml N-Neuraminidase-inhibitor (all obtained from SIGMA). Final concentrations were mixed in sterile 0.1M phosphate buffer (PH 7.4) and 5µl of the final mixture were injected through the sclera into the vitreous body of operated eyes with a pooled glass cappilary (opening tip diameter: 10 to 20 µm). The effective concentrations of the inhibitors were calculated according to the data and the bibliography presented in: Proteases and Biological Control, (eds. E. Reich, D. B. Rifkin, and E. Shaw), Cold Spring Harbor Conferences on cell proliferation, Vol. 2, 1975. The concentration of the irreversible inhibitor of calpain was calculated according to the references cited in: Mehdi, TIBS 16: 150-153 (1991) and Wang, TIPS, 11: 139-142 (1990).

Morphometry

The retinae obtained after optic nerve transection and subsequent degeneration *in situ* were viewed as whole-mounts. Fluorescent ganglion cells and microglia were observed within the fluorescein filter, since 4Di-10ASP fluoresces green-yellowish.

For quantification of the ganglion cells and microglia, each retina was divided into three concentric areas with radii of about 1 mm (central), 2 mm (middle) and more than 2 mm (peripheral) from the center of the optic nerve head as viewed in the whole-mounted retina. Ganglion cell and microglia densities were determined in each concentric field by measuring in each quadrant 30 to 40 randomly distributed microscope fields with the 20X lens. The data were averaged for each field and then to obtain densities of ganglion cells and microglia across the retinal surface. Since microglia show a staggered, bilaminated distribution at late stages of degeneration (Thanos et al., submitted), it was essential to measure the microglia within both layers, namely within the ganglion cell layer and within the deeper inner plexiform layer. Statistical analysis of the data obtained for each interval after axotomy was performed with the two-tailed student's t-test.

In the retinae used to study whether the axonal transport is intact after treatment with inhibitors, 4Di-10ASP was applied to the optic nerve stump 12 and 28 days after nerve transection. Two days later, the retinae were dissected and also viewed as whole-mounts, and the density of labelled ganglion cells but not of the unlabelled microglia, was determined and compared with the density of ganglion cells of control rats. The t-test was applied to verify statistical significance in the survival of ganglion cells capable of transporting the fluorescent dye.

Measuring of Fibers in the Retinal Explants

The retinal pieces cultured under the different conditions were scored for axonal growth 2 days after explantation by means of an inverted phase contrast microscope. Numbers of fibers were measured at a distance of 200 μm from the edge of each explant. Averaged numbers of axons from each group of explants were compared by means of the t-test. Calculation of the ability of the entire retinae to regenerate axons *in vitro* was made by multiplying the average numbers of fibers with 8, that is with the number of explants obtained from each retina.

RESULTS

Retrograde Labelling of Ganglion cells and Microglia

Deposition of the fluorescent dye 4Di-10ASP at the stump of the transected optic nerve of control rats which did not receive injection of protease inhibitors, and in control animals which received injection of 6 ul phosphate buffer resulted after 2 days in retrograde labelling of 740 ± 40 cells/mm^2 (12 rats), which corresponds to about 30% of the total population of ganglion cells in the rat retina (Perry, 1979). When the animals were killed at later stages after axotomy and labelling, the ganglion cells were intenselly labelled, indicating a long-term persistence of the dye within the surviving neurons (Fig. 1).

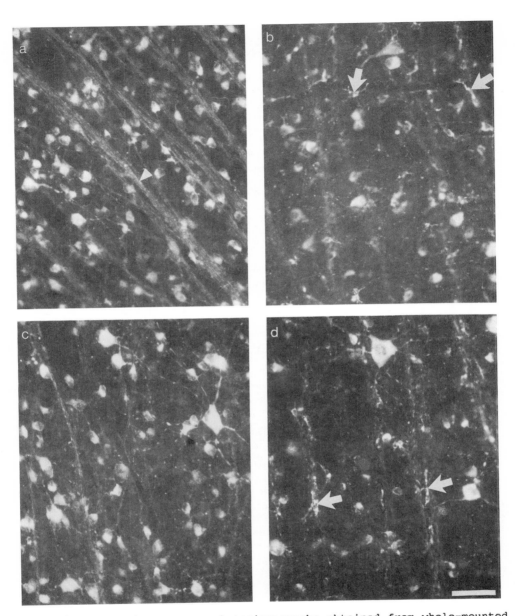

Figure 1. Fluorescence photomicrographs obtained from whole-mounted retinae 14 days after optic nerve transection and labelling. a, c) This eye received optic nerve transection, 4Di-10ASP at the nerve stump and intravitreal injection of protease inhibitors. Numerous fluorescent ganglion cell bodies are seen directly underneath the optic fiber fascicles (arrows) in the central (a) and in the peripheral retina (c), which has fewer and larger cell bodies and fewer axonal fascicles. b, d) This retina received optic nerve transection and 4Di-10ASP, but not protease inhibitors. The central field seen in (b) corresponds to that seen in the inhibitor-treated retina in (a), whereas that in (d) corresponds to the field seen in (c). There is substantial reduction of ganglion cell bodies and axonal fascicles. In addition, labelled microglial cells (arrows) appeared both in the central and in the peripheral retina. Scale bar: 50 μm.

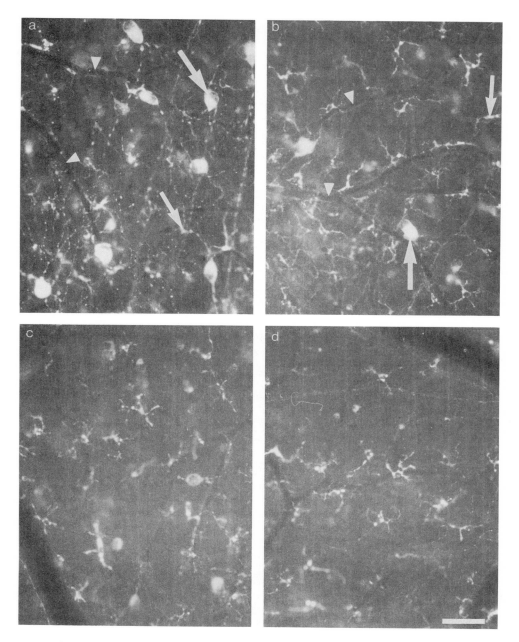

Figure 2. Fluorescence photomicrographs taken from inhibitor-treated (left photographs) and control retinae (right photographs) 50 (a, b) and 90 days (c, d) after surgery and labelling with the dye. a), b): Direct comparison between treated and untreated retina (same eccentricity as visible on the basis of the blood vessel calibers which are indicated with arrowheads). There are substantially more ganglion cells with enlarged cell bodies (large arrows) in treated than in the control retinae. Microglial cells (small arrows) are present in both retinae. c), d): Treated and control retinae 90 days after surgery. Ganglion cells are accassionally observed in both retinae, whereas the densities of microglial cells are identical. Scale bar: 50 µm.

The maximum persistence of the dye within ganglion cells observed was 6 months (data not shown). Morphologically, cells which survived axotomy always resembled those shown in Figures 1 and 2. Since axotomy causes a protracted degeneration of ganglion cells, the densities of these cells declined as expected with time elapsed after axotomy to approximately 20 ± 4 labelled cells/mm^2 at the end of the first, and to 10 ± 2 labelled cells/mm^2 at the end of the 3rd month after lesion (Figs. 2 and 3).

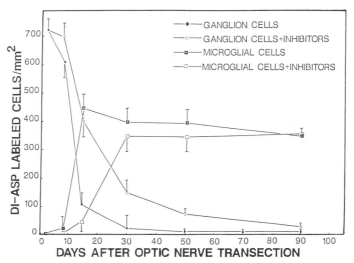

Figure 3. Kinetics of ganglion cell degeneration and effects of protease inhibitors. Retardation of ganglion cell degradation in the presence of protease inhibitors was significant at all stages of measuring ($P<0.01$) except of the end of the third month after surgery. The appearance and increase of transcellularly labelled microglial cells was also significantly delayed ($P<0.05$) at 14, but not after 30 days ($P>0.05$) after surgery. The data represent means and SEM.

In conjunction with the course of ganglion cell disappearance, non-ganglionic cells (Figs. 1 and 2), identified with different techniques as microglial cells (Thanos et al., submitted), first appeared in the optic fiber layer and ganglion cell layer on the 8th day after lesion, and their density increased in the GCL with time elapsed from lesion to peak at 14 days (Figs. 1, 2 and 3), and to decline to 350 ± 25 cells/mm^2 30 days and 50 days after optic nerve transection (Fig. 3). This microglial density remained stable throughout the time of investigation that covered three months after lesion (Fig. 3). At this and later stages after optic nerve transection, microglia displayed a strong territorial arrangement within the ganglion cell and inner plexiform layers, and staggered, bilaminated distribution within the two layers (Thanos et al., submitted).

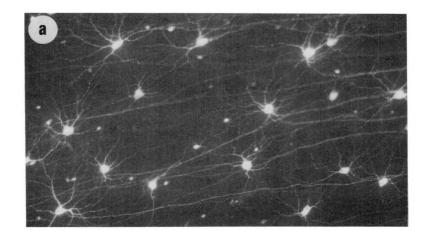

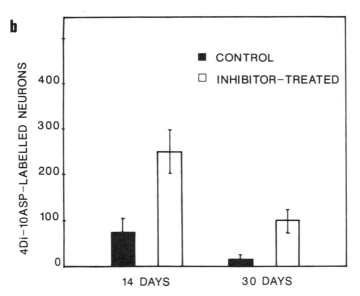

Figure 4. Viability of ganglion cells in the retina. a): Fluorescence photomicrograph demonstrating the morphologies of ganglion cells which survived axotomy in inhibitor-treated retina and were labelled 2 days before the animal's death by depositing 4Di-10ASP at the intraorbital optic nerve stump. b) Quantification of the densities of ganglion cells which survived axotomy 14 and 30 days revealed significant differences between inhibitor-treated and untreated retinae ($P<0.01$) for both stages. Four retinae were used for each stage and group, whereas several thousands cells were counted in each retina. The data give means and SEM.

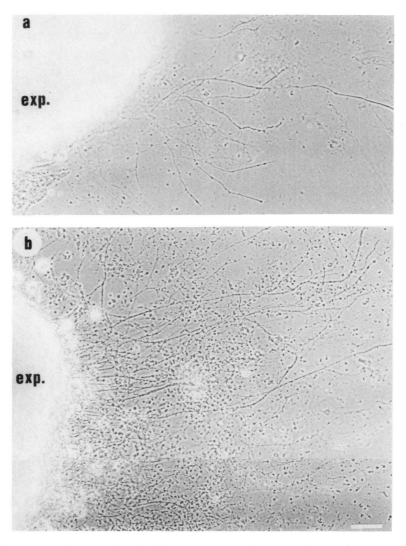

Figure 5. Outgrowth of fibers from retinal explants in culture. a): This retinal explant (exp.) was obtained from precrushed and untreated retina and was was cultured with bFGF added at the time of explantation. Individual outgrowing axons were photographed after 2 days in culture. b): This explant was taken from a retina which received intravitreal injection of protease inhibitors at the time of optic nerve crush. The explants were not substituted with any neurotrophic factors while in culture. There is a massive outgrowth of axons in comparison with control explants. Scale bar: 50 μm.

Retrograde labelling of the axotomized ganglion cells and simultaneous injection of protease inhibitors into the vitreous body resulted in a different course of ganglion cell depletion and microglial labelling in the retina observed 14 to 90 days after surgery (Fig. 1 and 2). At 14 days, the numbers of ganglion cells with intact perikaryal and dendritic morphologies were about 4-fold higher than in animals without injection of inhibitors (Fig.3). Parallel to the reduction of ganglion cells, the densities of labelled microglial cells were significantly lower than in controls during the first month after lesion (Fig. 3). Repetitive injections of protease inhibitors weekly after optic nerve transection led to not significantly higher densities of surviving ganglion cells and lower densities of microglial cells (in preparation).

Axonal Transport in Injured Ganglion Cells

Since the appearance of more fluorescent ganglion cells within the axotomized and inhibitor-treated retinae does not necessarily document that they were alive, as they can be dead, but non-phagocytosed cells, vital functions of the neurons were essential confirming their viability. The ability of cells to retrogradely trasport the fluorescent dye within their axons was taken as one of the indices of viability. Deposition of 4Di-10ASP at the optic nerve stump 14 and 30 days after transection proved whether ganglion cell bodies were labelled. The labelling of ganglion cell bodies and dendrites (Fig. 4a) revealed that numerous cells were capable of transporting the dye. Quantitative evaluation of the numbers of labelled cells revealed significant differences compared to the control retinae (Fig. 4b). Morphologically, labelled ganglion cells had almost normal dendritic morphologies in the inhibitor-treated retina (Fig.4a), indicating that dendritic retraction and degradation (Thanos, 1988) may be reduced when proteolytic activity is blocked.

Ability of Ganglion Cells to Regenerate Axons in Vitro

To further assess whether growth properties of neurons are influenced by the presence of protease inhibitors, retinal explants were prepared 1 week after optic nerve transection and intravitreal PI-injection and cultured in a chemically defined medium not containing neurotrophic agents (Thanos et al. 1989). Massive regrowth of axons 2 days after explantation (Fig. 5) was significantly higher when the retinae were taken from eyes injected with protease inhibitors (Fig.5). Figure 5 compares the efficacy of axonal growth between an explant cultured in the presence of bFGF (Fig. 5a) with the growth observed in an explant from retina treated with protease inhibitors during the axotomy in situ (Fig. 5b). In the explant shown in Figure 5b, 775 single axons grew out at the second day after explantation. Substitution of the cultures with different potent neurotrophic factors like brain-derived neurotrophic factor (BDNF), with basic fibroblast growth factor (Barde et al. 1982), or with sciatic nerve-derived exudate (Thanos et al. 1989) was less efficient than pretreatment with protease inhibitors. Sixty-four explants obtained from 8 retinae treated with protease inhibitors gave rise to an average of 650±120 axons/explant on polylysine/laminin. This efficacy of growth per explant corresponds to an incidence of regeneration that approaches 5% of the total population of ganglion cells when extrapolated to the entire retina. This incidence is higher than that estimated in vivo, when retinal neurites grew into transplanted peripheral nerve segments (Vidal-Sanz et al. 1987). The results indicate therefore that retardation of neuronal degeneration results in considerable outgrowth of axons.

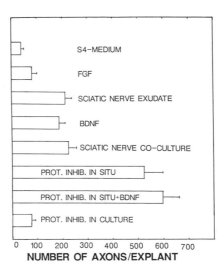

Figure 6. Quantification of the numbers of axons which grew out in control retinae and in those obtained after intravitreal injection with protease inhibitors *in situ*. The number of fibers growing out in the chemically-defined, serum-free medium can be doubled by adding bFGF or by adding protease inhibitors at the time of explantation. Further increase of the numbers of axons has been achieved by adding BDNF or sciatic nerve-derived conditioned exudate, or by co-culturing retinal pieces with cells from the precrushed sciatic nerve. Maximum numbers of axons were observed when the explants were cultured after *in situ* treatment of the retina with protease inhibitors ($P<0.05$ compared with each control). Addition of BDNF in pretreated retinae revealed a slight, not significant ($P>0.05$) increase in the number of axons.

DISCUSSION

The interruption of ganglion cell axons within the optic nerve of adult rats leads to a cascade of neuronal and environmental responses which culminate in the progressive and protracted depopulation of the retinal ganglion cell layer. Degenerating ganglion cells are phagocytosed by retinal microglial cells which become activated soon after injury and remove cell debris in a strong chrono-topological sequence that parallels the course of the neuronal degradation (Thanos et al. submitted). The principal new finding of the present study was that severed retinal neurons become enzymatically degraded by common proteases, whose activity can be specifically blocked, resulting in retardation of the degenerative events initiated by the axotomy.

The marked reduction of ganglion cells following transection of the optic nerve in mammals is one of the major impediments to rescuing and reconnecting these neurons with central target cells in sufficient quanity and in a topographic fashion that ensures functional significance. Consequently, increasing the number of neurons which survive the axotomy and those which contribute to the regrowth of axons, are interdependent prerequisites for restoring function in the retinofugal system. Cell survival after injury essentially co-regulates the efficacy of subsequent axonal regeneration. Thus, understanding of the mechanisms which contribute to the destruction of lesioned neurons, and the development of strategies for manipulating these mechanisms in order to rescue cells from degradation, will help to achieve both goals, that of preventing cell death, and that of promoting axonal regeneration.

As consistently documented in experiments using peripheral nerve grafts to allow axons to regenerate within the growth-supporting Schwann's cell environment and reach central targets, ganglion cells making use of the opportunity to grow (Tello, 1907; Politis and Spencer, 1986; Vidal-Sanz et al. 1987) can be rescued from cell death (Villegas-Perez et al. 1989). This intrinsic ability of lesioned ganglion cells to regrow their axons in favourable environments can also be used in organ cultures devoid of inhibiting central glial influences (Thanos et al. 1989). In addition, the intrinsic ability to regrow in vitro can be externally supported by using the peripheral nerve-derived growth supporting factors which significantly accelerate axonal elongation (Thanos et al. 1989). The major implication of these findings was that the axotomy-initiated cascade of degeneration can be, in principle, manipulated, indicating that insufficient influence of neurotrophic agents in situ is one of the factors which co-determine the fate of lesioned neurons. Among the molecules which can prevent cell death and promote axonal growth, brain-derived neurotrophic factor (BDNF, Barde et al. 1982; Thanos et al. 1989) and basic fibroblast growth factor (bFGF, Sievers et al. 1987) have been so far shown to influence ganglion cell survival. Similar effects have also been reported after repetitive intraocular injections of large amounts of nerve growth factor (NGF, Carmignoto et al. 1989), even though the numbers of rescued ganglion cells were lower than those obtained with bFGF (Sievers et al. 1987). The target cells of neurotrophic factors may be, however, different than the ganglion cells, since localization of receptors still remains obscure.

The major findings of the present work were that, in addition to the described strategies of rescuing cells with trophic agents and promoting growth with neurotrophic molecules, pharmacological blockade of the enzymes which degrade lesioned neurons can substantially contribute to the retardation of neuronal degeneration. Combined specific transcellular tracing of the neurophagic cells and manipulation of proteolytic activities in the retrogradely degenerating retina document highly specialized mechanisms which are initiated by axotomy and are devoted to the destruction of neurons (=neurophagy). In concert, the interactions between microglial cells and other retinal glial cells like the astrocytes and the Müller's cells (Bignami and Dahl, 1979) are probably part of this cascade of responses. Such microglial-macroglial interactions may be mediated by astrocytic activating molecules, like the interleukines which stimulate the astrocytes to proliferate (Giulian et al. 1989; Giulian, 1987) and to form the so-called gliosis. However, localization of the proteolytic enzymes remains to be demonstrated. Inasmuchas the present data permit a conjunction with the function of the microglial cells, they may indicate that microglial proteases (for review, see Giulian, 1990) are induced to degrade ganglion cells. Also the observations of Stoll et al. (1989) in the lesioned optic nerve demonstrated that optic nerve macrophages, which are correlates of retinal microglia, use proteases to perform myelinolysis and axonal degradation within the lesioned optic nerve. This would imply that microglial cells either become activated to secrete proteases or they directly attack the lesioned ganglion cells to degrade, and then to phagocytose the produced debris. The present data do not distinguish between secretable and cell-associated proteases. Alternatively, the findings are also consistent with the possibility that intraganglionic lysosomal activity can be blocked, thus resulting in retardation of cell death. Less likely, but not impossible, is that protease inhibitors are potent neurotrophic substances directly acting on the ganglion cells. Since, however, protease inhibitors are enzymes involved in catalyzing chemical reactions in dependence on specific substrates (Rich, 1986; Powers, 1986; Schnebli, 1975), the possibility to also act as neurotrophic agents is less likely. In addition to the described features of protease inhibitors (Schnebli, 1975; Rich, 1986; Powers, 1986), the only present experimental evidence opposing this possibility is that administration of protease inhibitors to the organ cultures during the procedure of explantation does not enhance outgrowth of axons, as injection of inhibitors during the procedure of optic nerve transection does on the other hand. An alternative explanation for the site of action of inhibitors is that they block the intracellular, lysosomal proteases which digest already degraded and endocytosed neuronal material. Although possible and not excluded, such an explanation was not confirmed by the present study, since it documents a blockade of degradation at an earlier level prior to the endocytosis. The spectrum of proteolytic activities which have been blocked with the inhibitors covers the major proteases used to degrade living cells (see Table 1). The spectrum can be certainly extended to more stable proteases, since pepstatin and leupeptin are less stable (Schnebli, 1975; Rich, 1986; Powers, 1986). In addition, the dose of protease can be optimized, for example by repeating injections of small amounts of protease inhibitors (in preparation). Also the combined inhibition of proteases and the promotion of axonal growth with neurotrophic agents and anti-inflamatory substances in vivo will be of considerable importance for the process of regeneration.

Apposition of peripheral nerve pieces at the ocular stump of the optic nerve in order to provide suitable guides for transected axons to grow and reach their targets (Politis and Spencer, 1982; Vidal-Sanz et al. 1987; Villegas-Perez et al. 1988; Thanos and Vanselow, 1989) has helped document the intrinsic ability of lesioned ganglion cells to regenerate their axons and to form synaptic contacts (Keirstead et al. 1989). However, the low numbers of neurons available for recruiting axons to regenerate is one of the circumstances that hitherto limited restoration of the retinocollicular pathway in adulthood. The critical role of the protease inhibitors, and probably of other substances which suppress inflamation (Perry and Gordon, 1988; Lampson, 1987) and (micro-)

glial activation seem to consist in being effective soon after nerve lesion. It will be of considerable importance to maintain optimal inhibition of proteases over the critical period of posttraumatic axonal growth, which covers a few weeks (Vidal-Sanz et al. 1987; Thanos and Vanselow, 1990). Exploration of the sequence of interdependent events which are initiated by axotomy and retrograde transport of axotomy-induced signals (Singer et al. 1982) is of crucial importance in determining their reversibility, which might be beneficial for the lesioned neurons. The massive, protracted macroglial response (Bignami and Dahl, 1979; Perry and Gordon, 1988; Streit and Kreutzberg, 1988; Streit et al. 1990) and the hypertrophy of microglia (Schnitzer and Scherer, 1990), as well as recruitment of macrophages to carry out myelinolysis and removal of axonal debris in the optic nerve (Stoll et al. 1989), are evidence that these groups of cells are responsible for most of the posttraumatic activities in the retina.

SUMMARY

Adult retinal ganglion cells of mammals respond to injuries with rapid anterograde and protracted retrograde (Wallerian) degeneration. To monitor the cascade of events initiated by neuronal injuries, and to explore whether and how neighbouring glial cells contribute to degrade lesioned neurons, axotomy-induced ganglion cell degeneration was investigated in adult rats. The experiment aimed at blocking degradation of axotomized ganglion cells with enzymes which inhibit proteolytic activities within the retina (protease inhibitors) and employed a new fluorescent technique to assess both the fate of debris produced by dying cells and the efficacy of the protease inhibitors in preventing cell death. Injection of protease inhibitors into the vitreous body of the animals whose optic nerves were transected protected ganglion cells from degradation and decreased the number of fluorescently labelled microglia. Two major functions of rescued ganglion cells proved their viability: (1) The retained intraaxonal transport of fluorescent dye revealed a higher incidence of cell survival compared to control retinae. (2) The numbers of ganglion cell axons emanated from in vitro cultured retinal stripes explanted 1 week after axotomy, were significantly higher when the retinal pieces originated from retinae pretreated with protease inhibitors at the time of optic nerve transection. The results assigned to the retinal proteases, which are presumably localized in microglial cells, an important function in eliminating severed neurons in the functionally and structurally disturbed retina.

ACKNOWLEDGEMENTS: The author thanks Dr. Y.A. Barde for providing the BDNF and Dr. W. Risau for providing the bFGF used in the cultures. The technical assistance of M. Wild is gratefully acknowledged. T. Rice proof-read the manuscript and the photographic team from our department helped in preparing the photographs. The work was supported by the Deutsche Forschungsgemeinschaft (grant Th 386 2-1).

REFERENCES

Barde, Y.A., D. Edgar, and H. Thoenen,1982, Purification of a new neurotrophic factor from mammalian brain. EMBO-J. 1:549-553.
Barron, K.D., M. P. Dentinger, G. Lrohel, S.K.Easton, and R. Mankes, 1986, Qualitative and ultrastructaral observations on retinal ganglion cell layer of rat after intraorbital nerve crush. J. Neurocytol. 15: 345-362.

Bignami, A., and D. Dahl, 1979, The radial glia of Müller and their response to injury. An Immunofluorescence study with antibodies to the glial fibrillary acidic (GFA) protein. Exp. Eye Res. 28: 63-69.

Cajal, R. y. S., 1928, Degeneration and regeneration of the nervous system. (R.M. May. Trans.) University Press, London and New York.

Cammermeyer, J.,1970, The life history of the microglia cell: A light microscopic study. In: S. Ehrenpreis and O. C. Solnitzky (eds): Neurosciences Research, Vol. 3, Academic Press, New York, pp. 44-129.

Carmignoto, G., L. Maffei, P. Candeo, R. Canella and C. Comelli, 1989, Effect of NGF on the survival of rat retinal ganglion cells following optic nerve section. J. Neurosci. 9: 1263-1272.

del Rio-Hortega, P., 1932, Microglia. In: Cytology and Cellular Pathology of the nervous system (eds. Penfield W.), pp. 482-534. Paul B. Hoeber, New York.

Grafstein, B., and N.A. Ingoglia, 1982, Intracranial transection of the optic nerve in adult mice: Preliminary observations. Exp. Neurol. 76: 318-330.

Giulian, D., 1987, Ameboid microglia as effectors of inlamation in the central nervous system. J. Neurosci. Res. 18:155-171.

Giulian, D., J. Chen, J. E. Ingeman, J. K. George, and M. Noponen, 1989, The role of mononuclear phagocytes in wound-healing after traumatic injury to adult mammalian brain. J.Neurosci. 9(12): 4416-4429.

Giulian, D., 1990, Microglia and tissue damage in the central nervous system. In: Differentation and functioning of Glial cells, Ed. Levi, Alan R. Liss, pp. 379-389.

Hickey, W.F., and H. Kimura, 1988, Perivascular microglial cells of the CNS are bone-derived and present antigen in vivo. Science, 239:290-292.

Gebhard, W., H. Tschesche, and H. Fritz, 1986, Biochemistry of aprotinin and aprotinin-like inhibitors. In: proteinase inhibitors (A. J. Barrett and J. Salvesen, eds), Elsevier, pp. 375-378.

James, G. R., 1933, Degeneration of ganglion cell following axonal injury. Arch. Ophthalmol. 9: 338-343.

Keirstead, S.A., M. Rasminsky, Y. Fukuda, D.A. Carter, A.J.Aguayo and M. Vidal-Sanz, 1989, Electrophysiological responses in hamster superior colliculus evoked by regenerating retinal axons. Science, 246: 255-257.

Lampson, L.A., 1987, Molecular basis of the immune response to neural antigens. TINS 10: 211-216.

Lieberman, A. R., 1971, The axon reaction: A review of the principal features of perikaryal responses to axon injury. Int. Rev. Neurobiol. 14: 49-124.

Murabe, Y., and Y. Sano, 1981, Thiaminepyrophosphatase activity in the plasma membrane of microglia. Histochem. 71: 45-52.

Perry, V. H., 1979, The ganglion cell layer in the retina of the rat. Proc. R. Soc. Lond. B204: 363-375.

Perry, V. H., and S. Gordon, 1988, Macrophages and microglia in the nervous system. TINS, Vol. 11, No. 6, 273-277.

Politis, M.J., and P. S. Spencer, 1986, Regeneration of rat optic axons into peripheral nerve grafts. Exp. Neurol. 91: 52-59.

Powers, C. J. and J. W. Harper, 1986, Inhibitors of serine proteases. In: Proteinase inhibitors (A. J. Barrett and G. S. Salvesen, eds) Elsevier, pp. 55-152.

Rich, D. H., 1986, Inhibitors of cysteine proteinases. In: proteinase inhibitors (A. J. Barrett and G. salvesen, eds.) Elsevier, pp. 179-217.

Schnebli, H. P., 1975, The effects of protease inhibitors on cells in vitro. In: Proteases and Biological Control. (Eds. E. Reich, D. B. Rifkin and E. Shaw), Cold Spring Harbor Conferences on cell proliferation. pp. 785-794.

Schnitzer J. and J. Scherer, 1990, Microglial cell responses in the rabbit retina following transection of the optic nerve. J. Comp. Neurol. 302: 779-791.

Schwab, M.E. and P. Caroni, 1988, Oligodendrocytes and CNS myelin are non-permissive for neurite growth and fibroblast spreading in vitro. J. Neurosci. 8: 2381-2393.

Sievers, J., Hausmann, B., Unsicker, K., and M. Berry, 1987, Fibroblast growth factors promote the survival of adult rat retinal ganglion cells after transection of the optic nerve. Neurosci. Lett. 76: 157-162.

Singer, P.A., S. Mehler, and H. L. Fernandez, 1982, Blockade of retrograde axonal transport delays the onset of metabolic and morphologic changes induced by axotomy. J. Neurosci. 2: 1299-1306.

Stoll, G., B.D. Trapp, and J.W. Griffin, 1989, Macrophage function during Wallerian degeneration of the rat optic nerve: Clearance of degenerating myelin and Ia expression. J. Neurosci. 9: 2327-2335.

Streit, W.J., M.B. Graeber and G.W. Kreutzberg, 1990, Functional plasticity of microglia: a review GLIA, 1(5) 301-307.

Tello, F., 1907, La regeneration de voies optigues. Trab. Lab. Invest. Biol. 5: 237-248.

Thanos, S., 1988, Alterations in the morphology of ganglion cell dendrites in the adult rat retina after optic nerve transection and grafting of peripheral nerve segements. Cell Tiss. Res. 259: 599-609.

Thanos, S., M. Bähr, Y. A. Barde, and J. Vanselow, 1989, Survival and axonal elongation of adult rat retinal ganglion cells. In vitro effects of lesioned sciatic nerve and brain derived-neurotrophic factor. E. J. Neurosci. 1: 19-26.

Thanos, S. and J. Vanselow, 1990, Fetal tectal transplants in the cortex of adult rats become innervated both by retinal ganglion cell axons regenerating through peripheral nerve grafts and by cortical neurons. Rest. Neurol. Neurosci. 2: 63-75.

Vanselow, J., M. E. Schwab and S. Thanos, 1990, Responses of regenerating rat retinal ganglion cell axons to contacts with central nervous myelin in vitro. E.J. Neurosci. 2: 121-125.

Vidal-Sanz, M., G. M. Bray, M. P. Villegas-Perez, S. Thanos and A. J. Aguayo, 1987, Axonal regeneration and synapse formation in the superior colliculus by retinal ganglion cells in the adult rat. J. Neurosci. 7: 2894-2909.

Villegas-Perez, M. P., Vidal-Sanz, M., G. M. Bray and Albert Aguayo, 1988, Influences of peripheral nerve grafts on the survival and regrowth of axotomized retinal ganglion cells in adult rats. J. Neurosci. 8(1): 265-280.

ORGANIZATION AND DEVELOPMENT OF SPARSELY DISTRIBUTED WIDE-FIELD AMACRINE CELLS IN THE RABBIT RETINA

Nicholas C. Brecha[1], Giovanni Casini[2] and Dennis Rickman[3]

Departments of Anatomy & Cell Biology[1] and Medicine[1,2]
Brain Research Institute[1], Jules Stein Eye Institute[1] and CURE-DDC[1], UCLA School of Medicine and VAMC West Los Angeles
Los Angeles, California 90073, USA and
Department of Anatomy & Cell Biology[3], USC School of
Medicine, Los Angeles, California 90034, USA

INTRODUCTION

The retina is characterized by six major neuronal cell classes: photoreceptor, bipolar, horizontal, interplexiform, amacrine and ganglion cells. These can be further divided into multiple subclasses, as defined by their cellular morphology, number, distribution, and histochemical phenotype (Cajal, 1893; Boycott and Dowling, 1969; Kolb et al., 1981; Brecha, 1983; Karten and Brecha, 1983). Amacrine cells are located in the proximal inner nuclear layer (INL) and ganglion cell layer (GCL), and their processes mainly innervate the inner plexiform layer (IPL). These cells form numerous presynaptic and postsynaptic contacts with bipolar, interplexiform and ganglion cells, as well as with other amacrine cells (Dowling and Boycott, 1966). Physiologically, they can be broadly classified into transient or sustained types based on their responses to light stimuli (see Kolb et al., 1988, Djamgoz et al., 1990, and Bloomfield, 1991, for references). Anatomical and physiological investigations indicate that amacrine cells participate in multiple pathways in the processing of visual information through the retina.

Amacrine cells have been recognized for about one hundred years as a diverse group of neurons characterized by cell bodies of various sizes and processes that are distributed to various levels or laminae of the IPL (Cajal, 1893). Early studies, based on the Golgi technique, identified many distinct cell types which ramify either in a single lamina or more diffusely in multiple laminae of the IPL. On this basis, Cajal described multiple amacrine cell types in several vertebrate retinas. Numerous morphologically distinct amacrine cell types have been recognized in turtle (Kolb, 1982; Kolb et al., 1988), cat (Kolb et al., 1981) and monkey (Rodieck, 1988; Mariani, 1990) retina using the Golgi technique, and a large diversity of amacrine cell types is now accepted as a general feature of all vertebrate retinas.

Histochemical and immunohistochemical studies have shown that many of these morphologically distinct types of amacrine cells also can be distinguished by their expression of one or more "classical" transmitters, neuroactive peptides or transmitter-related enzymes (see Brecha, 1983, and Vaney, 1990, for reviews). The use of histochemical and intracellular labeling methods (Tauchi and Masland, 1984) with quantitative approaches (Wässle and Riemann, 1978) has provided a better understanding of amacrine cells in general by allowing the evaluation of the spatial

The Changing Visual System, Edited by P. Bagnoli and
W. Hodos, Plenum Press, New York, 1991

organization of individual cell populations. Indeed, using these approaches we now have a more accurate understanding of amacrine cell morphology and cell number, density and distribution.

Overall, amacrine cells can be placed into two broad morphological categories, narrow- and wide-field, based on the lateral spread of their processes in the IPL. Both groups have numerous cell types that can be differentiated on the basis of cell body size, arborization and stratification patterns of their processes in the IPL, and cell number and density. In general, narrow-field amacrine cells, as exemplified by A II amacrines, have restricted fields and high cell population densities (Famiglietti and Kolb, 1975; Vaney, 1985; Mills and Massey, 1991) . These attributes suggest that narrow-field cells are likely to have important roles in the direct transmission of visual information through the retina.

In contrast, wide-field amacrine cells are considerably more heterogeneous, with marked differences in cell number and density, and the size of the retinal fields that they innervate (Kolb et al., 1981; Brecha et al., 1984; Tauchi and Masland, 1984; Sandell and Masland, 1986; Wässle et al., 1987; Rodieck, 1988; Vaney et al., 1988; Casini and Brecha, 1991a). Masland (1988) recently extended this classification scheme and proposed that wide-field amacrine cells can be further differentiated into two broad groups based on cell population densities and mosaics. One group has a high cell density across the retina and widely ramifying processes. This anatomical arrangement results in an extensive overlapping of cellular processes, which form a dense network in selected laminae of the IPL. In the case of cholinergic/GABAergic amacrine cells, any single point on the retina, depending on the region studied, is covered by processes of 30 to 70 cells (Tauchi and Masland, 1984). The second wide-field amacrine cell group has a sparse distribution of cell bodies with widely ramifying and overlapping processes. Numerous distinct cell types can be placed into this group. Examples are the tyrosine hydroxylase (TH), vasoactive intestinal polypeptide (VIP) and somatostatin (SRIF) immunoreactive amacrine cells of the rabbit retina (Brecha et al., 1984; Sagar, 1987a, b; Mitrofanis et al., 1988b; Rickman et al., 1986; Rickman and Brecha, 1989; Tauchi et al., 1990; Casini and Brecha, 1991a). The distribution of fibers of these cells results in widely spaced networks in specific IPL laminae. On the basis of these morphological observations, sparsely distributed wide-field amacrine cells may have diffuse, regulatory or modulatory functions in the retina (Masland, 1988).

Amacrine cells, like other retinal neurons, develop in a central to peripheral gradient, and their genesis encompasses a relatively long prenatal and early postnatal period (see Stone, 1988, for references; Schnitzer, 1990). Ultrastructural investigations have shown that most amacrine cell synaptic connections are formed postnatally at about the time of eye opening in rabbit and cat retina (McArdle et al., 1977; Morrison, 1982). Furthermore, the maturation of different components of several amacrine cell transmitter systems are reported to span the first 2 to 3 postnatal weeks in rabbit retina (Kong et al., 1980; Lam et al., 1980, 1981; Parkinson and Rando, 1984). Less is known about the ontogeny of specific amacrine cell populations, and recent investigations have focused on the development of the cholinergic/GABAergic, TH and SRIF immunoreactive cell populations, principally in the rat, rabbit and cat retina (Ferriero and Sagar, 1987; Mitrofanis et al., 1988a, 1989; Dann, 1989; Martin-Martinelli et al., 1989; Wong and Collin, 1989; Wang et al., 1990; Casini and Brecha, 1991c; Rickman et al., 1991). These studies have begun to address several developmental issues concerned with the ontogeny of amacrine cells, including assessments of 1) cellular outgrowth and differentiation, 2) cell density and distribution, and 3) timing of the expression of transmitter phenotypes. We have initiated a series of investigations to confront some of these issues by examining the TH and SRIF immunoreactive amacrine cells. We have chosen to study the sparsely distributed wide-field amacrine cell group because of the significant amount of immunohistochemical and morphological background information that we have available for several of its members. This includes knowledge of their cellular morphologies, population mosaics and adult transmitter phenotypes. An additional advantage of studying cells of this group is the virtue of their sparse distributions, which allow for some ease in quantitative analyses.

The present report describes our recent studies of TH, VIP and SRIF immunoreactive amacrine cells in the adult rabbit retina, and of TH and SRIF immunoreactive cells in the developing rabbit retina, as representatives of the sparsely distributed wide-field amacrine cell group. Some of these studies have been previously reported (Brecha et al., 1984; Rickman et al., 1986, 1991; Rickman and Brecha, 1989; Casini et al., 1990; Casini and Brecha, 1991a, b, c). Additional information is from the unpublished Ph.D. dissertation of Dennis Rickman.

METHODS

Tissue Preparation. These investigations have used adult New Zealand albino rabbits of either sex, timed-pregnant females and newborn pups, all of which were obtained from commercial sources. Care and handling of the animals were approved by the Animal Research Committee of the VAMC-West Los Angeles in accordance with all NIH animal guidelines.

The retinas, some previously exposed to colchicine (Casini and Brecha, 1991a), were fixed in a paraformaldehyde solution, washed, sectioned with a cryostat perpendicularly to the vitreal surface at 10-15 μm or processed as whole mounts (Casini and Brecha, 1991a). For studies of fetal retina, whole heads were fixed, washed and sectioned with a cryostat in the horizontal plane at 10-15 μm.

Immunohistochemical procedures. Tissue sections or whole mounts were processed for immunohistochemistry using antibodies directed to TH (#15A, #15B, #16, and clone 2/40/15 [Boehringer-Mannheim, Indianapolis, IN]), VIP (#7913, #7916) or SRIF (S8) and immunofluorescence, peroxidase anti-peroxidase or avidin-biotin-peroxidase techniques (Brecha et al., 1984; Rickman and Brecha, 1989; Casini and Brecha, 1991a). Specificity of the immune reactions was assessed by substitution of the primary antibodies with normal mouse or rabbit serum, or by preadsorption of the antibodies with the appropriate antigen.

Quantitative analysis. Cell densities were measured in different retinal regions. Retinal area coverage was calculated as cell density x cell field area. Average cell spacing and nearest neighbor analysis, including a determination of the degree of regularity (mean cell spacing / standard deviation of cell spacing) (Wässle and Riemann, 1978), were performed on homogeneously-stained retinal areas where immunoreactive cell density was relatively constant. Corrections for shrinkage were not made since the retinal whole mounts were attached to the slides before dehydration.

ORGANIZATION OF TH, VIP AND SRIF IMMUNOREACTIVE AMACRINE CELLS IN THE RABBIT RETINA

TH Immunoreactive Cells

Dopamine is the principal catecholamine found in the rabbit retina (see Brecha, 1983, and Nguyen-Legros, 1988, for reviews). Initial studies using the Falck-Hillarp histofluorescence method demonstrated catecholamine fluorescent neurons in the rabbit retina (Ehinger and Falck, 1969). Subsequent studies using autoradiography with the high affinity uptake of dopamine or immunohistochemistry with antibodies directed to TH, the rate limiting enzyme for the synthesis of dopamine, have confirmed these initial observations and have shown that these cells constitute a discrete population of amacrine cells (Brecha et al., 1984; Oyster et al., 1985; Voigt and Wässle, 1987; Dacey, 1990; Tauchi et al., 1990).

In the rabbit retina, TH immunoreactive cells are located in the proximal INL (Brecha et al., 1984; Mitrofanis et al., 1988b; Tauchi et al., 1990). They are characterized by pyriform shaped, medium to large cell bodies which are slightly smaller in central retinal regions (visual streak) than in the periphery (Table 1). TH

TABLE 1

	Cell Size	
	Area (μm^2)	Diameter (μm)
TH	119 (central)[1] 134 (peripheral)[1]	12.5[2]
VIP	51 (central)[5] 64 (peripheral)[5]	8-9 (central)[3] 9-10 (peripheral)[3] 6-8[4]
SRIF	140 (ventral)[6]	

[1]Brecha et al., 1984
[2]Tauchi et al., 1990
[3]Casini and Brecha, 1991a
[4]Pachter et al., 1990
[5]Sagar, 1987a
[6]Rickman and Brecha, 1989

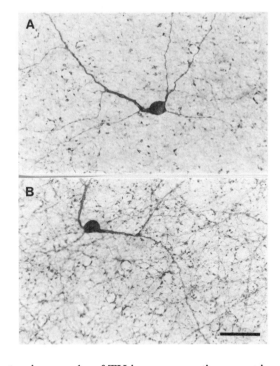

Figure 1. Photomicrographs of TH immunoreactive amacrine cells in a whole-mounted rabbit retina processed according to the avidin-biotin-peroxidase technique. TH immunoreactive processes are rich in varicosities and form a complicated network of fibers in lamina 1 of the IPL. A is from the ventral retina, B is from the visual streak. Scale bar: 50 μm

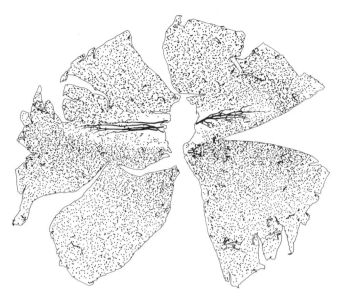

Figure 2. Reconstruction of a whole-mounted rabbit retina processed for TH immunoreactivity. TH-immunopositive somata are indicated by dots. The total retinal area is 436.7 mm^2, giving an average density of 19.4 cells/mm^2. The visual streak, which lies just ventral to the retinal blood vessels, has the highest cell density.

immunoreactive cells give rise to varicose processes that are distributed to lamina 1 of the IPL where they form an extensive plexus (Figure 1). In lamina 1 this meshwork consists of medium- to fine-caliber fibers, and there are examples of fibers that appear to form "rings" (Törk and Stone, 1979) around unlabeled cell bodies which may be A II amacrine cells, as demonstrated in the rat and cat retina (Pourcho, 1982; Voigt and Wässle, 1987). Immunoreactive fibers also are present in laminae 3 and 5 of the IPL, and are widely spaced as viewed in whole mount preparations. TH immunoreactive processes extend for considerable distances across the retina in lamina 1 of the IPL. These fields have been estimated, from intracellular staining studies using Lucifer Yellow, to be at least as large as 850 μm in diameter (Tauchi et al., 1990). However, because of the difficulties in visualizing labeled processes in immunohistochemical preparations or in obtaining completely labeled cellular processes using intracellular labeling methods (Voigt and Wässle, 1987), it is problematic to establish the full extent of these processes. Infrequent, sparsely distributed processes also are seen in the distal INL and in the outer plexiform layer (OPL). These appear to originate from both the fiber plexus in the IPL and in some cases from TH immunoreactive somata.

On the basis of these patterns, TH immunoreactive cells in the rabbit retina are classified as wide-field amacrine cells (Brecha et al., 1984; Mitrofanis et al., 1988b; Tauchi et al., 1990). The sparse number of TH processes observed in the OPL may be associated with a few TH immunoreactive interplexiform cells, as described in some species (Negishi et al., 1985; Oyster et al., 1985; Nguyen-Legros, 1988) or with TH immunoreactive amacrine cells (Voigt and Wässle, 1987; Dacey, 1990).

TH immunoreactive cells are observed in all retinal regions (Figure 2) with an overall cell density of about 19 cells/mm^2 (Brecha et al., 1984). Higher cell densities are observed in central, as compared to peripheral, retinal regions (Table 2) (Brecha et al., 1984). A similar gradient in cell density from peripheral to central retina has been reported in two other studies (Mitrofanis et al., 1988b; Tauchi et al., 1990). The total

TABLE 2

	Cell Number	Cell Density (cells/mm^2) Overall	Regional
TH	8492[1] 5613[2] 3780[3] 3810[3]	19.4[1] 13[3]	23 (central)[1] 13 (peripheral)[1]
VIP	11000[4]	25[4]	50 (central)[4] 12 (peripheral)[4] 40 (central)[5] 20 (peripheral)[5]
SRIF	1414[6] 1082[6] 877[7] 1256[7]	3-5[6]	

[1]Brecha et al., 1984
[2]Tauchi et al., 1990
[3]Mitrofanis et al., 1988b
[4]Casini and Brecha, 1991a
[5]Sagar, 1987a
[6]Rickman and Brecha, 1989
[7]Sagar, 1987b

number of TH immunoreactive cells counted in retinal whole mount preparations has been reported to be 8492 (Brecha et al., 1984) and 5613 (Tauchi et al., 1990). These values are somewhat higher than estimates of the total number of TH immunoreactive cells in the rabbit retina reported by Mitrofanis et al. (1988b).

The average nearest neighbor distances of TH immunoreactive cells in two retinas were found to be 143 μm and 172 μm (Brecha et al., 1984). Histograms of the distribution of these nearest neighbor distances are broad and skewed slightly towards higher nearest neighbor distances. These distributions do not fit a theoretical random distribution (according to Poisson probability rule) based on the same density of cells, suggesting that TH immunoreactive cells are non-randomly distributed (Wässle and Riemann, 1978; Brecha et al., 1984). The regularity indexes of cell distribution (mean / standard deviation of nearest neighbor distance) for these retinas are 3.2 and 3.9.

Considering an estimated diameter of 850 μm for TH immunoreactive cells from intracellular staining studies (Figure 3 in Tauchi et al., 1990) and an average TH immunoreactive cell density of 19 cells/mm^2 (Brecha et al., 1984), we calculate that this cell population has a retinal coverage (cell density x cell field area) of about 10.8.

A recent study using catecholamine uptake and intracellular labeling techniques has differentiated catecholamine-accumulating cells into two populations in the rabbit retina (Tauchi et al., 1990). The major cell population, called type 1, is probably identical to the TH immunoreactive amacrine cell population described above. These cells have large fields, which are confined to lamina 1 of the IPL. The second cell population, called type 2, is smaller in number than the type 1 cell population. Type 2 cells give rise to widely ramifying processes that are found in laminae 1, 3 and 5 of the IPL. Type 2 cells are thought to be incompletely stained using Falck-Hillarp histofluorescence or immunohistochemical methods, thus accounting for difficulties in demonstrating their presence in the retina. A detailed discussion of these two cell populations and a comparison to previously described TH immunoreactive patterns has been presented elsewhere (Tauchi et al., 1990) and is not reviewed here.

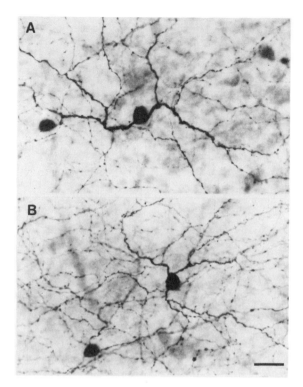

Figure 3. Photomicrographs of VIP immunoreactive amacrine cells in a whole-mounted retina processed according to the avidin-biotin-peroxidase technique. Immunostained cell bodies give rise to one, two (A) or three (B) primary processes which undergo further ramification. Photomicrographs are from the dorsal retina. Scale bar: 20 μm.

<u>VIP Immunoreactive Cells</u>

VIP is a 28 amino acid neuroactive peptide found throughout the nervous system (see Rostene, 1984, for review). Radioimmunoassay and immunohistochemical investigations have demonstrated the presence of VIP immunoreactivity in the retinas of many vertebrate species (Brecha, 1983; Sagar, 1987a; Pachter et al., 1989; see Casini and Brecha, 1991a, for references). In general, VIP immunoreactivity is localized to sparsely occurring amacrine cells with multistratified processes (see Casini and Brecha, 1991a, for references). In rabbit retina, VIP immunoreactive cells make up a distinct population of wide-field amacrine cells (Casini and Brecha, 1991a).

VIP immunoreactive amacrine cells are located in the proximal INL and, occasionally, in the GCL and IPL (Casini and Brecha, 1991a). They are characterized by small to medium cell bodies that are round to pyriform in shape. Cell body diameters in the visual streak are slightly smaller than those measured in the dorsal and ventral retina (Sagar, 1987a; Casini and Brecha, 1991a) (Table 1). Immunoreactive neurons have one to three thick primary processes that give rise to secondary processes and collaterals which are rich in varicosities (Figure 3). These processes ramify in the distal, middle and proximal portions of the IPL corresponding best to laminae 1, 3 and 5. VIP immunoreactive processes have a variable distribution in each of these laminae. For instance, primary and secondary processes may arborize within the same lamina. In other instances, single fibers may ramify and give rise to collaterals in one lamina and, in turn, enter and arborize in a different lamina. In addition, the same fiber can extend from one lamina to another without ramifying. The wide extent of the VIP-containing

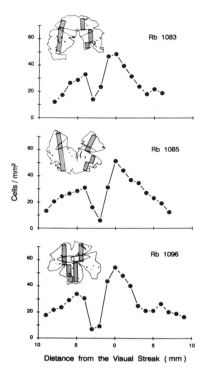

Figure 4. Density of VIP immunoreactive cell bodies along two vertical stripes oriented perpendicularly to the visual streak (shown in the insets) in three retinal whole-mounts. Each point represents the mean value calculated between corresponding locations of the two vertical stripes. Dorsal is on the left, ventral on the right. 0 mm represents the center of the visual streak.

arborizations produces a consistent overlap of processes of different cells, giving rise to a widely spaced and homogeneous meshwork across the retinal surface.

Generally, VIP-containing neurons in the dorsal retina possess wider arborizations with a lower degree of ramification as compared to those in central and ventral retina. Area values of the arbors range from 0.14 to 0.27 mm^2 in the dorsal retina, from 0.05 to 0.06 mm^2 in the visual streak and from 0.07 to 0.13 mm^2 in the ventral retina (Casini and Brecha, 1991a). These values are estimates, since these processes can not be completely traced through the plexus of immunostained fibers in the IPL.

Immunoreactive cells are present in all retinal regions (Figure 4) (Sagar, 1987a; Pachter et al., 1989; Casini and Brecha, 1991a) with an overall cell density of 25 cells/mm^2. The cell distribution shows a peak of about 50 cells/mm^2 in the visual streak and about 12 cells/mm^2 in peripheral retina (Sagar, 1987a; Casini and Brecha, 1991a). The total number of VIP-containing neurons is estimated to be about 11,000 (Table 2) (Casini and Brecha, 1991a).

The average nearest neighbor distances in two retinas were 99 μm and 109 μm in central retinal regions, and 124 μm and 170 μm in peripheral retinal regions (Casini and Brecha, 1991a). A comparison of the distribution of nearest neighbor distances to a theoretical random curve shows that these neurons are non-randomly spaced (Casini and Brecha, 1991a). The regularity value of cell distribution is about 3 in all retinal regions.

Estimated retinal coverage values for the VIP immunoreactive cell population, calculated from the cell density and cell field size measurements reported above, are

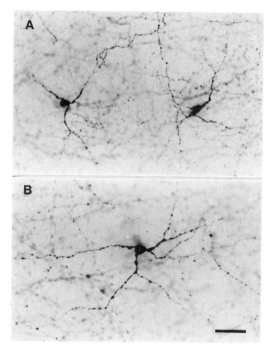

Figure 5. Photomicrographs of SRIF immunoreactive amacrine cells in a whole-mounted retina processed according to the avidin-biotin-peroxidase technique. A and B are both from the ventral retina. Immunoreactive cell bodies are located in the GCL and primary processes can be seen to arborize in lamina 5 of the IPL. The plexus of immunoreactive fibers in lamina 1 is out of focus. Scale bar: 50 μm.

about 3 in central and ventral retina, but values as high as 7 can be found in the dorsal retina.

SRIF Immunoreactive Cells

SRIF is a 14 amino acid neuroactive peptide that is found throughout the vertebrate nervous system (see Epelbaum, 1986, for review). Radioimmunoassay and chromatographic studies have demonstrated the presence of SRIF in retinal extracts, while immunohistochemical studies have shown that SRIF immunoreactivity is localized to neurons in the inner retina (Brecha, 1983; Sagar, 1987b; Sagar and Marshall, 1988; Rickman and Brecha, 1989; see White et al., 1990, for references).

In the adult rabbit retina, SRIF-containing somata are localized to the GCL and, rarely, to the INL of the ventral retina (Rickman et al., 1986; Sagar, 1987b; Rickman and Brecha, 1989). In addition, a high number of immunoreactive cells are located along the retinal margin adjacent to the ora serrata. In ventral retina, these cells are characterized by an ovoid or multipolar shape, medium to large size (140 μm²) and 2 to 5 primary processes which ramify in lamina 5 of the IPL (Table 1 and Figure 5). Primary processes are thick and give rise to a widely spaced meshwork of fine, beaded processes which arborize primarily in lamina 1. This network is present in both dorsal and ventral retina, providing complete coverage of the retinal surface. Frequently, a smooth, thin-caliber fiber can be observed to arise from a cell body or a primary process. These fibers can be followed for long distances across the retina in either the nerve fiber layer or lamina 1 of the IPL. A similar pattern of ramification of a long-range process has been described in human retina, although the process is located in the

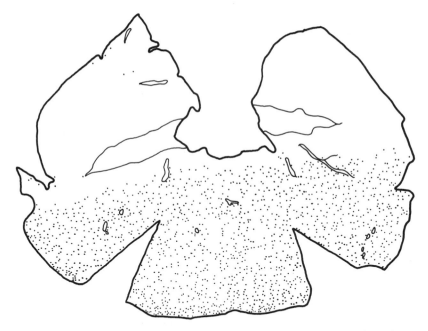

Figure 6. Reconstruction of a whole mount preparation of a rabbit retina demonstrating the location of every SRIF immunoreactive cell body. Labeled somata are confined almost exclusively to the ventral retina.

IPL adjacent to the GCL (Sagar and Marshall, 1988). Immunoreactive fibers also are observed in the OPL in both ventral and dorsal retina, and usually they can be traced to the plexus in lamina 1 of the IPL. SRIF immunoreactive fibers also have been noted in the OPL of rat, guinea pig and cat retina (Spira et al., 1984; Negishi et al., 1985; White et al., 1990). Finally, there is a dense accumulation of immunoreactive fibers along the retinal margin, which forms a circumferential band in all retinal regions (Rickman et al., 1986).

SRIF-containing cells are distributed predominantly to the ventral retina with a few scattered cells in the dorsal retina (Figure 6) (Rickman and Brecha, 1989). From the visual streak to far-peripheral ventral retina, the density of labeled somata is about 5 cells/mm^2 (Table 2) (Rickman and Brecha, 1989). As mentioned, there is a high number of cells located at the retinal margin. In one animal we estimated the density to be 19 cells/mm^2 along the ventral retinal margin. The total number of SRIF immunoreactive cells counted in the ventral retina of four whole mount preparations are 1,018 and 1,414 cells (Rickman and Brecha, 1989), and 877 and 1,256 cells (Sagar, 1987b).

The relatively large size of SRIF immunoreactive cell bodies, their location in the GCL and the presence of long-range processes suggest that these cells may be ganglion cells. This possibility was examined in animals in which one optic nerve was transected, and the animals were allowed to survive for several months (110 to 143 days), a sufficient time period for the elimination of most ganglion cells (Masland et al., 1984a; Brecha et al., 1987). In these retinas there was no change in the density of SRIF immunoreactive somata compared to the contralateral normal retina (Rickman and Brecha, 1989). Furthermore, when the sizes of stained somata were compared, no difference was noted between immunoreactive somata in retinas with an optic nerve transection and control retinas. Together, these observations indicate that there is no selective cell death or atrophic change in SRIF immunoreactive cells following optic nerve transection and suggest that SRIF immunoreactive cells are not ganglion cells.

SRIF-containing cells represent a class of wide-field amacrine cells whose cell bodies are mainly located in the GCL. However, since in rabbit retina there are many SRIF immunoreactive processes in the OPL, we cannot eliminate the possibility that at least some of these are interplexiform cells whose cell bodies are located in the GCL.

COMMENTS CONCERNING THE ORGANIZATION OF SPARSELY DISTRIBUTED WIDE-FIELD AMACRINE CELLS

Our studies, using as examples the TH, VIP and SRIF immunoreactive cell populations in the rabbit retina, have illustrated several characteristics of sparsely distributed wide-field amacrine cells. These include 1) the arborization and stratification patterns of their processes, 2) their cell number, density, distribution and mosaics, and 3) their transmitter phenotypes.

Sparsely distributed wide-field amacrine cells may be located in the INL, IPL or GCL. The majority of TH and VIP immunoreactive cells are localized to the proximal INL, while the majority of SRIF-containing cells are observed in the GCL (Brecha et al., 1984; Sagar, 1987a, b; Mitrofanis et al., 1988b; Rickman and Brecha, 1989; Pachter et al., 1990; Tauchi et al., 1990; Casini and Brecha, 1991a). All three of these cell types have widely ramifying processes that form large fields in specific laminae of the IPL. There is overlap of these processes such that widely spaced meshworks are found at all retinal eccentricities.

Our estimates of retinal coverage for the rabbit TH and VIP immunoreactive cells are comparable to those estimated for cat TH immunoreactive cells (Voigt and Wässle, 1987). The values of retinal coverage are considerably less than those of high cell density wide-field amacrine cells as exemplified by the cholinergic/GABAergic and the type 1 and 2 indoleamine-accumulating cell populations (Tauchi and Masland, 1984; Vaney, 1984; Sandell and Masland, 1986). Due to difficulties in tracing medium- and fine-caliber processes through a plexus of immunoreactive fibers, it is not possible to completely define the whole extent of TH, VIP and SRIF immunoreactive cell arborizations. Therefore, our estimates of arborization areas and retinal coverage are minimum values. A striking example of the uncertainty in determining field size is illustrated by SRIF-containing amacrine cells in the rabbit and cat retina (Sagar, 1987b; Rickman and Brecha, 1989; White et al., 1990; Chun et al., 1991). These cells are mainly located in the ventral retina, and undoubtedly some of their fibers innervate dorsal retinal regions. In the adult retina we cannot trace these processes to their somal origins because they become lost in the meshwork of processes in the IPL. However, in early postnatal rabbit retinas, where the immunoreactive plexus is not well developed, we can often follow processes from ventral into dorsal retinal regions. On this basis we suspect that the fields of the SRIF immunoreactive cells are asymmetric and very extensive. An asymmetric or very sparse distribution of processes, as illustrated for some cells in both Golgi (Figure 37 in Rodieck, 1988) and intracellularly labeled preparations (Figure 3 in Wässle et al., 1987), also would bias any estimates of retinal cell field area. Indeed, a measure of fiber density (fiber length/mm^2) is likely to be a better measure for these particular cell types.

A potential complication in defining the fields of wide-field amacrine cells is the suggestion that many have both "axon-like" and "dendritic" processes, which innervate different retinal fields (Mariani, 1982; Sagar, 1987b; Sagar and Marshall, 1988; Dacey, 1988, 1989, 1990). The identification of axons or "axon-like" fibers is based on light microscopic observations of Golgi, immunohistochemical and horseradish peroxidase (HRP) intracellularly labeled preparations, which show that fine- to very fine-caliber fibers arise from cell bodies or processes and innervate both local and distant regions. These fibers are characterized by a smooth appearance with some varicosities and few terminal branches. Often, these "axon-like" processes have considerably larger fields than "dendrites" and innervate retinal areas measuring many millimeters from their cell bodies (Dacey, 1988, 1989, 1990). In addition to the examples of HRP intracellularly labeled amacrine cells described in the cat and primate retina (Dacey, 1988, 1989, 1990), there are many other examples of sparsely distributed retinal cells having long-range processes, including long-range neurofibrillar-staining amacrine cells of the cat and rabbit retina (Vaney et al., 1988), sparsely branched indoleamine-accumulating amacrine cells of the cat retina (Wässle et al., 1987), associational nerve cells of the GCL of the dog and human retina (Gallego and Cruz, 1965), SRIF immunoreactive associational ganglion cells in the rabbit and human retina (Sagar, 1987b; Sagar and Marshall, 1988), NADPH-diaphorase (type 1 or ND 1) staining amacrine cells in the rabbit retina (Sagar, 1990) and proprioretinal cells of the chick retina (Catsicas et al., 1987). However, given the lack of any ultrastructural, biochemical or functional information, it is difficult to determine if the "axon-like" processes are axons, thin dendrites, or neurites having both axonal and dendritic properties. Until further information is available, we believe it is best to use more neutral terminology and to refer to these processes as long-range processes or fibers (Vaney et al., 1988).

TH-, VIP-, and SRIF-containing amacrine cellpopulations of the rabbit retina, like other sparsely distributed wide-field amacrine cell populationss (Oyster et al., 1985; Sagar, 1987b; Sagar and Marshall, 1988; Vaney and Young, 1988b; Vaney et al., 1988; Tauchi et al., 1990; White et al., 1990; Dacey, 1990), are low in overall cell density and absolute cell number. As illustrated by the TH and VIP immunoreactive cell populations, cell densities may be somewhat higher in central as compared to peripheral retinal regions (Brecha et al., 1984; Mitrofanis et al., 1988b; Vaney and Young, 1988b; Tauchi et al., 1990; Casini and Brecha, 1991a). In contrast, the SRIF immunoreactive cells are mainly distributed at a very low and even density in ventral retina, but there is a high concentration of cells along the retinal margin (Sagar, 1987b; Rickman and Brecha, 1989). At least for the TH and SRIF immunoreactive amacrines, their distribution patterns are similar in rabbit, cat and monkey retina (Brecha et al., 1984; Oyster et al., 1985; Sagar, 1987b; Rickman and Brecha, 1989; Dacey, 1990; White et al., 1990).

TH, VIP and SRIF immunoreactive cell populations are low in absolute cell number having a total of about 8,500 cells, 11,000 cells and 1,250 cells, respectively. Using a conservative estimate of 10^6 amacrine cells in the rabbit retina, then each of these cell populations make up about 1% or less of the total amacrine cell population. In comparison to other amacrine cell populations in the rabbit retina, the TH, VIP and SRIF immunoreactive cell populations are markedly smaller in number than the glycinergic (Kong et al., 1980), GABAergic (Vaney, 1990), cholinergic/GABAergic (Masland et al., 1984b), indoleamine-accumulating (Sandell and Masland, 1986) and NADPH-diaphorase (type ND 2) staining (Vaney and Young, 1988b) amacrine cells. For example, cholinergic/GABAergic and indoleamine-accumulating amacrines number 290,000 cells and 180,000 cells, respectively (Masland et al., 1984a; Sandell and Masland, 1986).

TH and VIP immunoreactive cell populations are not randomly distributed, and they have some regularity in their distributions (Brecha et al., 1984; Casini and Brecha, 1991a). That is, 1) the distribution of nearest neighbor distances of these cells does not match a theoretical random distribution (Wässle and Riemann, 1978) and 2) the index of regularity indicates some regularity in cell spacing. Interestingly, the TH and VIP immunoreactive cell populations, along with several other types of amacrine cells in the rabbit and cat retina, have similar degrees of regularity (Vaney et al., 1981; Brecha et al., 1984; Masland et al., 1984a; Oyster et al., 1985, Vaney, 1985; Sandell and Masland, 1986; Casini and Brecha, 1991a). Wide-field amacrine cells are less ordered as a group than either cat horizontal cells, or cat and monkey cones (Wässle and Riemann, 1978; Wässle et al., 1978).

The co-expression of GABA and a second neuroactive substance also is a feature of many wide-field amacrine cells (Brecha et al., 1988; Chun and Wässle, 1988; Pourcho and Goebel, 1988; Vaney and Young, 1988a, b; Vaney et al., 1989). In sparsely distributed wide-field amacrine cells, the co-expression of GABA with NADPH-diaphorase or TH has been demonstrated in several species including the rat, cat and rabbit retina (Kosaka et al., 1987; Versaux-Botteri et al., 1987; Vaney and Young, 1988b; Wässle and Chun, 1988; unpublished observations). Recently, the co-expression of GABA with VIP in both the rat and rabbit retina has been reported (Casini and Brecha, 1991b). In addition, all VIP immunoreactive cells in the rabbit retina contain peptide histidine isoleucine immunoreactivity (Pachter et al., 1989). A discussion of issues concerning the coexpression of neuroactive substances in neurons can be found elsewhere (Hökfelt et al., 1986).

Several populations of sparsely distributed, wide-field amacrine cells have been identified in the mammalian retina as discussed elsewhere in this chapter. In rabbit retina, the type 2 catecholamine-accumulating (Tauchi et al., 1990), NADPH-diaphorase-staining (type 1 or ND 1) (Vaney and Young, 1988b; Sagar, 1990) and long-range neurofibrillar-staining (Vaney et al., 1988) amacrine cells belong to this group. Undoubtedly, other cell populations will be included in this group in the future, since Golgi and reduced silver studies (Gallego and Cruz, 1965; Kolb et al., 1981; Rodieck, 1988; Mariani, 1990) have reported several amacrine cell types with widely ramifying processes in the mammalian retina, but these have not been studied in regards to their cell number, density, distribution and histochemistry.

Sparsely distributed wide-field amacrine cell types share many similarities in their general morphological and histochemical organization, but they also differ in several ways, including their somal distributions, absolute numbers, and perhaps most significantly, the laminar distribution of their processes in the IPL. This latter observation is evident from Golgi and reduced silver studies, (Gallego and Cruz, 1965; Kolb et al., 1981; Vaney et al., 1988; Mariani, 1990) and from immunohistochemical studies (Brecha et al., 1984; Rickman and Brecha, 1989; Tauchi et al., 1990; Vaney, 1990; Casini and Brecha, 1991a). Differences in the laminar distribution of processes may provide further clues as to distinct functional roles of these cells in the processing of visual information.

The influence of sparsely distributed wide-field amacrine cells on visual information processing is likely to be greater than suggested by their low density and small number, due to the wide spread distribution and overlap of their processes in all retinal regions. There are several hypotheses regarding the function of wide-field amacrine cells in visual information processing. However, before speculating on possible functional roles, it must be noted that there is a possibility that segments of amacrine cell processes are electrically isolated (Ellias and Stevens, 1980; Miller and Bloomfield, 1983) and that they may act independently (Masland et al., 1984b). In contrast, assuming the entire cell responds as described for many morphological types of rabbit amacrine cells (Bloomfield, 1991), then several suggestions have been put forth as to the function of wide-field amacrine cells. These include mediation of long-range interactions within the retina such as changing contrast or luminosity sensitivity over large retinal areas (McIllwain, 1964; Watanabe and Tasaki, 1980; Barlow et al., 1977; Dacey, 1988; Sagar and Marshall, 1988; White et al., 1990; Chun et al., 1991) and participation in directional selectivity (Mariani, 1982; Bloomfield, 1991). Wide-field cells also may have trophic effects, perhaps via actions of neurotransmitters or neuroactive peptides, which have a spectrum of non-transmitter effects on neurons (Bulloch, 1987; Lipton and Kater, 1989; Pincus et al., 1990). Whatever role these cells have in visual function, differences in 1) the laminar distribution of their processes, 2) their synaptic relationships in the IPL and 3) retinal responses after application of their putative transmitter substance to the retina (e.g. SRIF, Zalutsky and Miller, 1990; and dopamine, Thier and Alder, 1984; Jensen and Daw, 1986), indicate that sparsely distributed wide-field amacrine cells must have distinct, although admittedly poorly understood, roles in visual information processing.

ONTOGENY OF TH AND SRIF IMMUNOREACTIVE AMACRINE CELLS IN THE RABBIT RETINA

TH Immunoreactive Cells

The following section highlights some aspects of the development of TH immunoreactive cells. A more detailed description can be found in "Development of the tyrosine hydroxylase immunoreactive cell population in the rabbit retina" by G. Casini and N. C. Brecha in this volume.

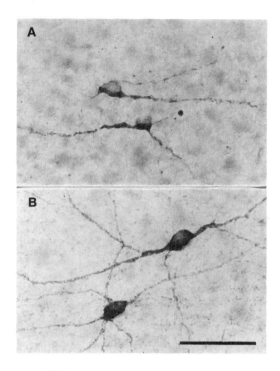

Figure 7. Examples of TH immunoreactive cells in whole-mounted rabbit retinas at PD-6 (A) and PD-12 (B). At the time of eye opening (about PD-12), a dense plexus of immunoreactive fibers is present in lamina 1 of the IPL. Scale bar: 50 μm.

TH immunoreactive neurons are present at postnatal day (PD) 0 (birth), the first day studied in this investigation (Casini and Brecha, 1991c). At birth, light immunoreactivity is confined to cell bodies located in the INL at the IPL border, and to developing processes located in the IPL adjacent to the INL. Immunoreactive cell bodies are widely spaced across the retina and are found in all retinal regions without any obvious central to peripheral gradient. From PD-0, they increase in number until about PD-19, when adult values are reached. Analysis of whole-mount preparations shows that TH immunoreactive cell bodies at PD-12 are non-randomly distributed, displaying low degrees of regularity typical of the adult.

At the earliest postnatal times studied, TH-containing processes are usually characterized by a short, truncated appearance, and often they give rise to several fine-caliber processes in lamina 1 of the IPL. From birth to eye opening (PD-12) there is a rapid growth of processes in laminae 1 of the IPL (Figure 7). These processes, many having growth cones, cross each other and form networks similar to those observed in the adult. At PD-6, fibers in lamina 3 of the IPL can also be seen. From eye opening to about PD-26, TH immunoreactive cells assume most of their adult characteristics.

SRIF Immunoreactive Cells

SRIF immunoreactivity is first detected at embryonic day 25 (ED-25), which is about 5 days prior to birth, in small, round to oval somata scattered throughout the INL of the ventral retina (Rickman et al., 1991). Occasional thick primary processes are observed entering the IPL, although overall there are few immunoreactive processes in the IPL. At ED-29, well stained somata are present in the proximal INL, IPL and GCL of the ventral retina. Some cells have a primary process located in the IPL which does not arborize extensively. These observations indicate that some SRIF immunoreactive cells have not yet reached their final adult positions in the GCL.

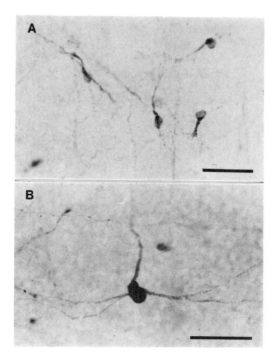

Figure 8. Examples of SRIF immunoreactive cells in whole-mounted rabbit retinas at PD-3 (A) and PD-10 (B). At PD-3, SRIF immunoreactive cells are characterized by processes which ramify in the IPL primarily near the GCL. At PD-10, fine processes are also observed in the IPL near the INL. Scale bars: 50 μm.

In early postnatal retinas (PD-3), SRIF immunoreactive somata are only located in the GCL and are restricted to the ventral retina (Figure 8A). Near the visual streak they are rare (about 1 cell/mm^2), while near the ventral edge they are numerous (72 cells/mm^2). SRIF immunoreactive processes are confined primarily to the IPL adjacent to the GCL, where they are beginning to form a meshwork. Rarely, stained processes are also located in the IPL adjacent to the INL, where they can be followed for only short distances. In both regions of the IPL, these processes often terminate in conspicuous growth cones.

At PD-10, SRIF immunoreactive cell density values have shifted to 5 cells/mm^2 near the visual streak and 26 cells/mm^2 at the ventral edge. At PD-10, many processes are observed in lamina 1 of the IPL, and they often have conspicuous growth cones (Figure 8B). Processes also can be traced in this region of the IPL from the ventral retina into the dorsal retina. By PD-31, the distribution of immunoreactive processes approximates that of the adult rabbit retina. In addition to the prominent processes seen in lamina 5 of the IPL, a fine, well-developed plexus is present in lamina 1 of the IPL. This plexus is also observed in the dorsal retina. Few growth cones are observed.

In addition to the population of SRIF immunoreactive neurons described above, which are likely to be the sparsely distributed wide-field amacrine cells described in the adult retina, we also observe a second group of SRIF immunoreactive cells during the perinatal period which disappears in the third postnatal week. These cells, also present in the GCL, are first observed at ED-29 and differ in morphology from the cells described above. They are characterized by large somata, dense perinuclear immunoreactivity and the lack of any stained processes. In whole mounts of early postnatal retinas (PD-3 and PD-10), this second group of cells is confined to the ventral retina, but is distributed in an apparently regular array with peak density in central retina and lower density in peripheral retina. There is a greater number of these cells at

PD-3 compared to PD-10. Some of these cells also are observed at PD-15, but by PD-20 they are not present in any retinal regions.

COMMENTS CONCERNING SOME ASPECTS OF THE ONTOGENY OF SPARSELY DISTRIBUTED WIDE-FIELD AMACRINE CELLS

In the rabbit retina, we first detected SRIF immunoreactivity at ED-25 in cell bodies located in the INL, IPL and GCL. We assume that these cells are the counterparts of the sparsely distributed, adult SRIF immunoreactive wide-field amacrine cells, which are principally located in the GCL. Our interpretation of the SRIF-containing cells observed in the INL and IPL at ED-25 is that they are undergoing migration to their final positions in the GCL. This interpretation is supported by observations on the following days which show that SRIF immunoreactive cells are mostly present in the IPL and GCL, and that by birth they are primarily located in the GCL (Rickman et al., 1991). An alternative explanation, which we can not rule out, is that the immunoreactive cells in the INL and IPL die by PD-0, since substantial numbers of pyknotic cells are present in the inner retina during this time period (Stone et al., 1985). We have not studied the TH immunoreactive cell population at prenatal periods, and therefore we do not have information regarding prenatal expression of TH immunoreactivity.

At birth, SRIF and TH immunoreactivities are present in a limited number of immature cells that are located at or near their adult laminar positions in the inner retina (Casini and Brecha, 1991c; Rickman et al., 1991). That is, TH immunoreactive cells are confined to the proximal INL in all retinal regions and SRIF immunoreactive neurons are mostly localized to the GCL of the ventral retina. These cells are widely spaced, usually characterized by weak immunoreactive staining and processes in the IPL bearing growth cones. These early expression patterns of TH and SRIF immunoreactivity match other reports in the cat retina (Mitrofanis et al., 1989; Wang et al., 1990) and are in contrast to the more advanced development of cholinergic/GABAergic amacrine cells in the rabbit GCL, and cat INL and GCL (Dann, 1989; Wong and Collin, 1989). There is a general increase in the number of TH immunoreactive cells (Casini and Brecha, 1991c) until adult values are reached at about PD-19. We do not have information about changes in the absolute number of SRIF immunoreactive cells.

The innervation of the IPL develops significantly during the first postnatal week, with an increase in the number of fibers and in the complexity of the immunoreactive plexus. Interestingly, TH and SRIF immunoreactive processes are only found in the IPL at the relative position in which they are observed in the adult retina. We suggest that these processes are guided into or restricted to the correct IPL laminae by the presence of factors that are specific to different strata of the IPL. Finally, the morphological characteristics of TH and SRIF immunoreactive cells seen at eye opening are similar to those of the adult retina suggesting that they are functional at this time. During later postnatal periods, the immunoreactive fiber network becomes more complex with cellular maturation apparently completed by the third or fourth week of age.

At birth, the number of cells expressing TH immunoreactivity is less than the number observed in adult retinas (Brecha et al., 1984; Casini and Brecha, 1991a), and there is a gradual increase in cell number during the first two postnatal weeks. The increase in cell number during the first postnatal week could be due to the genesis of new TH-containing amacrine cells, since neuronal proliferation in the rabbit INL continues during this time period after birth (Schnitzer, 1990). The lower number of TH immunoreactive cells at earlier postnatal times also may be explained by technical limitations of immunohistochemistry sensitivity, since at these times TH content is very low (Lam et al., 1981; Parkinson and Rando, 1984). Indeed, these technical limitations could account for TH immunoreactive cell number increase during the second and third postnatal weeks. This sequence of expression could be under strict genetic control. However, we can not exclude the interesting possibility that amacrine cells begin expressing TH immunoreactivity at different times after birth due to local environmental influences. In addition, there is an overall decrease in TH immunoreactive cell density that is likely due to retinal growth and stretch.

The genesis of the SRIF immunoreactive patterns is more complex (Rickman et al., 1991) due to the presence of two distinct cell populations. Cells that become the sparsely distributed wide-field amacrine cell population, identified on the basis of their distribution and appearance, appear to follow the same developmental pattern as the TH immunoreactive cells. The second, granular staining cells, transiently express SRIF immunoreactivity during the last prenatal and the first three postnatal weeks. Their morphology clearly distinguishes them from the other SRIF-containing cell population. We can not determine if these cells die or stop displaying SRIF immunoreactivity.

Although the role of this transient cell population during development is not known, the regular array of these cells suggests the presence of stable positional markers which may influence the direction of fiber outgrowth in the developing retina. A similar mechanism has been proposed for axonal guidance in the development of central visual connections (see Udin and Fawcett, 1988, and Harris and Holt, 1990, for reviews). An alternative, yet equally intriguing, possibility is that this transient cell population serves a scaffolding or "guidepost" function in the development of retinal mosaics.

Our studies show that TH immunoreactive neurons in the adult rabbit retina have some regularity in their distribution (Brecha et al., 1984). In contrast, at birth, TH immunoreactive cells have a very low degree of regularity (Casini and Brecha, 1991c). The shift towards a non-random distribution, with a degree of regularity characteristic of adult TH-containing cells, is likely due to several interacting events. These may include genetic mechanisms that influence cell location and environmental factors that modulate TH expression. Cell genesis and death in the INL during the first postnatal week (Schnitzer, 1990), and differential retinal growth (Robinson et al., 1989) also, undoubtedly, influence final cell position.

Rabbit TH and SRIF immunoreactive cells are immature at birth and develop over the first postnatal week (Casini and Brecha, 1991c; Rickman et al., 1991). In contrast, rabbit cholinergic/GABAergic amacrine cells located in the GCL already have their adult fiber branching pattern at birth (Wong and Collin, 1989). These observations indicate some variance in amacrine cell growth and innervation of the IPL.

Finally, wide-field amacrine cell processes grow extensively over the first postnatal week, and interactions among processes must be very permissive in order to obtain the overlap typical of fibers observed in adult retinas. Perhaps a plausible explanation for the development of these immunoreactive processes is that they are genetically programmed to grow to certain lengths and with certain patterns of ramification. The establishment of the adult organization of the TH immunoreactive meshwork would then depend on both fiber outgrowth patterns and the arrangement of the TH immunoreactive cell mosaic. In contrast, for the SRIF immunoreactive cells, cell body position would seem unimportant to the formation of the meshwork. This mode of formation of fiber plexuses is apparently quite different from dendritic field development of cat α-ganglion cells (Wässle et al., 1981). In this model, the mosaic of ganglion cell bodies would be formed first, and their processes would adapt to the available space--the arbor of one cell influencing the growth of arbors of nearby cells, resulting in very little overlap (Wässle et al., 1981).

The development of TH immunoreactive amacrine cells matches descriptions of the time course of the increase of dopamine and TH activities (Lam et al, 1981; Parkinson and Rando, 1984) in rabbit retina. There is not as much information available concerning the cholinergic/GABAergic, GABA-accumulating, glycine-accumulating or SRIF-containing amacrine cell systems (Kong et al., 1981; Lam et al., 1981; Wong and Collin, 1989; Rickman et al., 1991). Therefore it is difficult to compare these amacrine cell systems and to determine if there are differences in transmitter expression patterns of narrow-field and wide-field amacrine cells. The dramatic changes in the innervation of the IPL precede the period of greatest synaptogenesis in rabbit retina (McArdle et al., 1977). Overall, all of these changes occur just before the emergence of ganglion cell responsiveness and the formation of ganglion cell receptive field properties (Masland, 1977). Together, these observations suggest that the TH and SRIF immunoreactive amacrine cell populations are functional at about eye opening, although they continue their maturation for some time. Finally, it is intriguing to think that in addition to transmitter related functions, these cells may have trophic influences, as well, on the maturation of the developing retina.

ACKNOWLEDGEMENTS

We are grateful to Drs. A. W. Tank and N. Weiner for providing TH polyclonal antibodies, Dr. A. Buchan for providing the SRIF monoclonal antibody and Dr. J. Walsh and H. Wong for providing the VIP antibodies. We wish to thank Dr. C. Sternini for her helpful comments on this manuscript. Supported by National Institutes of Health grant EY 04067 and VA Medical Research Funds.

REFERENCES

Barlow, H.B., Derpingtion, A.M., Harris, L.R., and Lennie, P., 1977, The effects of remote retinal stimulation on the responses of cat retinal ganglion cells, J. Physiol. (Lond.), 269:177.

Bloomfield, S.A., 1991, Two types of orientation-sensitive responses of amacrine cells in the mammalian retina, Nature, 350:347.

Boycott, B.B., and Dowling, J.E., 1969, Organization of the primate retina: light microscopy, Phil. Trans. R. Soc. Lond. B, 255:109.

Brecha, N., 1983, Retinal neurotransmitters: histochemical and biochemical studies, in: "Chemical Neuroanatomy," P.C. Emson, ed., Raven Press, New York.

Brecha, N.C., Oyster, C.W., and Takahashi, E.S., 1984, Identification and characterization of tyrosine hydroxylase immunoreactive amacrine cells, Invest. Ophthalmol. Vis. Sci., 25:66.

Brecha, N.C., Johnson, D., Bolz, J., Sharma, S., Parnavelas, J.G., and Lieberman, A.R., 1987, Substance P-immunoreactive retinal ganglion cells and their central axon terminals in the rabbit, Nature, 6118:155.

Brecha, N., Johnson, D., Peichl, L., and Wässle, H., 1988, Cholinergic amacrine cells of the rabbit retina contain glutamate decarboxylase and γ-aminobutyrate immunoreactivity, Proc. Natl. Acad. Sci. USA, 85:6187.

Bulloch, A.G.M., 1987, Somatostatin enhances neurite outgrowth and electrical coupling of regenerating neurons in Helisoma, Brain Res., 412:6.

Cajal, S.R., 1893, La rétine des vertébré, Cellule, 9:17.

Casini, G., Brecha, N.C., Takahashi, E.S., and Oyster, C.W., 1990, Postnatal development of tyrosine hydroxylase-immunoreactive (TH-IR) neurons in the rabbit retina, Soc. Neurosci. Abs., 16:1075.

Casini, G., and Brecha, N.C., 1991a, Vasoactive intestinal polypeptide-containing cells in the rabbit retina: Immunohistochemical localization and quantitative analysis. J. Comp. Neurol., 305:313.

Casini, G., and Brecha, N.C., 1991b, Co-expression of vasoactive intestinal polypeptide (VIP) and other neurotransmitters in rat and rabbit retinas. Invest. Ophthalmol. Vis. Sci., 32:993.

Casini, G., and Brecha, N.C. 1991c, Morphological characterization of tyrosine hydroxylase (TH) immunoreactive neurons in the developing rabbit retina. Soc. Neurosci. Abs., 17: In press.

Catsicas, S., Catsicas, M., and Clarke, P.G.H., 1987, Long-distance intraretinal connections in birds, Nature, 326:186.

Chun, M.H., Brecha, N.C., and Wässle, H., 1991, Light and electron microscopic studies of the somatostatin immunoreactive plexus in the cat retina, Cell Tiss. Res., Submitted.

Dacey, D. M., 1988, Dopamine-accumulating retinal neurons revealed by in vitro fluorescence display a unique morphology, Science, 240:1196.

Dacey, D.M., 1989, Axon-bearing amacrine cells of the macaque monkey retina, J. Comp. Neurol., 284:275.

Dacey, D.M., 1990, The dopaminergic amacrine cell, J. Comp. Neurol., 301:461.

Dann, J.F., 1989, Cholinergic amacrine cells in the developing cat retina, J. Comp. Neurol., 289:143.

Djamgoz, M.B.A., Spadavecchia, L., Usai, C., and Vallerga, S., 1990, Variability of light-evoked response pattern and morphological characterization of amacrine cells in goldfish retina, J. Comp. Neurol., 301:171.

Dowling, J.E., and Boycott, B.B., 1966, Organization of the primate retina: electron microscopy, Proc. R. Soc. Lond. B, 166:80.

Ehinger, B., and Falck, B., 1969, Adrenergic retinal neurons of some New World monkeys, Zeitsch. Zellerforsc. Mikroskop. Anat., 100:364.

Ellias, S.A., and J.K. Stevens, 1980, The dendritic varicosity: a mechanism for electrically isolating the dendrites of cat retinal amacrine cells?, Brain Res., 196:365.

Epelbaum, J., 1986, Somatostatin in the central nervous system: physiology and pathological modifications, Progr. Neurobiol., 27: 63.

Famiglietti, E.V., and Kolb, H., 1975, A bistratified amacrine cell and synaptic circuitry in the inner plexiform layer of the retina, Brain Res., 84: 293.

Ferriero, D.M. and Sagar, S.M., 1987, Development of somatostatin immunoreactive neurons in rat retina, Brain Res., 431:207.

Gallego, A., and Cruz, J., 1965, Mammalian retina: associational nerve cells in ganglion cell layer, Science, 150:1313.

Harris, W.A. and Holt, C.E., 1990, Early events in the embryogenesis of the vertebrate visual system: cellular determination and pathfinding, Annu. Rev. Neurosci., 13:155.

Hökfelt, T., Holets, V.R., Staines, W., Meister, B., Melander, T., Schalling, M., Schultzberg, M., Freedman, J., Björklund, H., Olson, L., Lindh, B., Elfvin, L.-G., Lundberg, J.M., Lindgren, J.A., Samuelsson, B., Pernow, B., Terenius, L., Post, C., Everitt, B., and Goldstein, M., 1986, Coexistence of neuronal messengers - an overview, Progr. Brain Res., 68:33.

Jensen, R.J., and Daw, N.W., 1986, Effects of dopamine and its antagonists on the receptive field properties of ganglion cells in the rabbit retina, Neuroscience, 17:837.

Karten, H.J., and Brecha, N., 1983, Localization of neuroactive substances in the vertebrate retina: evidence for lamination in the inner plexiform layer, Vis. Res., 23:1197.

Kolb, H., Nelson, R., and Mariani, A., 1981, Amacrine cells, bipolar cells and ganglion cells of the cat retina: a Golgi study, Vis. Res., 21:1081.

Kolb, H., 1982, The morphology of the bipolar cells, amacrine cells, and ganglion cells in the retina of the turtle (Pseudemis scripta elegans), Phil. Trans. R. Soc. Lond. B, 298: 355.

Kolb, H., Perlman, I., and Normann, R.A., 1988, Neural organization of the retina of the turtle Mauremis caspica: a light microscope and Golgi study, Vis. Neurosci., 1:47.

Kong, Y.C., Fung, S.C. and Lam, D.M.K., 1980, The postnatal development of glycinergic neurons in rabbit retina, J. Comp. Neurol., 193:1127.

Kosaka, T., Kosaka, K., Hataguchi, Y., Nagatsu, I., Wu, J.-Y., Ottersen, O.P., Storm-Mathisen, J., and Hama, K., 1987, Catecholaminergic neurons containing GABA-like and/or glutamic acid decarboxylase-like immunoreactivities in various brain regions of the rat, Exp. Brain Res., 66:191.

Lam, D.M.K., Fung, S.C., and Kong, Y.C., 1980, The postnatal development of GABAergic neurons in the rabbit retina. J. Comp. Neurol., 193:89.

Lam, D.M.K., Fung, S.C., and Kong, Y.C., 1981, Postnatal development of dopaminergic neurons in the rabbit retina. J. Neurosci., 1:1117.

Lipton, S.A., and Kater, S.B., 1989, Neurotransmitter regulation of neuronal outgrowth, plasticity and survival, T.I.N.S., 12:265.

Mariani, A.P., 1982, Association amacrine cells could mediate directional selectivity in pigeon retina, Nature, 298:654.

Mariani, A.P., 1990, Amacrine cells of the rhesus monkey retina, J. Comp. Neurol., 301:382.

Martin-Martinelli, E., Simon, A., Vigny, A. and Nguyen-Legros, J., 1989, Postnatal development of tyrosine-hydroxylase-immunoreactive cells in the rat retina: morphology and distribution, Dev. Neurosci., 11:11.

Masland, R.H., 1977, Maturation of functions in the developing rabbit retina. J. Comp. Neurol., 175:286.

Masland, R.H., 1988, Amacrine cells, T.I.N.S., 11:405.

Masland, R.H., Mills, J.W., and Hayden, S.A., 1984a, Acetylcholine-synthesizing amacrine cells: identification and selective staining by using radioautography and fluorescent markers, Proc. R. Soc. Lond. B, 223:79.

Masland, R.H., Mills, J.W., and Cassidy, C., 1984b, The functions of acetylcholine in the rabbit retina, Proc. R. Soc. Lond. B, 223:121.

McArdle, C.B., Dowling, J.E., and Masland, R.H., 1977, Development of outer segments and synapses in the rabbit retina. J. Comp. Neurol., 175:253.

McIllwain, J.T., 1964, Receptive fields of optic tract axons and lateral geniculate cells; periphery extent and barbiturate sensitivity, J. Neurophysiol., 27:1154.

Miller, R.F., and Bloomfield, S.A., 1983, Electroanatomy of a unique amacrine cell in the rabbit retina, Proc. Natl. Acad. Sci. U.S.A., 80:3069.

Mills, S.L., and Massey, S.C., 1991, Labeling and distribution of A II amacrine cells in the rabbit retina, J. Comp. Neurol., 340:491.

Mitrofanis, J., Maslim, J., and Stone, J. , 1988a, Catecholaminergic and cholinergic neurons in the developing retina of the rat, J. Comp. Neurol., 276:343.

Mitrofanis, J., Vigny, A., and Stone, J., 1988b, Distribution of catecholaminergic cells in the retina of the rat, guinea pig, cat, and rabbit: independence from ganglion cell distribution, J. Comp. Neurol., 267:1.

Mitrofanis et al., 1989, Somatostatinergic neurones of the developing human and cat retinae, Neurosci. Lett., 104:209.

Morrison, J.D., 1982, Postnatal development of the area centralis in the kitten retina: an electron microscopic study, J. Anat., 135:255.

Negishi, K., Kato, S., Teranishi, T., Kiyama, H., Katayama, Y., and Tohyama, M., 1985, So-called interplexiform cells immunoreactive to tyrosine hydroxylase or somatostatin in rat retina, Brain Res., 346:136.

Nguyen-Legros, J., 1988, Morphology and distribution of catecholamine-neurons in mammalian retina, Progr. Ret. Res., 7:113.

Oyster, C.W., Takahashi, E.S., Cilluffo, M., and Brecha, N.C., 1985, Morphology and distribution of tyrosine hydroxylase-like immunoreactive neurons in the cat retina, Proc. Natl. Acad. Sci. USA, 82:6335.

Parkinson, D. and Rando, R.R., 1984, Ontogenesis of dopaminergic neurones in the postnatal rabbit retina: pre- and postsynaptic elements, Develop. Brain Res., 13:207.

Patcher, J.A., Marshak, D.W., Lam, D.M.K., and Fry, K.R., 1989, A peptide histidine isoleucine/peptide histidine methionine-like peptide in the rabbit retina: colocalization with vasoactive intestinal peptide, synaptic relationships and activation of adenylate cyclase activity, Neuroscience, 31:507.

Pincus, D.W., DiCicco-Bloom, E.M., and Black, I.B., 1990, Vasoactive intestinal peptide regulates mitosis, differentiation and survival of cultured sympathetic neuroblasts, Nature, 343:564.

Pourcho, R.G., 1982, Dopaminergic amacrine cells in the cat retina, Brain Res., 252:101.

Pourcho, R.G., and Goebel, D.J., 1988, Colocalization of substance P and γ-aminobutyric acid in amacrine cells of the cat retina, Brain Res., 447:164.

Rickman, D.W., Johnson, D., Sharma, S., and Brecha, N.C., 1986 Distribution of substance P and somatostatin immunoreactive cells in the rabbit retina. Soc. Neurosci. Abs., 12:641.

Rickman, D.W., and Brecha, N.C., 1989, Morphologies of somatostatin-immunoreactive neurons in the rabbit retina, in: "Neurobiology of the Inner Retina," R. Weiler and N.N. Osborne, eds., Springer-Verlag, Berlin Heidelberg.

Rickman, D.W., Brecha, N.C., and Blanks, J.C., 1991, Expression of somatostatin immunoreactivity (SRIF-IR) in the developing rabbit retina, Invest. Ophthalmol. Vis. Sci. 32:1129.

Robinson, S.R., Dreher, B., and McCall, M.J., 1989, Nonuniform retinal expansion during the formation of the rabbit's visual streak: Implications for the ontogeny of mammalian retinal topography. Vis. Neurosci., 2:201.

Rodieck, R.W., 1988, The primate retina, in "Comparative Primate Biology," Vol. 4: Neurosciences, Alan Liss Inc., New York.

Rostene, W.H., 1984, Neurobiological and neuroendocrine functions of the vasoactive intestinal peptide, Progr. Neurobiol., 22:103.

Sagar, S.M., 1987a, Vasoactive intestinal polypeptide (VIP) immunohistochemistry in the rabbit retina, Brain Res., 426:157.

Sagar, S.M., 1987b Somatostatin-like immunoreactive material in the rabbit retina: immunohistochemical staining using monoclonal antibodies, J. Comp. Neurol., 266:291.

Sagar, S.M., and Marshall, P.E., 1988, Somatostatin-like immunoreactive material in associational ganglion cells of human retina, Neurosci., 27:507.

Sagar, S.M., 1990, NADPH-diaphorase reactive neurons of the rabbit retina: differential sensitivity to excitotoxins and unusual morphologic features, J. Comp. Neurol., 300:309.

Sandell, J.H., and Masland, R.H., 1986, A system of indoleamine-accumulating neurons in the rabbit retina, J. Neurosci., 6:3331.

Schnitzer, J., 1990, Postnatal gliogenesis in the nerve fiber layer of the rabbit retina: an autoradiographic study, J. Comp. Neurol., 292:551.

Spira, A.W., Shimizu, Y., and Porstad, O.P., 1984, Localization, chromatographic characterization, and development of somatostatin-like immunoreactivity in the guinea pig retina, J. Neurosci., 4:3069.

Stone, J., 1988, The origins of the cells of vertebrate retina, Progr. Ret. Res., 7:1.

Stone, J., Egan, M. and Rapaport, D.H., 1985, The site of commencement of retinal maturation in the rabbit, Vis. Res., 1985, 25:309.

Tauchi, M., and Masland, R.H., 1984, The shape and arrangement of the cholinergic neurons in the rabbit retina, Proc. R. Soc. Lond. B, 223:101.

Tauchi, M., Madigan, N.K., and Masland, R.H., 1990, Shapes and distributions of the catecholamine-accumulating neurons in the rabbit retina, J. Comp. Neurol., 293:178.

Thier, P., and Alder, V., 1984, Action of iontophoretically applied dopamine on cat retinal ganglion cells, Brain Res., 292:109.

Török, I., and Stone, J., 1979, Morphology of catecholamine-containing amacrine cells in the cat's retina, as seen in retinal whole mounts, Brain Res., 169:261.

Udin, S. B. and Fawcett, J.W., 1988, Formation of topographic maps, Annu. Rev. Neurosci., 11:289.

Vaney, D.I., 1984, "Coronate" amacrine cells in the rabbit retina have the "starburst" dendritic morphology, Proc. R. Soc. Lond. B, 220:501.

Vaney, D.I., 1985, The morphology and topographic distribution of A II amacrine cells in the cat retina, Proc. R. Soc. Lond. B, 224:475.

Vaney, D.I., 1990, The mosaic of amacrine cells in the mammalian retina, Progr. Ret. Res., 9:49.

Vaney, D.I., Peichl, L., and Boycott, B.B., 1981, Matching populations of amacrine cells in the inner nuclear and ganglion cell layers of the rabbit retina, J. Comp. Neurol., 199:373.

Vaney, D.I., and Young, H.M., 1988a, GABA-like immunoreactivity in cholinergic amacrine cells of the rabbit retina, Brain Res., 438:369.

Vaney, D.I., and Young, H.M., 1988b, GABA-like immunoreactivity in NADPH-diaphorase amacrine cells of the rabbit retina, Brain Res., 474:380.

Vaney, D.I., Peichl, L., and B. B. Boycott, 1988, Neurofibrillar long-range amacrine cells in mammalian retinae, Proc. R. Soc. Lond. B, 235:203.

Vaney. D.I., Whitington, G.E., and Young, H.M., 1989, The morphology and topographic distribution of substance-P-like immunoreactive amacrine cells in the cat retina, Proc. R. Soc. Lond. B, 237:471.

Versaux-Botteri, C., Simon, A., Vigny, A., and Nguyen-Legros, J., 1987, Existence d' une immunoréactivité au GABA dans les cellules amacrines dopaminergiques de la rétine de rat. Comptes Rendus des Séances de l' Académie des Sciences, Paris, Série III, 305:381.

Voigt, T., and Wässle, H., 1987, Dopaminergic innervation of A II amacrine cells in mammalian retina, J. Neurosci., 7:4115.

Wang, H.-H., Cuenca, N. and Kolb, H., 1990, Development of morphological types and distribution patterns of amacrine cells immunoreactive to tyrosine hydroxylase in the cat retina, Vis. Neurosci., 4:159.

Wässle, H., and Riemann, H. J., 1978, The mosaic of nerve cells in the mammalian retina, Proc. R. Soc. Lond. B, 200:441.

Wässle, H., Peichl, L., and Boycott, B.B., 1978, Topography of horizontal cells in the retina of the domestic cat, Proc. R. Soc. Lond. B, 203:269.

Wässle, H., Peichl, L., and Boycott, B.B., 1981, Morphology and topography of on- and off-alpha ganglion cells in the cat retina. Proc. R. Soc. Lond. B, 212:157.

Wässle, H. and Chun, M.H., 1988, Dopaminergic and indoleamine-accumulating amacrine cells express GABA-like immunoreactivity in the cat retina, J. Neurosci., 8:3383.

Wässle, H., Voigt, T., and Patel, B., 1987, Morphological and immunocytochemical identification of indoleamine-accumulating neurons in the cat retina, J. Neurosci., 7:1574.

Wässle, H., and Chun, M.H., 1988, Dopaminergic and indoleamine-accumulating amacrine cells express GABA-like immunoreactivity in the cat retina, J. Neurosci., 8:3383.

Watanabe, J., and Tasaki, K., 1980, Shift-effect in the rabbit retinal ganglion cells, Brain Res., 181:198.

White, C.A., Chalupa, L.M., Johnson, D., and Brecha, N.C., 1990, Somatostatin-immunoreactive cells in the adult cat retina, J. Comp. Neurol., 293:134.

Wong, R.O.L. and Collin, S.P., 1989, Dendritic maturation of displaced putative cholinergic amacrine cells in the rabbit retina, J. Comp. Neurol., 287:164.

Zalutsky, R.A., and Miller, R.F., 1990, The physiology of somatostatin in the rabbit retina, J. Neurosci., 10:383.

AGING AND SPATIAL CONTRAST SENSITIVITY:

UNDERLYING MECHANISMS AND IMPLICATIONS FOR EVERYDAY LIFE

Cynthia Owsley and Kerri B. Burton

Departments of Ophthalmology and Psychology
School of Medicine/Eye Foundation Hospital
University of Alabama at Birmingham
Birmingham, Alabama 35294 U.S.A.

INTRODUCTION

With the percentage of older adults in our society on the increase, there is a pressing need to better understand the functional problems of the elderly, and to identify ways in which the quality of life can be maintained at a high level despite advancing age. One area of special concern is vision loss in later life, and how it impacts the performance of routine tasks that depend critically on vision. The goal of our laboratory over the past decade has been to use psychophysical techniques to not only describe the types of vision problems that older adults experience, but also to uncover the optical and neural mechanisms which underlie these deficits. In addition, our interest goes beyond simply measuring visual deficits in laboratory tasks; we are ultimately interested in discovering why many older adults have difficulty in performing everyday visual activities, such as driving, postural stability, navigating through the environment, and recognizing people.

The focus of our research has primarily been on older adults who are free from identifiable eye disease. Despite a clean bill of health, many older adults report that they experience significant visual problems which hamper routine daily activities (Kosnik et al., 1988). Our emphasis on the "ocular disease-free" elderly does not reflect our lack of interest in the serious functional problems stemming from eye diseases prevalent in old age, such as macular degeneration. Rather, several years ago we chose to focus on older adults free from eye disease because it was commonly believed, without empirical support, that this population was also free from visual functional problems. In the intervening years, several laboratories, including our own, have found that the normal aging process can itself be associated with vision loss.

It is important to stress that there is a fine and arbitrary line between what is considered to be good eye health in the elderly vs. the early stages of a pathological condition (Ludwig & Smoke, 1980; Johnson & Choy, 1987). There are many anatomical and physiological changes in the visual system in later adulthood (Weale, 1963, 1982, this volume). These changes in their minor forms are considered "normal" accompaniments to growing old, but in their more advanced stages, they can cause serious vision impairment and are consequently designated as "disease". For example, the crystalline lens in an older adult undergoes some degree of increased density and opacification. When this increased density progresses to where it causes significant functional problems, it is generally termed "cataract". A similar point can be made for the macular changes that typify many older retinae, such as pigmentary mottling and the appearance of drusen. When these changes become more serious and are accompanied by decreased acuity, a diagnosis of age-related macular degeneration is usually made. Thus, since these anatomical changes lie on a continuum rather than fall into dichotomous categories, the criteria for defining "normal eye health" in older adults are not easy to specify.

Despite the problem of defining normal aging, the study of visual function in adults free from significant eye disease is worthwhile. First, as mentioned earlier, many older adults never fall victim to ocular disease, yet still experience significant difficulty with daily visual activities such as mobility (e.g., driving). Second, ophthalmological tests of functional vision often require age-matched norms. If an older adult's performance is compared to norms generated from young adults, the older adult will often fall out of the normal range, and thus be viewed as "failing" the test, when in fact his/her performance may be the best that can be expected for that age. Third, many aging-related deficits in visual function can mimic the effects of ocular disease, and it is important to differentiate between the two whenever possible.

AGING-RELATED LOSSES IN SPATIAL CONTRAST SENSITIVITY

There are many aspects of visual function that can deteriorate during the aging process, and research on this broad topic has been reviewed in a number of chapters and volumes (e.g., Weale, 1963, 1982, this volume; Sekuler et al., 1982; Kline & Schieber, 1985; Owsley et al., 1986; Werner et al., 1990; Owsley & Sloane, 1990). The focus of much of our own work has been on aging-related changes in spatial contrast sensitivity. A primary function of the visual system is to process contrast information, which subserves our ability to see pattern in the environment. A useful way of characterizing the visual system's contrast perception capacities is to measure the system's modulation transfer function (MTF) (Campbell & Green, 1965), or in psychophysical parlance, the contrast sensitivity function. This function describes how an observer's contrast sensitivity (reciprocal of contrast threshold) varies as a function of the spatial frequency of a target. Over the past 20 years, contrast sensitivity techniques have proven useful in understanding early visual development (Banks, 1982) as well as disease processes (Bodis-Wollner & Camisa, 1980) in human vision, and thus it was a logical step to extend this analysis to the study of spatial vision in the late stages of life.

When we first became interested in the question of how aging affected spatial contrast sensitivity, we noted that there was tremendous disagreement among existing studies on this topic (Arden, 1978; Arden & Jacobsen, 1978; Arundale, 1978; Derefeldt et al., 1979; Sekuler et al., 1980; Skalka, 1980; McGrath & Morrison, 1981). Almost every conceivable type of spatial contrast sensitivity deficit had been reported, ranging from no loss, to a loss at selected frequencies, to a loss at all spatial frequencies. A detailed study of the literature revealed that the wide disagreement among studies was probably due to several methodological problems inherent in much of the previous work. First, many studies used relatively small sample sizes. Given the wide variability in functional and biological capabilities among the elderly (Ludwig & Smoke, 1980), use of a small N can lead to invalid inferences about characteristics of the population. Second, the effects of optical blur due to uncorrected refractive error were not controlled in several studies, which is of critical concern because of older adults' presbyopia and the common use of near test distances in psychophysical studies. In general, it cannot be assumed that the older adult's "walk-in" correction is the optimal correction. Observers must be individually refracted for the test distance. Third, it was unclear in the earlier studies whether subjects were screened for ocular pathology. Eye diseases, such as macular degeneration, glaucoma, cataract, and diabetic retinopathy, are relatively common in the elderly population (Leibowitz et al., 1980), and these conditions can significantly impair spatial contrast sensitivity. Thus, when the interest is in the aging process per se, it is crucial to identify the eye health characteristics of the sample, so that the confounding effects of significant eye disease can be parceled out.

In order to clarify the relationship between aging and spatial contrast sensitivity, we carried out a study designed to overcome many of these methodological problems (Owsley et al., 1983). The results of this study are illustrated in Figure 1. Targets were stationary sinusoidal gratings presented at a photopic level in central vision. All subjects had visual acuity no worse than 20/30. The results can be summarized as follows. Older adults on average tended to exhibit a contrast sensitivity loss at intermediate and higher spatial frequencies. The magnitude of this loss increased with increasing frequency. Since all subjects were refracted for the test distance, optical blur was not responsible for these aging-associated losses in contrast sensitivity. In addition, all subjects were free from identifiable eye disease, so these results were not mediated by serious sensitivity losses in a few subjects with clinically significant pathology. Rather, these results imply that contrast sensitivity loss can occur during the aging process itself, even in the absence of significant ocular pathology. This basic result has been confirmed by several other studies (Kline et al., 1983; Wright & Drasdo, 1985; Higgins et al., 1988; Tulunay-Kessey et al., 1988; Elliott et al., 1990). Electrophysiological studies on the visually-evoked potential in older adults are also consistent with this general pattern of results, indicating that the latency of the P100 component in the elderly is increased more for targets having high spatial frequency than having low spatial frequency (Sokol et al., 1981; Wright et al., 1985; Porciatti et al., 1991, this volume).

It is important to point out that while the average trend is for older adults to have some degree of loss in contrast sensitivity, there is substantial variability in older adults' contrast sensitivity abilities. Many older adults exhibit about a 0.5 log unit loss in sensitivity at higher spatial frequencies, while others perform well within the normal range for younger adults. This heterogeneity in the population calls into question the common practice of characterizing aging trends solely by group averages. The group mean is an idealization of some average older person, but does not adequately represent the breadth of biological diversity in the population. An alternative way of assessing aging trends is to consider what factors predispose one to "successful" aging vs. "unsuccessful" aging (Rowe & Kahn, 1987), so that risk factors can be identified and interventions developed if possible. In the present context, those who successfully age are those whose contrast sensitivity falls within some criterion level of satisfactory performance, and those who age unsuccessfully are the negative outliers. When planning future research efforts, it is important to recognize that this type of approach which tries to identify what factors distinguish these two groups is more likely to uncover the causes of visual functional disability in old age than is an approach relying on group averages.

One additional comment on variability is in order. Owsley et al. (1983) found that within age-group variability was much greater for older adults. For example, at a high spatial frequency, contrast sensitivity for a group in their 70's had a standard deviation about twice that for adults in their 20's. Furthermore, if the sample of older adults is restricted to persons with excellent acuity (20/20 or better), then the aging-related effect is minimal or disappears

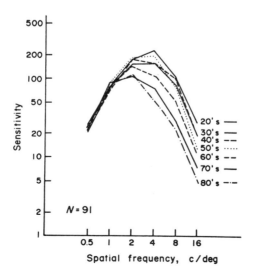

Fig. 1. Mean log spatial contrast sensitivity as a function of log spatial frequency for adults in their 20's to 80's. (From Owsley, Sekuler, & Siemsen, 1983)

entirely (Sturr & Taub, unpublished manuscript; Owsley et al., 1983). That is, contrast sensitivity in older adults with excellent acuity is typically similar to their younger counterparts. This finding makes sense given that acuity and sensitivity for higher spatial frequencies are theoretically linked. The practical implication of this finding is that the researcher can "direct" the magnitude of the aging effect by the strictness of the acuity criterion utilized for determining inclusion in the older adult sample.

The research discussed above demonstrates that many older adults have elevated contrast thresholds for *detecting* a spatial target. That is, compared to young persons, the elderly on average require greater contrast before they can just barely detect that "something" is present in a display, regardless of whether or not they can identify what it is. However, the literature is still unclear as to what extent they have problems seeing targets which are presented at *suprathreshold* contrast levels. There is evidence that these two aspects of spatial vision are mediated at least partially by separate mechanisms (Georgeson & Sullivan, 1975; Bowker, 1983), and thus it is possible that these two functions could be differentially affected by aging. Existing literature on this topic is sparse. Older adults require more contrast, compared to young adults, to discriminate and recognize complex targets typical of everyday life, such as faces and highway signs (Owsley, Sekuler, & Boldt, 1981; Owsley & Sloane, 1987). Using a more standard laboratory approach, Tulunay-Keesey et al. (1988) reported that older adults who exhibit contrast sensitivity losses do not, however, demonstrate deficits in a contrast-matching task performed at suprathreshold levels. They argued that this implies that aging does not affect a contrast compensation process in suprathreshold spatial vision, whether it is due to operation of a gain mechanism (e.g., Georgeson & Sullivan, 1975) or to a specialized mechanism for processing high contrast (e.g., Bobak et al., 1984). However, their oldest subject was only 67 years old, suggesting that there is still a possibility suprathreshold processing could be impaired at more advanced ages. Early and Smith (1990) examined the effect of aging on suprathreshold spatial vision by using a spatial frequency discrimination task. Their older adult sample included individuals as old as 81 years. They found that older adults had elevated discrimination thresholds for higher spatial frequencies, as compared to young adults. They speculated that these results could be due to increased noise levels in the activity of neurons in the older visual system. These results are consistent with those of Ball et al. (1986). Further work must clarify the relevance and extent of the differential aging effects in these suprathreshold laboratory tasks, given that many of our routine daily activities are carried out under high contrast conditions.

STUDYING UNDERLYING MECHANISMS

What are the mechanisms underlying the spatial contrast sensitivity loss exhibited by many older adults? There are a number of potential factors to be considered. First, the cognitive processes associated with making a decision as to whether a visual signal is present might be altered in older adults, as compared to young. For example, older adults may be more conservative in deciding when a grating is present, thus elevating their thresholds. However, studies utilizing criterion-free measures of threshold visibility with older adults have indicated that their contrast sensitivity loss is still present when criterion effects are taken into account (Higgins et al., 1988; Morrison & Reilly, 1986).

Another factor often blamed for older adults' contrast sensitivity loss is pupillary miosis, the tendency of the older adult's pupil to remain at a small diameter despite decreases in ambient illumination. Older adults' miotic pupil effectively reduces retinal illuminance which can decrease contrast sensitivity for high spatial frequencies (e.g., Van Nes & Bouman, 1967; De Valois et al., 1974). Thus, it seems like a natural candidate for the cause of older adults' contrast sensitivity difficulties. It is important to note, though, that pupillary miosis is not a special problem for older adults at high light levels (e.g., 100 cd/sq.m.), where contrast sensitivity losses have been found, since at high light levels pupil diameter is comparably small in both young and old adults (2 - 4 mm). The more pressing question is whether pupillary miosis is responsible for older adults' contrast sensitivity loss at *low* light levels. This is because as luminance decreases, the young adult's pupil increases in size, thereby increasing retinal illuminance. However, the older adult's pupil remains at a small, relatively fixed size, and thus places the elderly person at a selective disadvantage at low light levels, relative to young adults.

As Figure 2 illustrates, older adults' contrast sensitivity loss becomes more pronounced at low luminance levels (Sloane, Owsley, & Alvarez, 1988). This psychophysical result substantiates a common subjective complaint by older patients that they have increased difficulty with visual tasks under dim illumination (Kosnik et al., 1988). We next asked whether older adults' miotic pupils were responsible for their accentuated contrast sensitivity problem at low luminance. Under the conditions of this experiment, younger adults' pupil diameters were approximately 5 to 6 mm, whereas older adult's pupil diameters were about 3 to 4 mm. To examine the role of pupillary miosis in older adults' deficit, we pharmacologically increased each older adult's pupil diameter so that it matched the pupil diameter observed in younger subjects under the same viewing conditions (Sloane, Owsley, & Alvarez, 1988). The results were dramatic in that older adults' contrast sensitivity deficit did not disappear. In fact, older adults exhibited their best contrast sensitivity with their own miotic pupil. These results suggest that pupillary miosis is not responsible for older adults' spatial contrast sensitivity deficit. On the contrary, pupillary miosis may be a "hidden" asset in that it slightly improves contrast sensitivity in the elderly. Why might this be? One possibility may be related to the fact that the older eye has increased optical density of the ocular media, particularly the crystalline lens (Said & Weale, 1959). This increased optical density accentuates intraocular light scatter, thereby degrading the retinal image and reducing image contrast. A smaller pupil may actually be an asset under these circumstances, since it limits optical aberration and improves depth-of-focus, which facilitates image formation in the older eye.

Another feature of the aged eye that might contribute to contrast sensitivity problems in older adults is the crystalline lens, which, as just mentioned, increases in optical density and light scattering properties during adulthood (Said & Weale, 1959; Allen & Vos, 1967; Ijspeert et al., 1990). These changes in the lens could theoretically reduce the retinal illuminance and contrast of the retinal image in the aged eye. In our initial efforts to evaluate the role of the lens in older adults' contrast sensitivity loss (Owsley et al., 1985), we directed our attention to older adults with intraocular lenses (IOL). We measured contrast sensitivity in a group of older individuals who had previously undergone cataract extraction and IOL insertion. Since the crystalline lens had been removed in these individuals, we were presented with the opportunity to "bypass" the effects of the crystalline lens in examining how aging affects contrast sensitivity (see also Jay et al., 1987; Morrison & McGrath, 1985). The sample included only patients who were free from postoperative complications and who

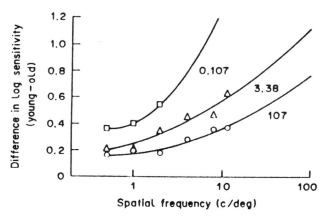

Fig. 2. Mean spatial contrast sensitivity loss in older adults (relative to young adults) at three light levels spanning a three log unit range (From Sloane, Owsley, & Alvarez, 1988)

had clear media at the time of testing. Contrast sensitivity data from these pseudophakic patients were then compared to data from older adults of the same age range who were in good ocular health and who had intact crystalline lenses. Their lenses exhibited the increased density characteristic of old age, but were not cataractous. A group of young adults in good eye health with intact crystalline lenses were also tested for comparison purposes. The logic behind this study was that, if changes in the crystalline lens contribute to the contrast sensitivity loss in older adults, one would expect that the IOL group would have better contrast sensitivity than the "old-normals". If the lens changes play little or no role in producing older adults' loss in contrast sensitivity, then contrast sensitivity should be similar in the two older groups.

Figure 3 illustrates the results of this study. Note that intermediate and high spatial frequency sensitivity is very similar in the old-normal and IOL groups. This implied to us at the time that the crystalline lens in older adults was not a major contributor to the contrast sensitivity loss of healthy older adults. These results are consistent with the Zuckerman et al. analysis (1973) that lens opacity must be fairly substantial (40% cataract) before image contrast is significantly reduced.

However, after further scrutinizing this study, we believe that there are two reasons why the use of an IOL control is not a straightforward method for "bypassing" the effects of the crystalline lens. First, cataract extraction and IOL implantation can lead to subtle retinal complications (e.g., retinal edema) that are not detected by standard clinical procedures. These changes could theoretically hurt contrast sensitivity, and could thus serve as a confounding factor. Second, the approach of using the IOL as a control for crystalline lens effects on contrast sensitivity makes the critical assumption that the MTF of the crystalline lens and the MTF of the IOL are highly similar, when they are not (Rosenblum & Block, unpublished data). Our own data in Figure 3 hint that the MTFs are different. Sensitivity at low spatial frequencies for the IOL group was significantly greater than in the old-normal group and the young group. This difference could not be attributed to optical magnification differences among the groups (see Owsley et al., 1985 more details). Therefore, owing to these considerations, we believe that the role of the crystalline lens cannot be adequately evaluated by IOL controls, and that the use of older subjects with IOLs does not actually permit one to bypass the optics of the eye when studying aging and visual function. Laser interferometric techniques are more appropriate for this purpose, which we will discuss later.

Another general technique for teasing apart the relative effects of optical and neural factors in older adults' deficits in contrast sensitivity is based on the use of psychophysical

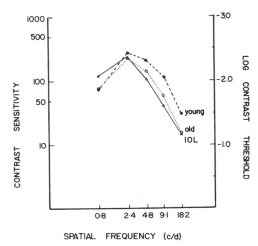

Fig. 3. Mean spatial contrast sensitivity at a photopic level for older adults with intact crystalline lenses, older adults with IOLs, and young adults with intact crystalline lenses. (From Owsley, Gardner, Sekuler, & Lieberman, 1985)

manipulations. Certain patterns of psychophysical data are best explained by models incorporating neural mechanisms (e.g., data generated by critical band masking), than by strictly optical explanations. These non-invasive techniques can also be useful in studying how the neural mechanisms which subserve spatial vision change during the aging process. For example, in a recent study (Sloane, Owsley, & Jackson, 1988), we were interested in how the function relating contrast sensitivity and background luminance could be used to determine whether optical factors (reduced retinal illuminance, increased intraocular light scatter) could alone account for older adults' loss in spatial contrast sensitivity. Figure 4 is a schematic diagram illustrating several hypotheses about the mechanism(s) underlying older adults' contrast sensitivity loss. Figure 4A illustrates how the function for contrast sensitivity versus luminance would differ for young and old adults if increased light absorption in the ocular media of the older eye were solely responsible for the sensitivity loss. In addition, Figure 4A is consistent with older adults' sensitivity loss being due to a decreased quantum-catching ability of photoreceptors, which could be the case given that there is evidence for age-related photoreceptor loss and disturbance of photoreceptor architecture (Marshall et al., 1980; Marshall & Laties, 1985; Smith et al., 1988; Curcio et al., 1990; Gao et al., 1990). Under either scenario, the function for older adults would be shifted rightward on the abscissa with no change in the slope.

Figure 4B illustrates how the sensitivity versus luminance function for young and old adults would appear if reduced retinal image contrast in the older eye were the sole cause of sensitivity loss in older adults. The function for the older adult would be displaced downward along the ordinate (contrast) axis, and there would be no slope change since the MTF of an optical system is invariant across changes in mean luminance.

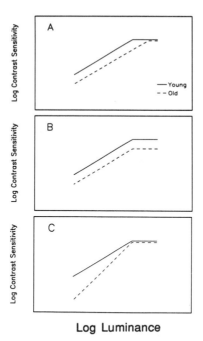

Fig. 4. Hypothetical functions illustrating how contrast sensitivity and luminance are related for younger and older adults: A, if increased light absorption in older eye were the sole cause of sensitivity loss in older adults (also if a decreased quantum-catching ability by older photoreceptors was sole cause); B, if reduced retinal contrast due to changes in the ocular media such as increased light scatter were the sole cause; C, if aging-related neural changes in the mechanisms underlying spatial vision were the sole cause. Spatial frequency distinctions are not incorporated. (From Sloane, Owsley, & Jackson, 1988)

A difference in slope between the functions for young and old adults would support the hypothesis that the decreased contrast sensitivity in older adults is at least partially due to an impairment in neural mechanisms subserving spatial vision. This possibility is illustrated in Figure 4C. Since retinal mechanisms are believed to control the change in sensitivity with decreasing light level (Barlow, 1972), this pattern of data would imply that changes in neural mechanisms during aging contribute to the impairment of spatial contrast sensitivity in the elderly. As discussed above, optical changes in the aged eye, such as reduced retinal illuminance and increased light scatter, would not predict a steeper slope in the sensitivity versus luminance function for older adults. Figure 5 shows the actual data from these measurements on a sample of young and old adults. Contrast thresholds were measured at two lower spatial frequencies, 0.5 and 2 c/d, so that we could measure thresholds at low light levels. The function for older adults had a steeper slope than that of young adults, and this trend was not only true for the group mean, but also for the slopes of the functions on individual subjects. These data do not rule out an optical contribution to older adults' loss in contrast sensitivity, but they do indicate that the neural mechanisms subserving spatial vision are at least partially involved in older adults' loss in spatial contrast sensitivity. The young-old difference is particularly obvious at the lowest light levels tested, suggesting that neural changes in the aged visual system may primarily hurt vision under dim illumination. We will return to this hypothesis later in this chapter.

Another technique for evaluating the relative contributions of optical and neural factors in older adults' contrast sensitivity loss is what we will term "optical simulations". The logic of this technique is to simulate in young adults the optical properties of some "typical" aged eye, through the use of specialized lenses, filters, or other optical manipulations (e.g., Owsley et al., 1983; Morrison & McGrath, 1985; Whitaker & Elliott, 1991). Spatial contrast sensitivity is then measured in these young adults, and if contrast sensitivity decreases toward the level exhibited by older adults, then it is concluded that optical factors must play some role in older adults' sensitivity deficit. If contrast sensitivity in young adults is unaffected by the optical simulation, then it is concluded that optical effects are not contributory to older adults' deficit. Although simulations can be instructive in developing preliminary hypotheses, there are a number of reasons why they cannot provide definitive answers about the relative contributions of optical vs. neural factors. First, the effect of optical simulation on young adults' contrast sensitivity, and the similarity between this simulation effect in young people and contrast sensitivity in older adults is basically a correlational relationship, and thus does not permit inferences about cause and effect. For example, while simulation studies on young adults imply that reduced illuminance due to increased lenticular density *could* underlie older adults' sensitivity loss, these experiments do not provide definitive answers but are often treated as if they do. Second, the simulations themselves assume that there is some typical aged eye, which has some highly representative set of optical properties applicable to all older adults. However, the optical characteristics (e.g., intraocular light scatter, pupillary diameter, lens density) of a sample of older eyes are quite variable, implying that a simulation approach based on an average optical model of the aged eye is overly simplistic. In addition, there is no reason to believe that the same mechanisms are responsible for spatial contrast sensitivity loss in all older adults.

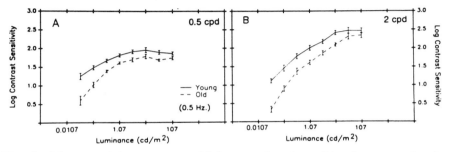

Fig. 5. Mean spatial contrast sensitivity as a function of luminance on log-log coordinates for young and older adults. Panel A, 0.5 c/d, Panel B 2 c/d. (From Sloane, Owsley, & Jackson, 1988)

A more direct method of examining the role of neural factors in older adults' spatial contrast sensitivity deficits is the use of laser interferometric techniques (e.g., Campbell & Green, 1965; Williams, 1985). Through these techniques, a grating produced by interference fringes is imaged on the retina such that it bypasses the optics of the eye. This enables the researcher to obtain a measure of "neural" contrast sensitivity which is uncontaminated by the quality of the eye's optics. Interferometic techniques may be especially useful in studying the aged visual system since they can parcel out the optical degradation characteristic of the aged eye. In addition, laser interferometry may prove useful in empirically validating Weale's theoretical argument (1975, 1982) that neural death and deterioration are the primary causes of acuity loss in old age.

Several earlier studies have used laser interferometry to examine the degree of neural contribution to older adults' spatial contrast sensitivity loss, but this research fails to present a cohesive answer to this question (e.g., Dressler & Rassow, 1981; Morrison & McGrath, 1985). Some of the disagreement among studies may be due to small samples and differences in inclusion criteria for subjects, but also may be attributable to the sheer difficulty in making threshold judgments in this task. Threshold measurements using laser interferometry are challenging for even the experienced psychophysical observer, let alone an older adult unaccustomed to the tedium and vigilance involved in a psychophysical task. In our own study using laser interferometry (Burton, Owsley, & Sloane, 1991), we took various steps to insure the reliability of our threshold estimates for young and old adults. All subjects received practice at four different spatial frequencies (spanning the range of test frequencies) before the actual threshold measurement runs were begun. Contrast threshold was measured using the method of constant stimuli with catch trials. In addition, half of our subjects returned to the lab for a second session, and given the difficulty of this task, test-retest reliability was reasonably good. Furthermore, we had two criteria for inclusion of a subject's data in the final analysis. First, the psychometric function which was fit to the data had to account for greater than 50% of the variance, and second, a subject's false alarm rate had to be less than 16%.

Figure 6 illustrates our interferometric contrast sensitivity data for samples of young and older adults. Older adults on average exhibited a small but statistically reliable loss in contrast sensitivity (about 0.2 log units) at all spatial frequencies tested. We did not measure contrast sensitivity in these same subjects using a "free-viewing" method with a conventional display. However, if we use the free-viewing sensitivity values from our earlier work (Owsley et al., 1983), we find that neural factors (as assessed by laser interferometry)

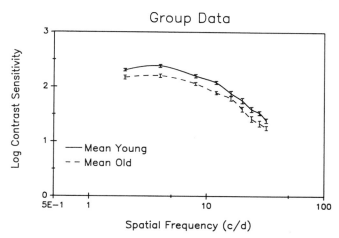

Fig. 6. Mean spatial contrast sensitivity at a photopic level for young and older adults as assessed by laser interferometry. (From Burton, Owsley, & Sloane, 1991)

account for most of the loss at intermediate spatial frequencies, but not quite half of the loss at higher spatial frequencies. Our data imply that there is a neural contribution to older adults' loss in spatial vision, but that optical factors also seem to be contributory, particularly at higher spatial frequencies. However, this issue is best addressed by performing both interferometric and "conventional display" contrast sensitivity measurements on the same subjects, a study currently underway in our laboratory.

Anatomical studies on the human visual system in later life are consistent with the notion that there could be some neural basis for the loss. There have been reports of aging-associated losses of photoreceptors (Marshall et al., 1980; Marshall & Laties, 1985; Yuodelis & Hendrickson, 1986; Marshall, 1987; Curcio et al., 1990; Gao et al., 1990), of ganglion cells (Balaszi et al., 1984; Drucker & Curcio, 1990), and of visual cortical neurons (Brody, 1955, 1973; Wisniewski & Terry, 1976; Strehler, 1976; Devaney & Johnson, 1980).

At present we cannot rule out another explanation of the age-associated loss in sensitivity. Williams (1985) has demonstrated that the use of purely coherent light in laser interferometry can lead to a spatial noise mask which can elevate contrast threshold. This mask is generated by the eye's own optics, and would be expected to be greater in the aged eye which has increased light scattering properties. Our laser interferometer is currently designed so that it uses only coherent light, and thus, we must consider the possibility that the contrast sensitivity loss in older adults depicted in Figure 6 may be generated by this spatial noise mask. Further work will investigate this competing explanation.

Another striking feature of our data is that while the older adults, as a group, average about a 0.2 log unit loss in sensitivity, there is actually considerable overlap between the performances of the young and old groups at all spatial frequencies tested. Figure 7 illustrates this overlap for two spatial frequencies. The contrast sensitivity values of many older adults fall within the range of values from young adults. As discussed earlier, it is important to consider this variability when characterizing aging trends.

To summarize, we have found that when assessed with laser interferometry older adults show a small loss in contrast sensitivity which averages about 0.2 log units, although it must also be pointed out that some older adults show no loss. This finding is in good agreement with five other interferometry studies using older subjects (Dressler & Rassow, 1981; Kayazawa et al., 1981; Elliott, 1987; Jankelovits et al., 1988; Sunness et al., 1991). This pattern of results differs from the interferometry studies of Nameda et al. (1989) and Morrison & McGrath (1985), which found substantial losses in spatial contrast sensitivity which increased in magnitude (up to about 1 log unit) with increasing spatial frequency. With

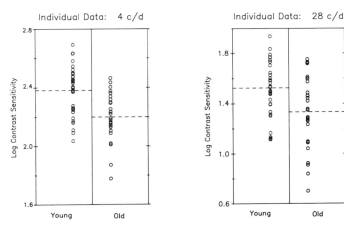

Fig. 7. Spatial contrast sensitivity measured by laser interferometry for individual young and old adults. On the left, data from 4 c/d; on the right, data from 28 c/d. Note overlap between age groups. (From Burton, Owsley, & Sloane, 1991)

respect to the Nameda et al. study (1989), it is not really surprising that they found a much larger loss in "neural" contrast sensitivity than in our work, since some of their older adults had acuity as low as 20/40. The Morrison & McGrath study (1985) is difficult to interpret for a number of reasons. For example, some of their contrast sensitivity values were exceedingly high (e.g., 10,000); older adults' loss in sensitivity was greatest at intermediate spatial frequencies, which does not agree with the vast majority of studies indicating maximal loss at higher frequencies; and they used pseudophakic subjects for some of their comparisons, which can be problematic as discussed earlier.

Although neural factors may account for only a small portion of the loss at photopic light levels (about 0.2 log units), there is reason to believe that older adults' vision problems under dim illumination may be largely due to neural deterioration in the aged visual system. First, older adults' loss in spatial vision is more pronounced at lower light levels than at photopic levels, as pointed out earlier (Sloane, Owsley, & Alvarez, 1988; Sloane, Owsley, & Jackson, 1988; Adams et al., 1988). These losses under dim illumination are not readily attributable to optical factors. Second, there is evidence that rod density decreases significantly in later life, whereas cone density does not (Curcio et al., 1990; Gao et al., 1990). Third, it is already known that temporal dark adaptation, primarily a retinally-mediated process (see Barlow, 1972), is affected by aging (McFarland et al., 1960; Sturr et al., 1991). Thus, there is indirect evidence that neural deterioration in the aging visual system may have its most deleterious effects on spatial vision at low luminance, a hypothesis which deserves further investigation.

UNDERSTANDING PROBLEMS IN EVERYDAY VISUAL TASKS

An ultimate goal of research on vision and aging is to understand why many older adults have difficulty performing routine visual activities, such as driving, wayfinding, and locating and recognizing objects in the environment. A surge of research during the past decade on visual sensory function in later adulthood has documented a vast array of visual deficits associated with aging (see Owsley & Sloane, 1990). However, there has been considerably less research on how these visual losses actually relate to performance difficulties by the elderly in everyday tasks which depend critically on vision. One area that has received some attention is to what extent contrast sensitivity in the elderly is predictive of their ability to perceive faces. We have shown that spatial contrast sensitivity is modestly associated with older adults' ability to identify faces, as assessed by the amount of contrast required to identify faces (Owsley & Sloane, 1987). Contrast sensitivity accounted for 18% of the variance in face identification, and 25% of the variance when the age of the perceiver was also considered. The inclusion of acuity as a predictor variable did not further improve the model. In a related study, Peli et al. (1989) found that face recognition could be improved for a significant number of patients through image contrast enhancement. More recently, Bullimore et al. (1991) reported a very strong relationship between contrast sensitivity and face recognition, accounting for 62% of the variance. The higher level of variance accounted for in this study may be attributable to their avoiding a restriction of range problem. Their sample had a much wider range of disease severity and functional ability (e.g., acuity) than in the Owsley and Sloane study (1987). Bullimore et al. pointed out that word-reading acuity was a stronger correlate than was contrast sensitivity, accounting for 92% of the variance in face recognition. The superiority of acuity as a predictor of face recognition problems in their study may be related to their use of a face recognition measure based on the distance required to successfully recognize a high-contrast face, rather than a contrast threshold measure for recognition as in the Owsley and Sloane study (1987). It could be that *suprathreshold* contrast tests are better predictors of face perception problems in real life, given that this perceptual activity is typically performed at relatively high contrast levels. This issue deserves further study. We may be overestimating older adults' deficits in contrast perception in everyday life by relying almost exclusively on tests of contrast *detection* abilities in the laboratory.

The face perception studies discussed above utilize outcome (dependent) measures that are analogs of real world tasks, but are not actual measures of face perception ability in a natural situation. In most of these studies, the face targets are constructed so that they embody strictly facial features, with distinctive personal characteristics removed such as hairstyle, hairline, spectacles, and moustaches/beards. On the one hand, it makes sense that these studies focus on the perception of the isolated facial features, since the emphasis is on what visual tests are best able to predict *face* perception problems per se. However, a major motivation for this research is to understand why individuals with vision loss report that they experience difficulty with face or person recognition in everyday situations. Under these circumstances, there are multiple sources of information about the face/person, such as information from other senses, as well as distinctive personal characteristics such as those mentioned above. Thus, it is important to recognize the limitations of the laboratory analog studies; while contrast sensitivity, acuity, or some other measure of visual sensory function, may be associated with a performance analog in the laboratory, the relationship between visual sensory function and the task in question may be quite different in a real-world situation where other sources of information are available (e.g., auditory cues, other visual cues) and where other characteristics of the observer are germane (e.g., cognitive abilities). Given the redundancy of information from multiple sensory systems, and the complexity of the recognition task from a psychological standpoint, an approach which studies visual sensory factors in isolation from other variables is necessarily limited if the ultimate goal is to identify why the elderly have problems in daily activities such as mobility and recognizing objects.

An alternative approach is to actually study natural outcome measures, i.e. performance in an everyday task. Of course there are many problems associated with defining and quantifying real-world behaviors, but this approach may be necessary for understanding older adults' problems in performing natural tasks. A case in point is driving a vehicle. An interesting question is whether visual dysfunction in older adults is associated with their driving problems. Older drivers in the U.S.A. have more accidents and traffic citations and incur more fatalities per miles driven than any other adult age group (NHTSA, 1989). Despite intuitions that older adults' impaired vision should be related to an increased risk for accidents, previous research has failed to establish a strong link between vision and driving in the elderly (Hills & Burg, 1977; Henderson & Burg, 1974; Shinar, 1977). There are a variety of reasons why the earlier work failed to demonstrate this link (Shinar & Schieber, 1991; Ball & Owsley, 1991). We believe that one crucial reason is that previous studies relied almost exclusively on visual sensory tests as the independent or predictor variables. Visual sensory tests, although quite appropriate for the clinical assessment of vision loss, do not by themselves reflect the visual complexity of an everyday visual task such as driving. The visual demands of functioning in a complex environment are quite intricate, involving a cluttered array, both primary and secondary visual tasks, and the simultaneous use of central and peripheral vision (Ball & Owsley, 1991). Contrast sensitivity tests, and other visual sensory tests, do not typically incorporate these features, but instead seek to minimize perceptual and cognitive influences. This approach is appropriate for the clinical management of eye disease, but can be inadequate by itself when applied to understanding visual performance in a complex task typical of everyday life. This is not to say that contrast sensitivity is not important in visual information processing. Rather, if we want to identify factors which predispose an older person to difficulties in visual tasks such as driving, contrast sensitivity and other tests of the visual sensory apparatus must be supplemented with additional assessments which evaluate the information processing system at higher levels.

We have adopted this general approach in our research program designed to determine the risk factors for vehicle accidents in older drivers. Thus in our efforts to develop a model to predict accident frequency in the elderly (Owsley et al., 1991), we have assessed the functional status of the visual information processing system at a number of different levels: health status of the visual system (e.g., presence of ocular disease); visual sensory function (e.g., contrast sensitivity, acuity, peripheral vision), visual attentional skills (a measure of early visual attention called the "useful field of view", see Ball et al., 1988); and mental status (cognitive skills such as memory, comprehension, orientation). We were particularly interested in evaluating visual attention, since earlier research indicated that some older adults have dramatic impairments in visual attentional abilities (Ball et al., 1990; Plude & Hoyer, 1988).

In addition to the battery of tests described above, on each of our 53 older drivers we obtained complete accident data from the State of Alabama for the previous five year period.

Since the goal of this study was to develop a predictive model of accident involvement based on measures from different levels of the visual information processing system, we utilized a regression analysis approach. Figure 8 illustrates the best-fitting model of the interrelationships among the variables, and how these variables related to accident frequency. Only statistically significant relationships are listed. If there is no arrow connecting two boxes, then there was no significant relationship between these two groups of variables (see Owsley et al., 1991 for details). To summarize this model, eye health and visual sensory function were unrelated to accident frequency. However, a measure of visual attention and mental status jointly accounted for 20% of the variance in accident frequency. A larger sample study from our lab, which avoided restriction of range problems, accounted for 27% of the accident variance (Ball et al., unpublished). This level of predictability is virtually unprecedented in previous research on older drivers which rarely accounted for more than 5% of the accident variance. Although eye health and visual sensory function such as contrast sensitivity abilities were not themselves directly related to accident frequency, they were related to visual attention. This was not really surprising, given that visual attention must depend to some extent on the integrity of visual signals entering the information processing system.

Our research on vision and driving identifies a potentially promising predictor of vehicle accidents in older drivers -- visual attention. Furthermore this line of research clearly illustrates that visual sensory function is an important ingredient in understanding performance limitation, but by itself it can be inadequate for understanding the problems older adults experience in everyday visual tasks, given the visual complexity of the environment, and multiplicity of problems intrinsic to the elderly individual. Our present perspective is that a complete model of why older adults face problems in everyday visual

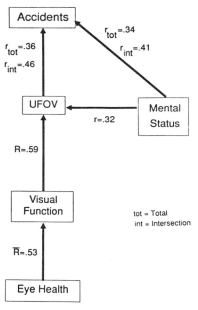

Fig. 8. Regression model illrustating significant predictors of accident frequency in our sample of older drivers. UFOV refers to a test of visual attention called the useful field of view. The numbers labelling each arrow refer to the strength of the relationship between different levels of the model. A model for predicting all types of vehicle accidents is represented by the subscript "tot"; a model for predicting intersection accidents only (a special problem for the elderly) is represented by the subscript "int". (From Owsley, Ball, Sloane, Roenker, & Bruni, 1991)

tasks must not only include visual sensory function such as contrast sensitivity, but must also incorporate higher-order properties of the information processing system such as visual attention.

SUMMARY

Older adults on average exhibit a deficit in spatial contrast sensitivity which increases in magnitude with increasing spatial frequency, and is more pronounced at lower light levels. This loss occurs even in older adults free from significant eye disease, suggesting that this decrease in sensitivity is part of what is typically referred to as the normal aging process of the human visual system. However, it must be emphasized that there is considerable variability in the extent of the deficit, with some older adults showing losses as large as 0.5 log units while others show no loss. This heterogeneity in the population calls into question the common practice of characterizing aging trends solely by group averages, and supports an alternative method of assessing aging trends in terms of a framework of "successful" vs. "unsuccessful" aging.

Research has clearly indicated that older adults' loss in spatial contrast sensitivity cannot be attributed to optical blur, pupillary miosis, or cognitive factors associated with decision-making in setting a sensory threshold. The specific roles of increased intraocular light scatter and reduced retinal illuminance in producing contrast sensitivity loss in older adults have not been clearly established, although it is reasonable to expect them to be contributory. However, studies using "indirect" psychophysical techniques suggest that aging-related changes in the neural mechanisms which subserve spatial vision contribute to older adults' loss in spatial vision. Studies using laser interferometry are consistent with this notion, implying that there is a small but reliable loss in "neural" contrast sensitivity at photopic levels in later life. Although neural factors may account for only a small portion of the loss at photopic light levels, a working hypothesis is that older adults' vision problems under dim illumination are largely neural in origin. In future work designed to examine the mechanisms underlying older adults' loss in spatial contrast sensitivity, it is important to consider that the same mechanisms may not be responsible for these deficits in all older adults, and that different mechanisms can contribute in varying degrees for different individuals. Another issue that deserves further investigation is the extent to which older adults' contrast sensitivity deficits extend to suprathreshold contrast levels.

In efforts to understand older adults' problems in performing everyday tasks which depend critically on vision, the best models are likely to be those which supplement tests of visual sensory function such as contrast sensitivity with tests evaluating higher-order properties of the visual information processing system, such as visual attention and cognitive abilities. This approach has proven fruitful in identifying predictors of driving problems in the elderly, and may also be useful in identifying risk factors for older adults' problems in other visually-guided tasks such ambulation, wayfinding, and object recognition.

ACKNOWLEDGEMENTS

Research in our laboratory is supported through NIH grants AG04212, EY06390, and EY03039, the AARP Andrus Foundation, the Rich Retinal Research Foundation, Helen Keller Eye Research Foundation, and a Department Development grant from Research to Prevent Blindness to the UAB Department of Ophthalmology. We thank Michael Sloane, Karlene Ball, and Christine Curcio for helpful comments on an earlier version of this paper.

REFERENCES

Adams A.J., Wang L.S., Wong L., and Gould B. (1988) Visual acuity changes with age: Some new perspectives. *American Journal of Optometry and Physiological Optics* **65**, 403-406.

Allen M. and Vos J.J. (1967) Ocular scattered light and visual performance as a function of age. *American Journal of Optometry and Physiological Optics* **44**, 717-727.

Arden G.B. (1978) The importance of measuring contrast sensitivity in cases of visual disturbance. *British Journal of Ophthalmology* **62**, 198-209.

Arden G.B. and Jacobsen J. (1978) A simple grating test for contrast sensitivity: Preliminary results indicate value for screening in glaucoma. *Investigative Ophthalmology & Visual Science* **17**, 23-32.

Arundale K. (1978) An investigation into the variation of human contrast sensitivity with age and ocular pathology. *British Journal of Ophthalmology* **62**, 213-215.

Balaszi A.G., Rootmen J., Drance S.M., Schulzer M., and Douglas G.R. (1984) The effect of age on the nerve fiber population of the human optic nerve. *American Journal of Ophthalmology* **97**, 760-766.

Ball K., Beard B.L., Roenker D.L., Miller R.L., and Griggs D.S. (1988) Age and visual search: Expanding the useful field of view. *Journal of the Optical Society of America A* **5**, 2210-2219.

Ball K. and Owsley C. (1991) Identifying correlates of accident involvement for the older driver. *Human Factors* (to appear in October 1991 issue).

Ball K., Owsley C., Sloane M.E., Roenker D.L., and Bruni J.R. (unpublished manuscript) Visual attention problems as a predictor of vehicle accidents among older drivers.

Ball K., Phillips G., and Sekuler R. (1986) Improved spatial frequency discrimination related to acuity and age. *Investigative Ophthalmology & Visual Science (Supplement)* **27**, 111.

Ball K., Roenker D.L., and Bruni J.R. (1990) Developmental changes in attention and visual search throughout adulthood. In J. Enns (Ed.) *Advances in Psychology* **69**, 489-508.

Banks M.S. (1982) The development of spatial and temporal contrast sensitivity. *Current Eye Research* **2**, 191-198.

Barlow H.B. (1972) Dark and light adaptation: Psychophysics. In D. Jameson and L.M. Hurvich (Eds.) *Handbook of Sensory Physiology Vol. VII/4, Visual Psychophysics*, pp. 1-55. New York: Springer-Verlag.

Bobak P., Bodis-Wollner, I., Harnois C., and Thorton J. (1984) VEP's in humans reveal high and low spatial contrast mechanisms. *Investigative Ophthalmology & Visual Science* **25**, 980-983.

Bodis-Wollner I. and Camisa J.M. (1980) Contrast sensitivity measurement in clinical diagnosis. In S. Lessell and J.T.W. van Dalen (Eds.) *Neuro-ophthalmology*, pp. 373-401. Amsterdam: Excerpta Medica.

Bowker D.O. (1983) Suprathreshold spatio-temporal response characteristics of the human visual system. *Journal of the Optical Society of America A* **73**, 436-441.

Brody H. (1955) Organization of the cerebral cortex. III. A study of aging in the human cerebral cortex. *Journal of Comparative Neurology* **102**, 511-566.

Brody H. (1973) Aging of the vertebrate brain. In M. Rockstein and M.L. Sussman (Eds.) *Development of Aging in the Nervous System*, pp. 121-133. New York: Academic Press.

Bullimore M.A., Bailey I.L., and Wacker R.T. (1991) Face recognition in age-related maculopathy. *Investigative Ophthalmology & Visual Science* **32**, 2020-2029.

Burton K.B., Owsley C., and Sloane M.E. (1991) Aging and "neural" spatial contrast sensitivity. *Investigative Ophthalmology & Visual Science (Supplement)* **32**, 1274.

Campbell F.W. and Green D.G. (1965) Optical and retinal factors affecting visual resolution. *Journal of Physiology (London)* **181**, 576-593.

Curcio C.A., Allen K.A., and Kalina R.E. (1990) Reorganization of the human photoreceptor mosaic following age-related rod loss. *Investigative Ophthalmology & Visual Science (Supplement)* **31**, 38.

Derefeldt G., Lennerstrand G., and Lundh B. (1979) Age variations in normal human contrast sensitivity. *Acta Ophthalmologica* **57**, 679-690.

De Valois R.L., Morgan H., and Snodderley D.M. (1974) Psychophysical studies of monkey vision III. Spatial luminance contrast sensitivity tests of macaque and human observers. *Vision Research* **14**, 75-81.

Devaney K.O. and Johnson H.A. (1980) Neuron loss in the aging visual cortex of man. *Journal of Gerontology* **35**, 836-841.

Dressler M. and Rassow B. (1981) Neural contrast sensitivity measurements with a laser interference system for clinical and screening application. *Investigative Ophthalmology & Visual Science* **21**, 737-744.

Drucker D.N. and Curcio C.A. (1990) Retinal ganglion cells are lost with aging but not in Alzheimer's disease. *Investigative Ophthalmology & Visual Science (Supplement)* **31**, 356.

Early F. and Smith A.T. (1990) Spatial frequency discrimination in normal ageing and in one case of Alzheimer's disease. *Clinical Vision Sciences* **6**, 59-64.

Elliott D.B. (1987) Contrast sensitivity decline with ageing: A neural or optical phenomenon? *Ophthalmic & Physiological Optics* **7**, 415-419.

Elliott D.B., Whitaker D., and MacVeigh D. (1990) Neural contribution to spatiotemporal contrast sensitivity decline in healthy eyes. *Vision Research* **30**, 541-547.

Gao H., Rayborn M.E., Myers K.M., and Hollyfield J.G. (1990) Differential loss of neurons during aging of human retina. *Investigative Ophthalmology & Visual Science (Supplement)* **31**, 357.

Georgeson M.A. and Sullivan G.D. (1975) Contrast constancy: deblurring in human vision by spatial frequency channels. *Journal of Physiology (London)* **252**, 627-656.

Henderson R. and Burg A. (1974) *Vision and audition in driving* (Tech. Rep. No. TM[L]-5297/000/00). Washington, D.C.: U.S. Department of Transportation.

Higgins K.E, Jaffe M.J., Caruso R.C., and deMonasterio F.M. (1988) Spatial contrast sensitivity: Effects of age, test-retest, and psychophysical method. *Journal of the Optical Society of America A* **5**, 2173-2180.

Hills B.L. and Burg A. (1977) *A re-analysis of California driver vision data: General findings* (Report 768). Crowthorne, England: Transport and Road Research Laboratory.

Ijspeert J.K., de Waard, P.W.T., van den Berg, T.J.T.P., and de Jong, P.T.V.M.(1990) The intraocular straylight function in 129 healthy volunteers; dependence on angle, age and pigmentation. *Vision Research* **30**, 699-707.

Jankelovits E.R., Lichtenstein S.J., Groll, S.L., Remijan P.W., and Hirsch, J. (1988) Assessment of retinal function in cataract patients by a combination of laser interferometry and conventional display methods to measure contrast sensitivity. *Applied Optics* **27**, 1057-1063.

Jay J.L., Mammo R.B., and Allan D. (1987) Effect of age on visual acuity after cataract extraction. *British Journal of Ophthalmology* **71**, 112-115.

Johnson M.A. and Choy D. (1987) On the definition of age-related norms for visual function testing. *Applied Optics* **26**, 1449-1454.

Kayazawa K., Yamamoto T., and Itoi M. (1981) Clinical measurement of contrast sensitivity function using laser generated sinusoidal grating. *Japanese Journal of Ophthalmology* **25**, 229-236.

Kline D.W. and Schieber F. (1985) Vision and aging. In J.E. Birren and K.W. Schaie (Eds.) *Handbook of the Psychology of Aging*, Ch. 12, pp. 296-331. New York: Van Nostrand Reinhold.

Kline D.W., Schieber, F., Abusamra L.C., and Coyne A.C. (1983) Age, the eye, and visual channels: Contrast sensitivity and response speed. *Journal of Gerontology* **38**, 211-216.

Kosnik W., Winslow L., Kline D., Rasinski K., and Sekuler R. (1988) Vision changes in daily life throughout adulthood. *Journal of Gerontology* **43**, 63-70.

Leibowitz H.M., Krueger D.E., Maunder L.R., Milton R.C., Kini M.M., Kahn H.A., Nickerson R.J., Pool J., Colton T.L., Ganley J.P., Loewenstein J.I., and Dawber T.R. (1980) The Framingham eye study monograph. *Survey of Ophthalmology (Supplement)* **24**, 335-610.

Ludwig F.C. and Smoke M.E. (1980) The measurement of biological aging. *Experimental Aging Research* **6**, 497-521.

Marshall, J. (1987) The ageing retina: physiology or pathology. *Eye* **1**, 282-295.

Marshall, J., Grindle J., Ansell P.L., and Borwein B. (1980) Convolution in human rods: an aging process. *British Journal of Ophthalmology* **63**, 181-187.

Marshall J. and Laties A. The special pathology of the aging macula. In M.M. La Vail, J.G. Hollyfield, and R.E. Anderson (Eds.) *Retinal Degeneration: Experimental and Clinical Studies.* New York: Liss.

McFarland R.A., Domey R.G., Warren A.B., and Ward D.C. (1960) Dark adaptation as a function of age: I. A statistical analysis. *Journal of Gerontology* **15**, 149-154.

McGrath C. and Morrison J.D. (1981) The effects of age on spatial frequency perception in human subjects. *Quarterly Journal of Experimental Physiology* **66**, 253-261.

Morrison J.D. and McGrath C. (1985) Assessment of the optical contributions to the age-related deterioration in vision. *Quarterly Journal of Experimental Physiology* **70**, 249-269.

Morrison J.D. and Reilly J. (1986) An assessment of decision-making as a possible factor in the the age-related loss of contrast sensitivity. *Perception* **15**, 541-552.

Nameda N., Kawara T., and Ohzu H. (1989) Human visual spatio-temporal frequency performance as a function of age. *Optometry and Vision Science* **66**, 760-765.

National Highway Traffic Safety Administration (1989) *Conference on Research and Development Needed to Improve Safety and Mobility of Older Drivers.* (Report Number DOT HS 807 554). Washington, D.C.: U.S. Department of Transportation.

Owsley C., Ball K., Sloane M.E., Roenker D.L., and Bruni J.R. (1991) Visual/cognitive correlates of vehicle accidents in older drivers. *Psychology and Aging* (to appear in September 1991 issue).

Owsley C., Gardner T, Sekuler R., and Lieberman H. (1985) Role of the crystalline lens in the spatial vision loss of the elderly. *Investigative Ophthalmology & Visual Science* **26**, 1165-1170.

Owsley C., Kline D, Werner J., Greenstein V., and Marshall J. (1986) Optical radiation effects on aging and visual perception. In M. Waxler, V. Hitchens (Eds.) *Optical Radiation and Visual Health*, pp. 125-136. Boca Raton FL: CRC Press.

Owsley C., Sekuler R, and Boldt C. (1981) Aging and low contrast vision: Face perception. *Investigative Ophthalmology & Visual Science* **21**, 362-365.

Owsley C., Sekuler R., and Siemsen D. (1983) Contrast sensitivity throughout adulthood. *Vision Research* **23**, 689-699.

Owsley C. and Sloane M.E. (1987) Contrast sensitivity and the perception of "real-world" targets. *British Journal of Ophthalmology* **71**, 791-796.

Owsley C. and Sloane M.E. (1990) Vision and aging. In F. Boller and J. Grafman (Eds.) *Handbook of Neuropsychology*, Vol. 4, pp. 229-249. The Netherlands: Elsevier.

Peli, E., Goldstein R.B., Trempe C.C. and Arend L.E. (1989) Image enhancement improves face recognition. In *Noninvasive Assessment of the Visual System, 1989 Technical Digest Series*, Vol. 7, pp. 64-67. Washington, D.C.: Optical Society of America.

Plude D. and Hoyer W. (1988) Attention and performance: Identifying and localizing age deficits. In N. Charness (Ed.) *Aging and Human Performance*, pp. 47-99. New York: Wiley.

Porciatti V., Fiorentini A., Morrone M.C., and Burr D. (1991) The effects of ageing on the pattern electroretinogram and visual evoked potential in humans. *Investigative Ophthamology & Visual Science (Supplement)* **32**, 910.

Porciatti V., Burr D.C., Fiorentini A., and Morrone C. (this volume) Spatio-temporal properties of the pattern ERG and VEP in the aged. In P. Bagnoli and W. Hodos (Eds.) *The Changing Visual System: Maturation and Aging in the Central Nervous System*, London: Plenum.

Rosenblum W.F. and Block M. (1991) Comparisons of the modulation transfer function in intraocular lenses and human crystalline lenses. Unpublished data.

Rowe J.W. and Kahn R.L. (1987) Human aging: usual and successful. *Science* **237**, 143-149.

Said F.S. and Weale R.A. (1959) The variation with age of the spectral tranmissivity of the living human crystalline lens. *Gerontologia* **3**, 213-231.

Sekuler R., Hutman L.P., and Owsley C. (1982) Human aging and spatial vision. *Science* **209**, 1255-1256.

Sekuler R., Kline D., and Dismukes K. (1980) *Aging and Human Visual Function.* New York: Liss.

Shinar D. (1977) *Driver visual limitations. Diagnosis and treatment* (Contract DOT-HS-5-1275). Washington, D.C.: U.S. Department of Transportation.

Shinar D. and Schieber F. (1991) Visual requirements for safety and mobility of older drivers. *Human Factors* (to appear in October 1991 issue).

Skalka H. W. (1980) Effect of age on Arden grating acuity. *British Journal of Ophthalmology* **64**, 21-23.

Sloane M.E., Owsley C., and Alvarez S.L. (1988) Aging, senile miosis and spatial contrast sensitivity at low luminance. *Vision Research* **28**, 1235-1246.

Sloane M.E., Owsley C., and Jackson C.A. (1988) Aging and luminance-adaptation effects on spatial contrast sensitivity. *Journal of the Optical Society of America A* **5**, 2181-2190.

Smith V.C., Pokorny J., and Diddie K.R. (1988) Color matching and the Stiles-Crawford effect in observers with early age-related macular changes. *Journal of the Optical Society of America A* **5**, 2113-2121.

Sokol S., Moskowitz A., and Towle V.L. (1981) Age related changes in the latency of the visual evoked potential: influence of check size. *Electroencephalography and Clinical Neurophysiology* **51**, 559-562.

Strehler B.L. (1976) Aging and the human brain. In R.D. Terry and S. Gershon (Eds.) *Neurobiology of Aging*, pp. 1 -22. New York: Raven Press.

Sturr J.F. and Taub H.A. (unpublished manuscript) Contrast threshold measures in the elderly: Methodological issues.

Sturr J.F., Taub H.A., and Hall B.A. (1991) Foveal early dark adaptation in young and older observers in good ocular health. *Clinical Vision Sciences* **6**, 257-260.

Sunness J.S., Rubin G.S., and Massof R.W. (1991) Conventional contrast sensitivity and laser interferometry in eyes with drusen. *Investigative Ophthalmology & Visual Science (Supplement)* **32**, 690.

Tulunay-Keesey U., Ver Hoeve J.N., and Terkla-McGrane C. (1988) Threshold and suprathreshold spatiotemporal response throughout adulthood. *Journal of the Optical Society of America A* **5**, 2191-2200.

Van Nes F.L. and Bouman M.A. (1967) Spatial modulation transfer in the human eye. *Journal of the Optical Society of America* **57**, 401-406.

Weale R.A. (1963) *The Aging Eye*. London: HK Lewis.

Weale R.A. (1975) Senile changes in visual acuity. *Transactions of the Ophthalmological Society, U.K.* **95**, 36-38.

Weale R.A. (1982) *A Biography of the Eye*. London: H.K. Lewis.

Weale R.A. (1982) Senile ocular changes, cell death, and vision. In R. Sekuler, D. Kline, and K. Dismukes (Eds.) *Aging and Human Visual Function*, pp. 161-171. New York: Liss.

Weale R.A. (this volume) Modern theories of aging and their application to ocular senescence. In P. Bagnoli and W. Hodos (Eds.) *The Changing Visual System: Maturation and Aging in the Central Nervous System*. London: Plenum.

Werner J.S., Peterzell D., and Scheetz, A.J. (1990) Light, vision, and aging. *Optometry and Vision Science* **67**, 214-229.

Whitaker D. and Elliott D.B. (1991) The effect of simulating optical changes associated with ocular ageing. *Investigative Ophthalmology & Visual Science (Supplement)* **32**, 1275.

Williams D.R. (1985) Visibility of interference fringes near the resolution limit. *Journal of the Optical Society of America A* **2**, 1087-1093.

Wisniewski H.M. and Terry R.D. (1976) Neuropathology of aging brain. In R.D. Terry and S. Gershon (Eds.) *Neurobiology of Aging*, pp. 265-280. New York: Raven Press.

Wright C.E. and Drasdo N. (1985) The influence of age on the spatial and temporal contrast sensitivity function. *Documenta Ophthalmologica* **59**, 385-395.

Wright C.E., Williams D.E., Drasdo N., and Harding G.F.A.(1985) The influence of age on the electroretinogram and the visual evoked potential. *Documenta Ophthalmologica* **59**, 365-384.

Yuodelis C. and Hendrickson A. (1986) A qualitative and quantitative analysis of the human fovea during development. *Vision Research* **26**, 847-855.

Zuckerman J.L., Miller D., Dyes W., and Keller M. (1973) Degradation of vision through a simulated cataract. *Investigative Ophthalmology & Visual Science* **12**, 213-224.

LIFE-SPAN CHANGES IN THE VISUAL ACUITY AND RETINA IN BIRDS

W. Hodos and R. F. Miller

Dept. of Psychology, Univ. of Maryland
College Park, MD 20742-4411 USA

K. V. Fite

Dept. of Psychology, Univ. of Massachusetts
Amherst, MA 01003, USA

V. Porciatti

Istituto di Neurofisiologia del CNR
Via S. Zeno 51, 56127 Pisa, Italy

A. L. Holden, J.-Y. Lee and M. B. A. Djamgoz

Dept. of Biology, Imperial College
London, SW7 2BB, UK

Birds offer a number of important advantages for the study of life-span development of the visual system. Their vision is excellent (Hodos, et al., 1985; Wright, 1972; Blough, 1956) and their life span often is considerably shorter than that of humans (Altman and Ditman, 1974). They also are relatively inexpensive to obtain and maintain, especially domesticated species such as pigeons, canaries, chickens, budgerigars and quail from which individuals at nearly all stages of the life span can frequently be obtained. In the article that follows we shall describe a series of anatomical, behavioral and electrophysiological studies we have carried out on pigeons (*Columba livia*) and Japanese quail (*Coturnix coturnix japonica*). The behavioral studies consisted of the measurement of visual acuity with operant-conditioning techniques as a function of age. The electrophysiological studies evaluated the retina's contribution to life-span changes in acuity by means of the flash electroretinogram and the pattern electroretinogram. The anatomical studies investigated life-span changes in cellular components of the retina in birds of known visual acuity.

The Changing Visual System, Edited by P. Bagnoli and
W. Hodos, Plenum Press, New York, 1991

VISUAL ACUITY IN PIGEONS

Behavioral Acuity

Pigeons were trained to peck the center key of a conventional three-key pigeon operant-conditioning chamber that had been modified by the addition of a motorized filter wheel behind the center key (Hodos, et al. 1976; 1985; 1991). The wheel contained a series of square-wave optical gratings, each of which was matched to a glass, neutral-density filter to within 0.01 log unit of luminous transmission. The gratings ranged in spatial frequency from 1-20 lines/mm. The gratings were viewed directly through the center key, which had been fabricated from optically neutral glass, against a uniformly illuminated screen.

The psychophysical procedure was a variation of the method of constant stimuli in which the pigeon was required to discriminate the presence of a grating from its matched neutral-density filter. After a series of pecks on the center key to maximize the likelihood that the bird was paying attention to the target, the pigeon was then required to make a single peck on one of the two side keys. One key was "correct" if the grating had been present and the other was "correct" if the blank had been present. Correct responses were rewarded with grain; incorrect response were mildly punished by a short delay in the progress of the experiment and an obligatory repetition of the trial. Such correction repetitions were not included in the calculation of the bird's percentage of correct responses to each grating frequency.

At the end of each testing session, the data were plotted to form a psychometric function of the percentage of correct responses at each grating frequency. The bird's visual acuity was taken to be that spatial frequency at which the psychometric function had a value of 75% correct, which is the midpoint between chance performance and perfect detection of the grating. Testing was continued until the pigeons performance satisfied a criterion of stability. The birds were periodically videotaped as they performed in the chamber from which the distance from the eye to the target could be determined, This permitted us to convert acuity in lines/mm to acuity in degrees of visual angle subtended by the least resolvable bar or cycles per degree, which is the number of just detectable lines and adjacent spaces per degree of visual angle.

Data were collected from 20 pigeons that ranged in age from 2-16 years. Two-year-old pigeons are regarded by breeders as prime breeding stock. Pigeons generally are culled from commercial breeding stock at 5-7 years because of a decline in reproductive efficiency. Sixteen-year-old pigeons show signs of aging such as dullness of the scales of the feet and occasional stiffness of leg joints. An important feature of this research project was that the breeder (Palmetto Pigeon Plant, Sumter, SC, USA) attaches a leg ring to all of its breeding pigeons that identifies the bird with a unique number and gives the year of its birth.

The results of this study are shown in Figure 1, which indicates a progressive decline in acuity from an average of 15 cycles/degree (18-19 cycles/degree in the best of the young old birds) to approximately 3 cycles/degree in the oldest birds. The acuity of the youngest pigeons is not far from the normal acuity of untrained human observers (30 cycles/degree). But a human with a visual acuity of 3 cycles/degree would be able to resolve only the largest letter on the Snellen eye chart and would be eligible for social-security benefits in many countries. As a further indication of their visual impairment, when offered grains of various sizes scattered across the floor, the oldest pigeons tend to select only the larger grains whereas the younger ones tend to select the closer grains irrespective of size. We have concluded that the deficit is not cognitive because the pigeons show little change in the detection of coarse gratings. Moreover the deficit may be specific for spatial vision, because the birds are virtually unimpaired on a luminance-difference task that uses the identical procedure as the acuity task except that the stimulus is a uniformly illuminated field (Kurkjian and Hodos, 1990).

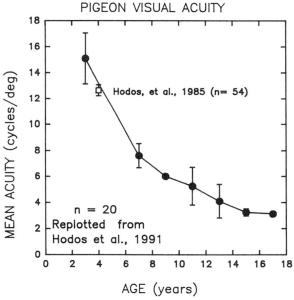

Fig. 1. *Mean visual acuity of 20 pigeons as a function of age collected in a cross-sectional design. The open square represents normative data from 54 pigeons aged 3-5 years (Hodos et al.,1985). Error bars indicate standard errors of the mean.*

A possible confounding factor in age-dependent losses in visual acuity could be senile miosis; i.e., the decrease in maximal pupil diameter with increasing age. A smaller pupil would admit less light to the retina with a consequent loss of visual acuity. Our measurements of the pigeon pupil as a function of age indicated a 37% reduction in retinal illumination equivalent to 0.2 log unit (Hodos, et al, 1991). This reduction in the luminosity of the retinal image, however, should reduce acuity only by about 0.6 cycles/degree (Hodos, et al., 1986). Moreover, a modest optical benefit of a decreased pupillary diameter is an increased depth of focus that occurred as a function of age. Other factors that were ruled out as contributing to the deficit were presbyopia (age-dependent loss of accommodation), refractive errors and increased density of the crystalline lens or cornea.

Morphological Changes

A factor that did change with age in the Hodos et al. (1991) study was retinal morphology. Both total photoreceptor nuclei and numbers of ganglion cells showed an approximately 1/3 reduction in their numbers between the youngest and the oldest pigeons. When the cones were studied in detail according to type, we observed that only those cones that contained a colorless or yellow oil droplet (Bowmaker, 1977; Mariani and Leure-Duprée, 1978) were reduced in number. The numbers of other cone types, which contained red or orange droplets, did not show an age-related decline.

Electroretinography

In order to determine the extent to which the retina is involved in age-dependent visual-acuity loss in pigeons, we recorded both the flash electroretinogram (FERG) and the pattern electroretinogram (PERG) in two groups of pigeons, two years old and ten years old (Porciatti et al., 1991). Both of these techniques have been extensively used for evaluating retinal pathology (Armington, 1974), for the functions of various retinal layers (Holden and Vaegan, 1983a), changes in these functions with age (Bagolini, et al., 1988) and early development (Bagnoli, et al., 1985; Porciatti, et al., 1988). The ERG was recorded from a small, stainless-steel electrode inserted into the conjunctiva.

Flash Electroretinogram. For the FERG , the pigeon's head was placed inside of a Ganzfeld bowl and a series of light flashes were delivered with a strobe lamp at various intensities. The intensity of the flash was controlled by neutral density filters. The amplitude of the a-wave as a function of intensity rose more steeply in the young birds than in the old. Moreover, the a-wave function of the young birds saturated at the highest intensities whereas that of the old birds did not. The amplitude-intensity function of the b-wave saturated at the highest intensities for both age groups, but the saturation amplitude was higher for the young pigeons than for the old. The b-wave data were subjected to a Naka-Rushton analysis (Naka and Rushton, 1966), which suggested a general reduction in retinal gain probably due to a dysfunction or reduction in the number of b-wave generators, but no difference in retinal sensitivity or preretinal light absorption. The FERG results led to the conclusion that increased age resulted in changes both in the outer retina (a-wave) and middle retina (b-wave).

Pattern Electroretinogram. The stimuli for the PERG were high-contrast, phase-reversing, square-wave gratings presented at various spatial frequencies. The PERG is generated whenever a local luminance change occurs in the photoreceptor plane of the retina (Holden and Vaegan, 1983b). Such a luminance change occurs when the dark bar of the grating is exchanged with a light bar during phase reversal. A PERG is generated at each transition from dark to light bars. Because the amplitude of the

PERG diminishes as the spatial frequency increases, that spatial frequency at which the amplitude-frequency function reaches zero indicates the limits of the retina to resolve the bars; i.e., it's visual acuity. Porciatti et al. level of physiological noise may be taken as an indicator of the ability of (1991) reported that the PERG acuity of the two-year-old pigeons was 20 cycles/degree, but only 7.8 cycles/degree for the ten-year-old birds. Moreover, we were able to rule out optical blur as a possible cause of the acuity loss. Since optical blur removes the high-frequency components of a stimulus, an effect due solely to optical blur would have produced spatial-frequency tuning curves that were the same at the low-frequency end but that differed at the high-frequency end. The old pigeons that we studied differed equally at both low and high spatial frequencies, which is indicative of a deficiency of the inner retina in the processing of frequency information.

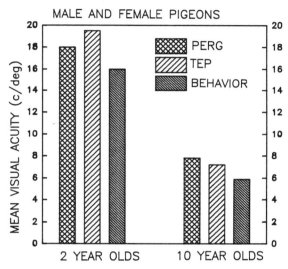

Fig. 2. Mean visual acuity young and old pigeons determined from pattern electroretinograms (PERG), tectal evoked potentials (TEP) and behavioral psychophysics. The behavioral data are from Hodos, et al., 1991 and the PERG and TEP data are from Porciatti et al., 1991.

Tectal Evoked Potentials. In order to determine whether these age-dependent differences in retinal responsiveness were being passed on to the brain, we recorded evoked potentials from the optic tectum (TEP) to the same grating frequencies as had been used for the PERG (Porciatti et al., 1991). These TEPs, like the PERGs, had a roughly sinusoidal wave form with a period equal to the reversal rate of the gratings. The visual acuity estimated by the TEP was approximately the same as that for the PERG. Figure 2 presents a comparison of the three acuity-assessment methods: PERG, TEP and behavioral psychophysics for the two age groups of pigeons. The data for the three techniques are consistent within each age group.

VISUAL ACUITY IN QUAIL

Behavioral Acuity

The data described above for pigeons were collected on unsexed animals. Since pigeons have no obvious sexual dimorphism, their sex could be determined with confidence only by post-mortem examination (or if an isolated bird laid an egg). This option often was not available because birds of specific ages that were borrowed from other experiments and other laboratories to have their vision tested were returned safely home. In contrast, Japanese quail are sexually dimorphic and indeed the females are reported to live for considerably shorter periods than the males if they are maintained on long days (12 hours or more of illumination) under which conditions they are continuously ovulating (Woodard and Abplanalp, 1971). In contrast to pigeons, quail, which are sexually mature one month after hatching, generally are retired from breeding and egg production after only 12-15 months under conditions of continuous long-day illumination.

Our initial attempts to measure visual acuity in female quail were with long-day birds. We decided to take advantage of their short life span and to test their acuity in a longitudinal design in which the same bird is periodically tested over a long period of time. Our efforts were frustrated by the high frequency of death after one year of age in these birds. We therefore changed our subject population to short-day (10 hours of illumination) quail and were able to continuously test three females until age 39 months at which time the birds were sacrificed to examine their retinas for signs of pathology, although they were still quite healthy and showed only early

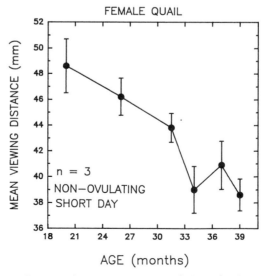

Fig. 3. Mean viewing distance (cornea to target) of three freely moving female quail during a visual acuity task. Error bars indicate standard errors of the mean.

signs of somatic aging. The apparatus and procedure were identical to those used to measure the pigeons' visual acuity described above with the addition of a small platform so that the quail, which are much smaller birds than pigeons, could reach the pecking keys and see the stimuli. The results of this study were consistent with our cross-sectional study of pigeon acuity; i.e., the acuity of the female quail showed a decline from 6.8 cycles/degree to 4.2 cycles/degree (see Fig. 5, bottom). An important difference, however, was that unlike the pigeons, the quail showed an initial increase in acuity from about 5 cycles/degree at 16-18 months to the peak at 6.8 cycles per degree at 22-24 months. A similar increase in visual acuity in the early phases of the human life span has been described by Weale (1982; see also Fig. 3 in the chapter by Hodos, this volume) and by Pitts (1982). These increases in acuity are not likely to be due to learning because of the long time course. Moreover, our finding of a similar initial increase in acuity at the level of the retina, as measured by the PERG (described below), would seem to argue against an explanation based on learning in the conventional sense, unless one were able to document that the retina alone is capable of learning.

Whether the absence of an initial increase in acuity in pigeons reflects a fundamental difference in the life-span development of visual acuity in pigeons and quail or is the result of our failure to study pigeons younger than two years is an open question. Our suspicion is that studies of the acuity of pigeons less than two years old will reveal a similar rise in spatial resolution to a peak as seen in humans and in quail.

A possible morphological basis for this peak in acuity may be found in the data of Rakic and coworkers (Rakic, this volume; Rakic, et al., 1986) who reported peaks in synaptic density in various cortical regions, including primary visual cortex, in monkeys at approximately 2-4 months after birth. Thereafter, synaptic density shows a progressive decline throughout the life span.

A possible histochemical correlate of the life-span fluctuations in visual acuity may be dopamine, which has been shown to influence the lateral spread of electrical activity within the retina (Djamgoz and Wagner, in press). For example, Harnois and Di Paolo (1990) have described decreased dopamine levels in the retinas of patients with Parkinson's disease. Moreover, Domenici et al. (1985) have reported that contrast sensitivity can be improved in human volunteers by the administration of L-dopa, a drug that increases dopamine levels.

Another difference between the pigeons and the quail emerged from an examination of the data on the distances from which the birds viewed the grating targets. The quail, like the pigeons, were videotaped periodically during their testing sessions so that we could measure their viewing distance in order to calculate the number of bars per degree of visual angle contained within the images of the gratings on the retina. The mean progressive changes in the viewing distance of three short-day, female quail are shown in Figure 3. Unlike the pigeons, which showed an increase in viewing distance with age that is indicative of a slight presbyopia, the quail decreased their viewing distance, which would suggest a progressively increasing myopia (near-sightedness). Since the quail tended to view the target with their lower visual fields, this decreased viewing distance may be indicative of an increase in the lower-field myopia phenomenon described by Fitzke et al.,(1985) and Hodos and Erichsen (1990) and may not signify an increase in myopia in the frontal or lateral visual fields.

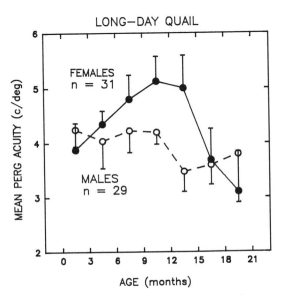

Fig. 4. Visual acuity measurements derived from the pattern electroretinogram (PERG) for male and female quail as a function of age. The birds were maintained on long days and were sexually active. Error bars indicate standard errors of the mean.

Pattern Electroretinogram

The PERG acuity of long-day quail, both males and females, was measured using methods similar to those used by Porciatti et al. (1991). Since the females were being maintained on long days, they were continually ovulating. The recordings were made using a cross-sectional design; i.e., many cases of different ages were studied over a relatively short time span rather than following a relatively few cases over a long period as in the longitudinal method. The research is still in progress at the time of writing this article and so the results reported here are incomplete. They reveal, however, a very different pattern of life-span development of visual acuity in males and females as may be seen in Figure 4. The males have an initial mean acuity of about 4.2 cycles/degree that remains virtually constant acuity during the first 12 months of life followed by a modest decline of about 0.5 cycle/degree over the next nine months. The females, on the other hand, initially have an acuity that is slightly below that of the males (3.8 cycles/degree). Over the course of the next nine months, however, their acuity showed a rapid rise to 5 cycles/degree. where it remained for about six months followed by a sharp decline to 3 cycles/degree. The decline in acuity after 12-15 months, which corresponds to the age at which quail generally are retired from breeding and commercial egg production, may be related to declining levels of steroid hormones (Ottinger, et al., 1983).

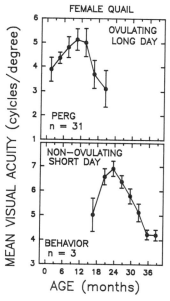

Fig. 5. (Top) Visual-acuity measurements (derived from PERGs in a cross-sectional design) from long-day, ovulating female quail as a function of age. (Bottom) Behavioral visual-acuity measurements (in a longitudinal design) in short-day, non-ovulating female quail. Error bars indicate standard errors of the mean.

The decline in acuity after 12-15 months in the ovulating, long-day females is in sharp contrast to the much delayed decline in acuity of their short-day, non-ovulating counterparts. Figure 5 (top) shows the behavioral acuity of the short-day females (bottom). A comparison of PERG-acuity data of the long-day females plotted on the same scale indicates the same general form in both. Porciatti et al. (1991) reported a good correspondence between behavioral acuity and PERG acuity in young and old pigeons. The main difference between the short-day (non-ovulating) females and the long-day (ovulating) females is the location of the peak of the acuity-age function, which is at 9-15 months for the long-day females and 21-24 months for the short-day females; i.e., the long-day females are in the depths of their acuity decline when the short-day females are just achieving their peak. We suspect that we may not be able to extend the long-day female graph much further because of the higher age-specific mortality of the females than the males under conditions of long-day illumination (Woodward and Abplanalp, 1971).

CONCLUSIONS

By reducing day length, which, among other changes, reduces the activity of the neuro-endocrine reproductive system as seen in the decline in ovulation (Ottinger, in press), we have delayed the onset of the visual-acuity decline. In other words, short day length decreases the rate of aging of the visual system in female Japanese quail (see chapter by Hodos, this volume). This finding suggests a relationship between age-specific levels of steroid hormones and their consequent interaction with neurochemical processes in the aging of those components of the visual system that are involved in high-contrast spatial vision. These data also are consistent with the disposable-soma theory of aging proposed by Kirkwood (1981, 1990) which predicts that organisms that invest a large proportion of their body's resources in reproduction (usually because the inhabit high-risk environments) have fewer remaining resources left to provide for repair and maintenance of their own somatic cells and therefore age more rapidly than those that invest less in reproduction.

ACKNOWLEDGEMENTS

The research reported in this article was supported by the US National Eye Institute through grants EY-00735 (W. H.), EY-04742 (W. H.) and EY-07370 (K. V. F.) and by Fight for Sight, UK (M. B. A. D.). Portions of the research were carried out while the first author was a Visiting Professor at the Department of Biology, Imperial College, London, England.

REFERENCES

Altman, P. L. and Dittman, D. S., 1974, "Biology Data Book," Federation of Societies of Experimental Biology, Bethesda, Maryland.

Armington, J. C., 1974, "The Electroretinogram", Academic Press, New York.

Bagolini, B., Porciatti, V., Falsini, B., Scalia, G., Neroni, M. and Moretti, M., 1988, Macular electroretinogram as a function of age of subjects. Doc. Ophthalmol., 70:37-43.

Blough, D. S., 1956, Dark adaptation in the pigeon. J. Opt. Soc. Amer., 49:425-430.

Bowmaker, J. K., 1977, Visual pigments, oil droplets and spectral sensitivity of the pigeon. Vis. Res., 17:1112-1138.

Djamgoz, M. B. A. and Wagner, H. -J., in press, Localization and function of dopamine in the adult vertebrate retina. Neurochem. Int.

Domenici, L., Trimarchi, C., Piccolino, M., Fiorentini, A. and Maffei, L., 1985, Dopaminergic drugs improve human visual contrast sensitivity. Human Neurobiol., 4:195-197.

Fitzke, F. W., Hayes, B. P., Hodos, W., Holden, A. L. and Low, J. C., 1985, Refractive sectors in the visual field of the pigeon eye. J. Physiol., (London), 369:17-31.

Harnois, C. and Di Paolo, T., 1990, Decreased dopamine in the retinas of patients with Parkinson's disease. Invest. Ophthal. Vis. Sci., 31:2437-2475.

Hodos, W., in press, Animal models of life-span development, in "The Changing Visual System: Maturation and Aging in the Central Nervous System," P. Bagnoli and W. Hodos, eds., Plenum, New York.

Hodos, W., Bessette, B. B., Macko, K. A. and Weiss, S. R. B., 1985, Normative data for pigeon vision. Vision Res., 25:1525-1527.

Hodos, W. and Erichsen, J. T., 1990, Lower-field myopia in birds: An adaptation that keeps they ground in focus. Vis. Res., 30:653-657.

Hodos, W., Leibowitz, R. W. and Bonbright, J. C., 1976, Near field visual acuity of pigeons: effects of head position and stimulus luminance. J. Exp. Anal. Behav., 25:129-141.

Hodos, W., Miller, R. F. and Fite, K. V., 1991, Age-dependent changes in visual acuity and retinal morphology in pigeons. Vision Res., 31:669-677.

Holden, A. L. and Vaegan, 1983a, Vitreal and intraretinal responses to contrast reversing patterns in the pigeon eye. Vis. Res., 23:561-572.

Holden, A. L. and Vaegan, 1983b, Comparison of the focal electroretinogram and the pattern electroretinogram in the pigeon. J. Physiol. (London), 334:11-23.

Kirkwood, T. B. L., 1981, Repair and its evolution: survival versus reproduction, in "Physiological Ecology: An Evolutionary Approach to Resource Use," C. R. Townsend and P. Calow, eds., Blackwell, Oxford.

Kirkwood, T. B. L., 1990, The disposable soma theory of aging, in "Genetic Effects on Aging II," D. E. Harrison, ed., Telford, Caldwell, NJ.

Kurkjian, M. L. and Hodos, W.,1990, Age-dependent changes in visual intensity difference threshold in pigeons. Neuroscience Abstracts, 16:1161.

Mariani, A. and Leure-Dupree, A. E., 1978, Photoreceptors and oil droplet colors in the red area of the pigeon retina. J. Comp. Neurol., 182:821-838.

Naka, K. I. and Rushton, W. A. H., 1966, S-potentials from color units in the retina of fish (Cyprinidae). J. Physiol. (London), 85:536-555.

Ottinger, M. A. Neuroendocrine and behavioral determinants of reproductive aging. Poultry Biol., in press.

Ottinger, M. A., Duchala, C. S. and Masson, M., 1983, Age-related reproductive decline in male Japanese quail. Hormones and Behav., 17:197-207.

Pitts, D. G. 1982, The effects of aging on selected visual functions: Dark adaptation, visual acuity, stereopsis, and brightness contrast, in "Aging and Human Visual Function", R. Sekuler, D. Kline and K. Dismukes, eds., Alan R. Liss, New York.

Porciattti , V., Falsini, B., Scalia, G., Fadda, A. and Fontanesi, G., 1988, Doc. Ophthal., 70:117-122.

Porciatti, V. Hodos, W., Signorini, G. and Bramanti, F., 1991, Electroretinographic changes in aged pigeons. Vis. Res., 31:661-668.

Rakic, P., Bourgeois, J. -P., Eckenhoff, M, Zecevic, N. and Goldman-Rakic, P.S., 1986, Concurrent overproduction of synapses in diverse regions of primate cerebral cortex. <u>Science,</u> 232:232-235.

Rakic, P., in press, Development of the primate visual system throughout life, <u>in</u> "The Changing Visual System: Maturation and Aging in the Central Nervous System," P. Bagnoli and W. Hodos, eds., Plenum, New York.

Woodard, A. E. and Abplanalp, H., 1971, Longevity and reproduction in Japanese quail maintained under stimulative lighting. <u>Poul. Sci.,</u>50:688-692.

Wright, A. A., 1972, Psychometric and psychophysical hue discrimination functions for the pigeon. <u>Vis. Res.,</u> 12:1447-1464.

SYNAPTIC PLASTICITY IN THE ADULT VERTEBRATE RETINA:

A ROLE FOR ENDOGENOUS DOPAMINE

Mustafa B.A. Djamgoz

Neurobiology Group, Department of Biology
Imperial College of Science
Technology & Medicine, London SW7 2BB, U.K.

INTRODUCTION

The nervous system, in concert with the endocrine and the immune systems, controls the main functions of the body. Neuronal organization is known to be 'plastic' in early development whereby the wiring of neuronal subsets is significantly affected by environmental factors. However, beyond the "critical period" and increasingly in adult life, the system is thought to lose its plasticity and gradually become 'hard-wired'. The nervous systems of lower vertebrates generally remain changeable for longer periods and parts of the central nervous system (CNS) can regenerate completely after damage or surgery. Another set of major changes occurs in the nervous system during the process of ageing. Ageing has been shown to involve structural changes in neurones including loss of synaptic connections, decrease in levels of neurotransmitter substances, as well as complete disappearance of neurones. In between maturation and beginning of ageing, the nervous system may be thought to be functioning optimally. Interestingly, even during this major phase of adult life the apparently hard-wired nature of the neuronal connections may still be modifiable to some extent so as to sustain the expediency of neural networks in performing their controlling role. The main aim of this article is to review our recent progress in understanding synaptic plasticity in the adult vertebrate retina, concentrating on chromatic signalling and in particular the horizontal cell → cone photoreceptor feedback interaction in teleost fish.

The Changing Visual System, Edited by P. Bagnoli and
W. Hodos, Plenum Press, New York, 1991

149

The retina is essentially an outgrowth of the CNS, projecting from forebrain during development, and comprises a network of six main types of neurones and their sub-types (Djamgoz & Wagner, 1987). Images of the external world are focussed upon the retinal layer lining the back of the eye and aspects of the visual information present in the image are 'extracted' by retinal neurones via their specialised receptive fields. The receptive field of a neurone is that part of the retina which, when illuminated by appropriate stimuli, will elicit a response in the neurone. A given receptive field is constructed from a combination of the neurone's intrinsic membrane properties and synaptic connectivity (Djamgoz & Yamada, 1990).

HORIZONTAL CELL RECEPTIVE FIELDS AND CONNECTIVITY WITH CONES

Horizontal cells (HCs) are second-order retinal neurones receiving synaptic inputs from photoreceptors. In the cyprinid fish retina, a set of HCs selectively contact cones at 'central' and 'lateral' sites around synaptic ribbons within cone pedicles (Stell et al.,1975). HCs are intimately involved in processing of chromatic information and have been extensively studied in the cyprinid fish retina for a number of reasons (Douglas & Djamgoz, 1990). Firstly, cyprinid fish possess well-developed tri- or even tetra-chromatic vision and extremely large and morphologically well-characterised HC types. Secondly, the different spectral types of cone photoreceptor in these fish can be recognized by morphological and ultrastructural characteristics; consequently their chromatic connectivity to the HC types can be readily determined (e.g. Scholes, 1975; Stell & Harosi, 1976; Bowmaker, 1984, 1990; Downing et al.,1986). Thirdly, there is a wealth of other information about fish HCs, thus making it possible to reach an integrated understanding of their functional organization (e.g. Kaneko, 1987; Dowling, 1987; Djamgoz & Yamada, 1990).

HCs respond to increasing areas of illumination with increasing amplitudes of response over most of the retina i.e. their receptive fields are very broad (Norton et al.,1968). According to their spectral characteristics, cone-driven HCs have been divided into two main classes, as follows (Svaetichin & MacNichol, 1958).

1. **Luminosity:** (L-type) units which generate hyperpolarizing responses to all spectral stimuli. The most common L-type unit is mainly red-sensitive (L/H1 type) (Fig. 1a).

2. **Chromaticity**: (C-type) units which hyperpolarize to some wavelengths and depolarize to others. A major subtype of C-unit (C_b/H2 type) generates biphasic responses, depolarizing to long- and hyperpolarizing to middle- and short-wavelength lights (Fig. 1b). Triphasic and even tetraphasic C-type responses have also been described (Tomita, 1965; Naka & Rushton, 1966c; Tamura & Niwa, 1967; Mitarai et al.,1974; Djamgoz, 1984; Hashimoto et al.,1976, 1988).

This article is concerned with synaptic plasticity in the retinal circuit involving L/H1 and C_b/H2 HCs.

Ultrastructural characteristics of cone inputs to photopic luminosity (L-type) and biphasic/chromaticity (C_b-type) HCs in the roach retina have been determined by Downing and Djamgoz (1989). The cone connectivity patterns of these cells are as follows.

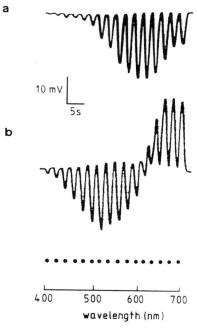

Fig. 1   Two common types of cone-driven S-potential in the retina of the cyprinid fish, roach (<u>Rutilus rutilus</u>). (a) Red-sensitive luminosity (L) - type response generated by H1 HCs. (b) Biphasic, chromaticity (C_b) type response generated by H2 HCs. Sixteen different spectral stimuli (20 nm intervals) of near-equal quantum content were presented in sequence (dots on bottom of figure) to cover the spectral range from 400 nm to 700 nm (inclusive).

L-type HCs have H1-like morphologies (Stell & Lightfoot, 1975) and contact on average 14 cone pedicles over a retinal area of some 1030 μm^2. Most of the contacted pedicles are those of red (R)- and green (G)-sensitive cones (roughly in equal numbers), although some cells also contact a blue (B)-sensitive cone. The distribution of L/H1 HC dendritic endings relative to the synaptic ribbons of different spectral cone pedicles is highly consistent. Most (78%) of the HC dendrites contact the synaptic ribbons in the 'lateral' position. Of these, the majority (71%) are within R-cone pedicles; the rest are mostly within G-cones (29%); only a very small percentage (<<1%) of the contacts are within B-cone pedicles. 93% of the HC contacts 'central' to the ribbons are within R-cones, but a few are also found within G- and B-cone pedicles (6% and 1%, respectively). Importantly, most HC 'lateral' contacts exhibit pronounced "spinules" (finger-like extensions) on their surfaces away from the synaptic ribbon and ridge (see next section).

C_b-type horizontal cells have H2-like morphologies and also contact 14 cone pedicles, on average. However the density of these contacts is less than half that of the L/H1 cells, the contacted pedicles occurring over some 2090 μm^2. C_b/H2 HCs contact G- and B-sensitive cones with equal frequency, on average. Importantly, C_b/H2 HCs do not contact any R-sensitive cones. The ultrastructural connectivity patterns of these HCs show somewhat greater variability. On average, most (77%) of their dendritic contacts are 'central' to synaptic ribbons. Of these, 73% are made within G-cone pedicles, whilst the rest (27%) are made within B-cone pedicles. Laterally positioned contacts make up some 23% of the total number of ribbon contacts; the majority (71%) of these are in B-cone pedicles, the rest (27%) in G-cone pedicles. Again most 'lateral' HC contacts have spinules projecting into the pedicle cytoplasm on the surface away from synaptic ridge.

Correlation of the ultrastructural findings (i.e. the positions of HC dendritic terminals in chromatic subtypes of cone pedicles) with the spectral characteristics of the HCs leads to the following structure-function relationships.

1) All centrally positioned HC dendrites are post-synaptic to the cones as suggested originally by Stell et al. (1975).

2) Each laterally positioned dendrite has a dual function in those cone pedicles from which the cell receives direct hyperpolarizing/feed-forward input.

One possibility is that at least selective 'lateral' dendrites are post-synaptic next to the ribbon in the synaptic ridge, whilst their spinules are pre-synaptic to the cones away from the ridge. In accordance with this hypothesis, we have frequently observed Ω-shaped perturbations in cone plasma membranes directly apposing labelled HC 'lateral' dendrites (Downing & Djamgoz, 1989). These profiles resemble synaptic vesicles caught in the process of exocytosis (Heuser & Reese, 1981), and have been observed also in retinae of the goldfish (Stell et al.,1982), the turtle (Lasansky, 1971), and the toad (Witkovsky & Powell, 1981; Nagy & Witkovsky, 1981). Furthermore, ethanolic-phosphotungstic acid (EPTA), recognized as a selective marker for synaptic membrane proteins (Pfenninger, 1973; Bloom & Aghajanian, 1973), stains the membranes of HC dendrites in close proximity to the synaptic ridge for both 'central' and 'lateral' HC contacts (Wagner, 1978, 1980; Stell et al.,1982). Intra-membraneous particles reminiscent of synaptic receptor proteins and/or receptor-ionophore complexes have been observed at both sites of EPTA staining (Stell et al., 1982). An intracleft 'matrix' has also been found between both 'central' and 'lateral' dendrites and the synaptic ridge. In the goldfish retina, this 'matrix' appears to be coextensive with the arciform density, its closely related band of vesicle discharge sites on the synaptic ridge and the apposing EPTA-positive sub-membraneous thickenings of HC dendrites (Stell et al.,1982). The existence of such an ultrastructural coextension implies that the sub-membraneous thickenings of HC dendrites immediately opposite the synaptic ridge have a role such as binding of transmitter molecules (Stell, 1976; Stell et al.,1982). The similarity of the paramembraneous structures and configurations observed for both 'central' and 'lateral' sites of HC contacts suggests similar functional properties of the two types of contact i.e., they may both be post-synaptic. Furthermore, the cleft matrix is characteristic of Gray Type I (i.e., excitatory) synapses (Gray, 1969).

CHANGE IN HORIZONTAL CELL SPECTRAL RESPONSE DURING LIGHT ADAPTATION

The cone-HC connectivity data reviewed in the preceding section can explain the generation of the R-sensitive depolarizing response in C_b/H2 HCs if it is assumed that L/H1 cells make an inhibitory synapse (i.e. negative feedback) upon G-sensitive cones in accordance with the idea originally put forward by Fuortes and Simon (1974) in turtle, and Stell and Lightfoot (1975) and Stell et al.(1975) in goldfish. An interesting property of this feedback interaction in the cyprinid fish retina is its light-dependent plasticity. This characteristic has been studied most extensively for the L/H1 and C_b/H2 HCs in roach and carp retinae (Djamgoz, 1984; Weiler & Wagner, 1984; Djamgoz et al., 1985, 1988; Kirsch et al.,1990, 1991).

We originally noted that HCs generating purely hyperpolarizing spectral responses (i.e. apparent L-type units) in the roach retina could be made to depolarize to long-wavelength stimuli following brief laser irradiation; these were referred to as "hidden C-type responses" (Djamgoz & Ruddock, 1978). In a subsequent intracellular staining study, the cellular origins of such responses were confirmed indeed to be H2 HCs (Djamgoz et al.,1985). During more systematic recordings from roach retinae gradually light adapting in the mesopic state, H2 HCs were found, in fact, to generate a variable spectral response (Fig. 2). In response to

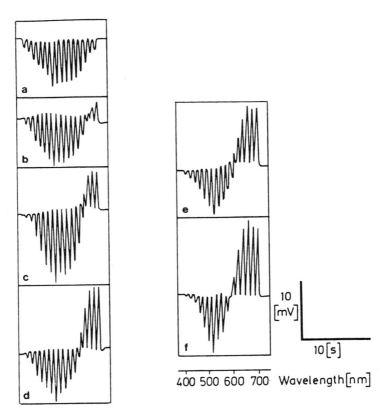

Fig. 2   The range of spectral responses recorded from Cb/H2 HCs during light adaptation (a → f) in the roach retina. The red-sensitive depolarizing component is absent in the fully dark-adapted retina (a) and gradually becomes prominent with light adaptation to give a well-balanced spectrally opponent response (e & f).   Stimuli, as in Fig. 1 legend.

a long-wavelength (674 nm) criterion stimulus, H2 HCs (identified morphologically by intracellular marking) mostly generated a hyperpolarizing response early on in the recordings when retinae were relatively dark adapted (Djamgoz et al.,1988). With gradual light adaptation, however, an increasingly greater proportion of H2 units generating depolarizing responses to the 674 nm stimulus were found. The degree of depolarization in C_b/H2 HCs has been quantified as the "neutral wavelength" (λ_o), i.e. the wavelength of transition from hyperpolarizing to depolarizing responses. Fig. 3 shows the time course of λ_o in H2 HCs during light adaptation in the presence of a background white light of moderate intensity (3×10^{-4} candela). Clearly, λ_o has a value of some 658 nm at the beginning, and this shifts to 609 nm after 40 minutes of light adaptation. Interestingly, λ_o subsequently rises to 640 nm, possibly as a result of a desensitization process involved in prolonged light adaptation (see also later). Thus, C_b/H2 HCs selectively lose the R-sensitive

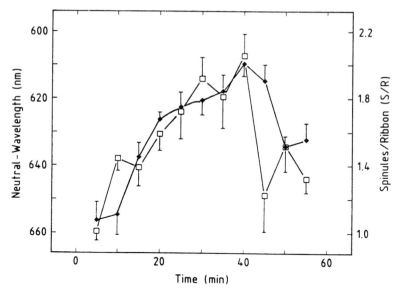

Fig. 3   Time courses of the 'neutral wavelength' (nm; left-hand ordinate/ open squares) and 'spinule/ribbon ratio' (S/R; right-hand ordinate/ filled diamonds) in the roach retina. Both parameters have been plotted on the same time scale for comparison. Each data point denotes the mean ± SEM (n > 7 for each data point). The two parameters are clearly closely related in time. From Kirsch et al. (1990).

depolarizing component of their spectral response in the dark and regain it following light adaptation. During the whole of this process, the L/H1 HC spectral response was 'normal', thereby indicating that R-cones were fully functional. It would appear, therefore, that the feedback pathways are suppressed in dark-adapted retinae and are reactivated during light adaptation.

CHANGE IN HORIZONTAL CELL DENDRITIC ARCHITECTURE DURING LIGHT ADAPTATION

A profound change occurs in the dendritic architecture of 'lateral' dendrites of HCs during light adaptation. In the dark-adapted state, the 'lateral' dendrites of HCs have rounded profiles away from the synaptic ridge. During light-adaptation, however, these terminals give rise to finger-like extensions called "spinules" which progressively penetrate the cone cytoplasm (Fig. 4). The number of spinules around each synaptic ribbon (S/R) increases in number over 50 minutes of light adaptation from about 0.7 (just above the fully dark-adapted level) to 2.0, the maximal light-adapted value being about 2.8 (Fig. 3). Spinules have cytological characteristics which suggest that they may function as synaptic terminals. The available ultrastructural evidence for this is as follows:

1.   Spinules are also EPTA-positive, thus resembling synaptic membranes generally (Wagner, 1980; Stell et al.,1982). However, the paramembraneous configuration at spinules is different than that close to the synaptic ridge. It is made up of brief, triangular, periodic regions, as opposed to a continuous structure.

2.   Unlike HC dendrites at either position around the synaptic ridge, the E-face intramembraneous particles are not noticeably specialised at spinules (Stell et al.,1982).

3.   No intracleft matrix has been observed in the extracellular space opposite spinules.

In the above three respects, spinules differ from membranes of HC dendrites around the synaptic ridge. We have concluded, therefore, that the respective sites within a given HC 'lateral' process have different functional characteristics. One possibility is that cone transmission around the synaptic ridge is excitatory, as noted above, whilst spinules mediate the inhibitory (i.e. negative) feedback interaction between HCs and cones. Interestingly, few or no vesicles have been observed by ultrastructural examination of laterally positioned dendrites or spinules

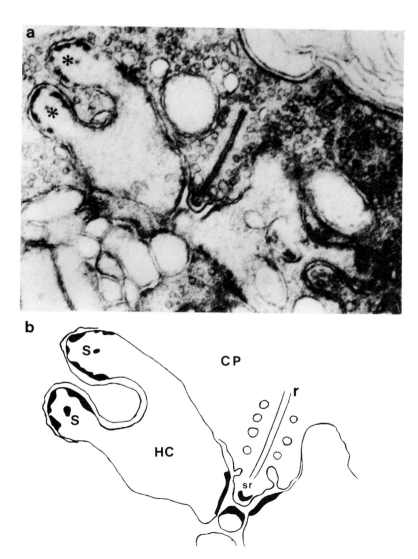

Fig. 4 Typical electron micrograph (a) and partial schematic drawing (b) of a ribbon synapse within a cone pedicle (CP) in the roach retina fixed in the mesopic state. Spinules (S; marked by asterisks in a) are clearly seen projecting from horizontal cell (HC) dendrites positioned laterally with respect to the synaptic ribbon (r) and synaptic ridge. x 80,000 (a). Schematic drawing by J.E.G. Downing. Adapted from Downing et al. (1986).

of HCs, contrary to what one would expect of chemically transmitting presynaptic terminals (Stell et al.,1982). Lack of vesicles may have two implications. On the one hand, it may correspond to release of gamma-aminobutyric acid (GABA) from HCs as being largely non-vesicular and Ca^{2+}-independent (Yazulla & Kleinschmidt, 1983; Ayoub & Lam, 1984, 1985). A considerable body of evidence suggests that GABA is the transmitter of L/H1 horizontal cells (Lam et al.,1980; Yazulla, 1986) and that HC → cone negative feedback is GABAergic (Prince et al.,1987). Alternatively, the negative feedback may be electrotonic (i.e. non-chemical), as proposed by Byzov et al.(1977) and Byzov & Shura-Bura, 1986).

CORRELATION OF ELECTROPHYSIOLOGICAL AND ULTRASTRUCTURAL ASPECTS OF HORIZONTAL CELL SPECTRAL PLASTICITY

The evidence reviewed so far clearly suggests that HCs are 'plastic' both in electrophysiological (spectral) and ultrastructural respects. Possible correlation of the two light-dependent charateristics has been investigated in a variety of ways (Kirsch et al.,1990, 1991).

Global analysis

For this analysis, λ_os were sampled during light adaptation up to 60 min after dissection of the retinae (roach). The recordings were terminated after different durations of light adaptation and the retinae fixed for electron microscopy (EM). The S/R values were determined for the different times. The measured values (λ_o and S/R) were combined separately in 5 min time-bins and plotted against time for comparison (Fig. 3). Clearly, the decrease in the λ_o values and the increase in the number of spinules per ribbon (S/R) during light adaptation followed very similar time courses. Interestingly, after about 40 min of adaptation the S/R value showed a decrease. The reason(s) for this is not known but some 'desensitization' phenomenon becoming apparent at latter stages of light adaptation may be involved. Irrespective of the underlying cause(s), however, λ_o also showed a corresponding increase towards dark-adapted values, indicating a close parallel between the two parameters.

In order to test more closely the correlation of the two parameters studied, S/R values were plotted against λ_o values recorded during the last 5 min before fixation. This analysis is shown in Fig. 5a. Although there is considerable scatter in the data points, on the whole λ_o gets shorter as S/R increases.

Single-cell analysis

The correlation between the degree of spinule formation and spectral plasticity was tested directly by collecting the data from single $C_b/H2$ HCs, i.e. by determining λ_o for a given cell and then staining with horseradish peroxidase and fixing the retina immediately for EM (Kirsch et al.,1990). As the morphological measure of HC feedback, we used a weighted spinule number (S^*), defined as follows:

$$S^* = \text{Unlabelled spinules} / (\text{central + lateral processes}).$$

This term essentially represents a morphological measure of feedback strength, taking into account the relative magnitudes of feed-forward (nominator) and feedback (denominator) effects within G-sensitive cone pedicles where the feed-back interaction occurs (Downing & Djamgoz, 1989).

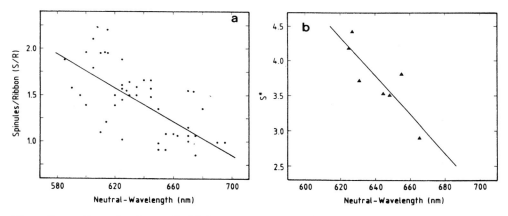

Fig. 5 Correlation of light-dependent spinule dynamics with spectral response (feedback) plasticity in $C_{b/H2}$ HCs of the roach retina. (a) Global approach. Relation of spinule/ribbon ratio (S/R) to neutral wavelength (nm). Data were obtained from 72 cells (37 retinae). The straight line denotes the best fit from linear regression analysis and has a correlation coefficient of 0.68. (b) Single-cell approach. Direct relationship between S* and neutral wavelength (nm) for individual cells from a sample of 7 Cb/H2 HCs. S* is the weighted term for spinules, representing the morphological correlate of negative feedback. The points can be fitted by a straight line from a linear regression with a correlation coefficient of 0.84. From Kirsch et al. (1990).

As this parameter is based on morphological data from individually labelled C_b/H2 HCs, it could not be calculated in the 'global' approach. Fig. 5b shows the result of the single-cell analysis. Clearly, there is a highly significant, inverse correlation between S^* and λ_o in the range 625–665 nm.

The results of these analyses taken together suggest that there is a strong parallel between the light-dependent number of spinules present within cone pedicles and the degree of the negative feedback interaction mediated by HCs as judged by λ_o.

NEUROCHEMICAL SIGNALS IN HORIZONTAL CELL SYNAPTIC PLASTICITY

The experimental evidence reviewed so far demonstrates that during light adaptation of the cyprinid fish retina HC dendrites positioned laterally at cone ribbon synapses form finger-like extensions ("spinules") and concomittantly the HC → cone feedback pathway is strengthened thereby leading to a corresponding decrease in the value of λ_o in C_b/H2 HC responses. We have also investigated the neurochemical basis of this phenomenon. There is now abundant evidence that dopamine (DA) is involved in light/dark adaptation and release of DA may, in fact, initiate light adaptation in the teleost retina (see Djamgoz & Wagner, 1991, for a recent review). In the teleost retina, DA is contained in a sub-type of interplexiform cell which synapses onto HCs (Dowling & Ehinger, 1975, 1978). We, therefore, tested by several different kinds of experiment the possibility that light-induced spinule formation in the roach retina involves DA release (Kirsch et al.,1991).

1) Application of DA to retinae maintained in darkness indeed caused spinule formation in a dose-dependent mannner. 0.1 mM DA gave the maximal effect, the S/R value reaching 2.5, just below the level achieved by fully light adapting the retina; 10–20 µM DA were required to achieve a half-maximal effect. These concentration (µM) effects are indicative of D_1 receptors; D_2 receptors are activated by nM DA (Bradford, 1986). The effect of light itself on S/R and λ_o could be blocked by pre-treating the retina with the dopaminergic antagonist haloperidol (Djamgoz et al.,1989). Thus, it appears that light-induced DA release could cause spinule formation and bring about a decrease in λ_o.

2) Destruction of the dopaminergic interplexiform cells in the retina using the neurotoxin 6-hydroxydopamine (6-OHDA) prevented the effect of light adaptation in forming spinules and shifting λ_o to shorter values. However, both effects could still be induced in such retinae by applying DA exogenously.

3) The effect of exogenous DA in forming spinules could be blocked to different extents by various DA antagonists. The rank order of potency of the antagonists tested was as follows:

SCH23390 > cis-flupentixol > fluphenazine > sulpiride.

This pharmacological profile is again strongly indicative of D_1 receptors.

4) Extracellular application of dibutyryl-cAMP (membrane-permeant analogue of cAMP) to dark dark-adapted retina caused significant spinule formation. This further supports the view that the DA-induced spinule formation involves D_1 receptors and cAMP as second messenger.

The available evidence taken together suggests the following sequence of cellular and molecular events in light-induced formation of HC spinules and feedback plasticity in the cyprinid fish retina:

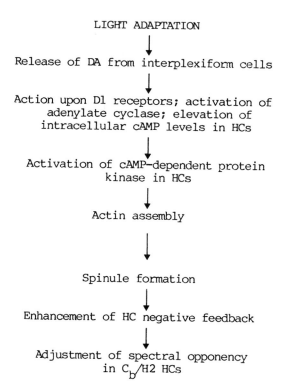

LIGHT ADAPTATION
↓
Release of DA from interplexiform cells
↓
Action upon D1 receptors; activation of adenylate cyclase; elevation of intracellular cAMP levels in HCs
↓
Activation of cAMP-dependent protein kinase in HCs
↓
Actin assembly
↓
Spinule formation
↓
Enhancement of HC negative feedback
↓
Adjustment of spectral opponency in C_b/H2 HCs

The least understood stage of the proposed sequence is the process leading from cAMP accumulation in HCs to actin assembly (i.e. polymerization of actin), presumably by phosphorylation. HCs are known to contain a cAMP-dependent protein kinase (Lasater, 1987; Liman et al.,1989) and are also abundant in F-actin (Drenckhahn & Wagner, 1985; Vaughan & Lasater, 1990). Actin assembly is necessary for spinule formation since cytochalasin (a drug that prevents this process) blocks light-evoked spinule formation, as well as the shift in λ_o (A. Ter-Markarian & M.B.A. Djamgoz - in preparation).

BEHAVIOURAL AND ECOLOGICAL CONSEQUENCES OF HORIZONTAL CELL SPECTRAL PLASTICITY

The available evidence would suggest that the kind of HC plasticity described here may occur specifically in fish and not in higher vertebrates. A summary of the relevant HC characteristics in teleosts and mammals is shown below.

Characteristics	Teleost	Mammal
HC - cone connectivity	highly specific & hierarchical	non-specific
HC spectral feedback	yes	no (?)
HC spinules	yes	no
HC feedback plasticity	yes	no (?)

In the mammalian (including primate) retina, HC-cone connectivity appears to be non-specific i.e. all HCs contact nearby cones irrespective of their chromatic identity (Boycott et al.,1987; Wässle et al.,1989). This would imply that generation of spectral responses (if any) in mammalian HCs may not depend upon specific HC → cone negative feedback, unlike the situation in cyprinid fish. However, some mammalian HCs do contain the inhibitory neurotransmitter GABA (Chun & Wässle, 1989), so HC → cone feedback may be present but serve some other synaptic function (e.g. control of temporal aspects; formation of bipolar cell receptive field surrounds). Mammalian (in fact, all non-teleost) HCs do not form spinules (Wagner, 1980) and hence lack such a mechanism for modulating the feedback interaction. Thus, highly specific cone connectivity, spectral feedback, HC spinules and plasticity would appear to be exceptionally well developed in cyprinid fish retinae. Although the amphibian retina contains C-type

HCs (e.g. Stone et al.,1990), their cone connectivity has not yet been elucidated. Selective cone-HC connectivity and HC → cone feedback do occur in the turtle retina (Fuortes & Simon, 1974; Leeper, 1978a,b), but there is no evidence for feedback plasticity. It would appear, therefore, that at least some of the HC characteristics listed above are not so developed in higher vertebrates and may be absent in mammals. Although the reason(s) for this apparent distinction is not clear at present, it would seem attractive to consider that it may be related to the chromatic conditions experienced by fish within aquatic environments. The chromatic world underwater is most certainly much richer and more dynamic compared with terrestrial conditions (Loew & McFarland, 1990). The colour of the water changes in space and time, depending on (i) its contents; (ii) the season; (iii) depth; and (iv) the angle of viewing at a given depth and time. Thus, HC spectral plasticity probably exists in fish to ensure maximal visual efficiency underwater.

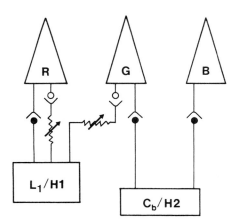

Fig. 6 A functional wiring model summarising our current knowledge of the cone connectivity of L/H1 and C_b/H2 HCs. R, G, B, red-, green- and blue-sensitive cones, respectively. Inverted arrowheads denote pre-synaptic terminals : dark, excitatory; light, inhibitory. Inhibitory feedback from L/H1 HCs onto R- and G-cones are 'plastic' (as indicated by the variable resistor in each pathway) being suppressed in the dark and potentiated by light adaptation of the retina. The circuitry involving the output(s) of the Cb/H2 HC and possible feedback onto B-cones are not shown as these are currently under investigation. From Djamgoz et al. (1988).

The plasticity in the generation of colour-coded HC responses in cyprinid fish retinae could explain why red/green-antagonistic ganglion cell responses are also absent in the dark-adapted retina, but reappear upon light adaptation (Raynauld et al. 1979). Thus, this phenomenon is not restricted to the retina and would appear, in fact, to be signalled to the brain. It would seem likely that fully functional colour processing would not be of much use to fish in reduced ambient illumination conditions. Thus, suppression of the feedback pathways in the dark would probably ensure economic synthesis and release of the feedback transmitter. Neumeyer (1986) has indeed shown that in dim light, goldfish lose the ability to discriminate between red and green stimuli. Another consequence of red-green opponency in C_b/H2 horizontal cells is relative enhancement of chromatic sensitivity in the far-red region of the spectrum - the so-called "pseudopigment" effect (Naka and Rushton, 1966a-c). This is thought to be ecologically expedient as it would result in better matching of retinal spectral sensitivity to the colour of the water (Lythgoe & Northmore, 1973; Beauchamp & Rowe, 1977; Cameron, 1982; Wheeler, 1982; Djamgoz, 1984; Neumeyer, 1984; Douglas, 1986). It would follow, therefore, that a variable negative feedback effect would enable fish to constantly adjust and optimize their spectral sensitivity, in accordance with the dynamic lighting conditions found within aquatic environments.

CONCLUDING REMARKS

This article concentrated upon the plasticity of the HC → cone negative feedback synapse in cyprinid fish retinae, its neurochemical basis and possible role in processing of chromatic visual information. This pathway is suppressed in the dark and becomes activated during light adaptation. It is likely that many other types of neuronal interaction in vertebrate retinae generally are also plastic. Retinal control of visual sensitivity, for example, is likely to involve synaptic plasticity within the process of network adaptation. Cat retinal ganglion cell receptive fields indeed lose their inhibitory surrounds during dark adaptation (Barlow et al., 1957). It would appear, in fact, that even adult vertebrate retinae are much less hard-wired than perhaps originally thought. Retinal synaptic organization is, therefore, highly dynamic and capable of undergoing light- (i.e. use-) dependent plasticity.

Acknowledgements

I am grateful to my collaborators, James Downing, Elizabeth

Greenstreet, Matthias Kirsch, Jochen Wagner and Masahiro Yamada, in the various aspects of the research outlined in this article.

REFERENCES

Ayoub, G.S. and Lam, D.M.K. (1984) The release of gamma-aminobutyric acid from horizontal cells of the goldfish (Carassius auratus) retina. J. Physiol., 355: 191-214.

Ayoub, G.S. and Lam, D.M.K. (1985) The content and release of endogenous GABA in isolated horizontal cells of the goldfish retina. Vision Res., 25: 1187-1193.

Barlow, H.B., Fitzhugh, R. and Kuffler, S.W. (1957) Change of organization of the receptive fields of the cat's retina during dark adaptation. J. Physiol., 137: 338-354.

Beauchamp, R.D. and Rowe, J. (1977) Goldfish spectral sensitivity: a conditioned heart rate measure in restrained or curarized fish. Vision Res. 17: 617-624.

Bloom, F.E., and Aghajanian, G.K. (1973) Fine structural and cytochemical analysis of the staining of synaptic junctions with phosphotungstic acid. J. Ultrastruct. Res. 22: 361-375.

Bowmaker, J.K. (1984) Microspectrophotometry of vertebrate photoreceptors. Vision Res., 24: 1641-1650.

Bowmaker, J.K. (1990) Visual pigments of fishes. In: The Visual System of Fish. Douglas, R.H. and Djamgoz, M.B.A., eds. Chapman and Hall, London. pp. 81-107.

Boycott, B.B., Hopkins, J.M. and Sperling, H.G. (1987) Cone connections of the horizontal cells of the rhesus monkey's retina. Proc. R. Soc. Lond. B, 229: 345-368.

Bradford, H.F. (1986) Chemical Neurobiology. An Introduction to Neurochemistry. W.H. Freeman, New York.

Byzov, A.L., Golubtzov, K.V. and Trifonov, Yu.A. (1977) The model of mechanism of feedback between horizontal cells and photoreceptors in vertebrate retina. In: Vertebrate Photoreception. Barlow, H.B. and Fatt, P., eds. Academic Press, London. pp. 265-274.

Byzov, A.L. and Shura-Bura, T.M. (1986) Electrical feedback mechanism in the processing of signals in the outer plexiform layer of the retina. Vision Res., 26: 33-44.

Cameron, N.E. (1982) The photopic spectral sensitivity of a dichromatic teleost fish (Perca fluviatilis). Vision Res., 22: 1341-1348.

Chun, M.H. and Wassle, H. (1989) GABA-like immunoreactivity in the cat retina: electron microscopy. J. Comp. Neurol., 279: 55–67.

Djamgoz, M.B.A. (1984) Electrophysiological characterization of the spectral sensitivities of horizontal cells in cyprinid fish retina. Vision Res., 24: 1677–1687.

Djamgoz, M.B.A. and Downing, J.E.G. (1988) A horizontal cell selectively contacts blue-sensitive cones in cyprinid fish retina: Intracellular staining with horseradish peroxidase. Proc. R. Soc. Lond. B, 235: 281–287.

Djamgoz, M.B.A., Downing, J.E.G. and Wagner, H.-J. (1985) The cellular origin of an unusual type of S-potential: an intracellular horseradish peroxidase study in a cyprinid fish retina. J. Neurocytol., 14: 469–486.

Djamgoz, M.B.A., Downing, J.E.G., Kirsch, M., Prince, D.J. and Wagner, H.-J. (1988) Light-dependent plasticity of horizontal cell functioning in cyprinid fish retina: effects of background illumination of moderate intensity. J. Neurocytol., 17: 701–710.

Djamgoz, M.B.A., Kirsch, M. and Wagner, H.-J. (1989) Haloperidol suppresses light-induced spinule formation and biphasic responses of horizontal cells in fish (roach) retina. Neurosci. Lett., 107: 200–204.

Djamgoz, M.B.A. and Ruddock, K.H. (1978) Changes in structure and electrophysiological function of retinal neurones induced by laser irradiation. Neurosci. Lett., 7: 251–256.

Djamgoz, M.B.A. and Wagner, H.-J. (1987) Intracellular staining of retinal neurones: applications to studies of functional organization. Prog. Retinal Res., 6: 85–150.

Djamgoz, M.B.A. and Wagner, H.-J. (1991) Localization and function of dopamine in the adult vertebrate retina. Neurochem. Int. In press.

Djamgoz, M.B.A. and Yamada, M. (1990) Electrophysiological characteristics of retinal neurones: synaptic interactions and functional outputs. In: The Visual System of Fish (R.H. Douglas & M.B.A. Djamgoz, eds.). Chapman & Hall, London. pp. 159–210.

Douglas, R.H. (1986) Photopic spectral sensitivity of a teleost fish, the roach (Rutilus rutilus), with special reference to its ultraviolet sensitivity. J. Comp. Physiol. A, 159: 415–421.

Douglas, R.H. & Djamgoz, M.B.A., eds. (1990) The Visual System of Fish. Chapman and Hall, London.

Dowling, J.E. (1987) The Retina. An Approachable Part of the Brain. The Belknap Press at Harvard University Press, Cambridge.

Dowling, J.E. & Ehinger, B. (1975) Synaptic organization of the amine containing interplexiform cells of the goldfish and cebus monkey retina. Science NY, 188: 270-273.

Dowling, J.E. & Ehinger, B. (1978) The interplexiform cell system. I. Synapses of the dopaminergic neurones of the goldfish retina. Proc. R. Soc. Lond. B, 201: 7-26.

Downing, J.E.G., Djamgoz, M.B.A. and Bowmaker, J.K. (1986) Photoreceptors of a cyprinid fish, the roach: morphological and spectral characteristics. J. Comp. Physiol A, 159: 859-868.

Downing, J.E.G. and Djamgoz, M.B.A. (1989) Quanatitative analysis of cone photoreceptor-horizontal cell connectivity patterns in the retina of a cyprinid fish: Electron microscopy of functionally identified and HRP-labelled horizontal cells. J. Comp. Neurol., 289: 537-553.

Drenckhahn, D. and Wagner, H.-J. (1985) Relation of retinomotor responses and contractile proteins in vertebrate retinas. Eur. J. Cell Biol., 37: 156-168.

Fuortes, M.G.F. and Simon, E.J. (1974) Interactions leading to horizontal cell responses in the turtle retina. J. Physiol., 240: 177-198.

Gray, E.G. (1969) Electron microscopy of excitatory and inhibitory synapses: a brief review. Prog. Brain Res., 31: 141-155.

Hashimoto, Y., Kato, A., Inokuchi, M. and Watanabe, K. (1976) Re-examination of horizontal cells in the carp retina with Procion Yellow electrode. Vision Res., 16: 25-29.

Hashimoto, Y., Harosi, F.I., Ueki, K. and Fukurotani, K.-I. (1988) Ultra-violet sensitive cones in the color-coding systems of cyprinid retinas. Neurosci. Res. Suppl. 8: S81-S95.

Heuser, J.E. and Reese, T.S. (1981) Synaptic vesicle exocytosis captured by quick freezing. In: The Neurosciences. Fourth Study Program. Schmitt, F.O. and Worden, F.G., eds. The MIT press, Cambridge. pp. 573-600.

Kaneko, A. (1987) The functional role of retinal horizontal cells. Jpn. J. Physiol. 37: 341-358.

Kirsch, M., Djamgoz, M.B.A. and Wagner, H.-J. (1990) Correlation of spinule dynamics and plasticity of the horizontal cell spectral response in cyprinid fish retina: Quantitative analysis. Cell Tissue Res., 260: 123-130.

Kirsch, M., Wagner, H.-J. and Djamgoz, M.B.A. (1991) Dopamine and plasticity of horizontal cell function in the teleost retina: regulation of a spectral mechanism through D1 receptors. Vision Res., 31: 401-412.

Lam, D.M.K., Su, Y.Y.T., Chin, C.-A., Brandon, C., Wu, J.W., Marc, R.E. and Lasater, E.M. (1980) GABAergic horizontal cells in the teleost retina. Brain Res. Bull., 5: 137-140.

Lasansky, A. (1971) Synaptic organization of cone cells in the turtle retina. Phil. Trans. R. Soc. Lond. B, 262: 365-381.

Leeper, H.F. (1978a) Horizontal cells of the turtle retina. I. Light microscopy of Golgi preparations. J. Comp. Neurol., 182: 777-794.

Leeper, H.F. (1978b) Horizontal cells of the turtle retina. II. Analyses of interconnections between photoreceptors and horizontal cells by light microscopy. J. Comp. Neurol., 182: 795-810.

Liman, E.R., Knapp, A.G. and Dowling, J.E. (1989) Enhancement of kainate-gated currents in retinal horizontal cells by cyclic AMP-dependent protein kinase. Brain Res., 481: 399-402.

Loew, E.R. and McFarland, W.N. (1990) The underwater visual environment. In: The Visual System of Fish (R.H. Douglas & M.B.A. Djamgoz, eds.). Chapman & Hall, London. pp. 1-43.

Lythgoe, J.N. and Northmore, D.P.M. (1973) Colours underwater. In: Colour 73. International Colour Association, London. pp.77-98.

Mitarai, G., Asano, T. and Miyake, Y. (1974) Identification of five types of S-potential and their corresponding generating sites in the horizontal cells of the carp retina. Jap. J. Ophthalmol., 18: 161-178.

Nagy, A.R. and Witkovsky, P. (1981) A freeze-fracture study of synaptogenesis in the distal retina of larval Xenopus. J. Neurocytol., 10: 161-176.

Naka, K.-I. and Rushton, W.A.H. (1966a) S-potentials from colour units in the retina of fish (Cyprinidae). J. Physiol., 185: 536-555.

Naka, K.-I. and Rushton, W.A.H. (1966b) An attempt to analyse colour reception by electrophysiology. J. Physiol., 185: 587-599.

Naka, K.-I. and Rushton, W.A.H. (1966c) S-potentials from luminosity units in the retina of fish (Cyprinidae). J. Physiol., 185: 587-599.

Neumeyer, C. (1984) On spectral sensitivity in the goldfish. Evidence for neural interactions between different "cone mechanisms". Vision Res., 24: 1223-1231.

Neumeyer, C. (1986) Wavelength discrimination in the goldfish. J. Comp. Physiol. A, 158: 203-213.

Norton, A.L., Spekreijse, H., Wolbarsht, M.W. and Wagner, H.G. (1968) Receptive field organization of the S-potential. Science NY, 160: 1021-1022.

Pfenninger, K.H. (1973) Synaptic morphology and cytochemistry. Prog. Histochem. Cytochem., 5: 1-86.

Prince, D.J., Djamgoz, M.B.A. and Karten, H.J. (1987) GABA transaminase in cyprinid fish retina: localization and effects of inhibitors on temporal characteristics of S-potentials. Neurochem. Int., 11: 23-30.

Raynauld, J.-P., Laviolette, J.R. and Wagner, H.-J. (1979) Goldfish retina: a correlate between cone activity and morphology of the cone horizontal cell in cone horizontal cells. Science NY, 204: 1436-1438.

Scholes, J.H. (1973) Colour receptors and their synaptic connections in the retina of a cyprinid fish. Phil. Trans. R. Soc. Lond. B, 270: 61-118.

Stell, W.K. (1976) Functional polarization of horizontal cell dendrites in goldfish retina. Invest. Ophthalmol. Visual Sci., 15: 895-908.

Stell, W.K. and Lightfoot, D.O. (1975) Color-specific interconnections of cones and horizontal cells in the retina of the goldfish. J. Comp. Neurol., 159: 473-502.

Stell, W.K., Lightfoot, D.O., Wheeler, T.G. and Leeper, H.F. (1975) Goldfish retina: functional polarization cone horizontal cell dendrites and synapses. Science NY, 190: 989-990.

Stell, W.K. and Harosi, F. (1976) Cone structure and visual pigment content in the retina of goldfish. Vision Res., 16: 647-657.

Stell, W.K., Kretz, R. and Lightfoot, D.O. (1982) Horizontal cell connectivity in goldfish. In: The S-potential. Drujan, B. and Laufer, M., eds. A.R. Liss, New York. pp. 51-75.

Stone, S., Witkovsky, P. and Schutte, M. (1990) A chromatic horizontal cell in the Xenopus retina: Intracellular staining and synaptic pharmacology. J. Neurophysiol., 64: 1683-1694.

Svaetichin, G. and MacNichol, E.F. Jr (1958) Retinal mechanisms for chromatic and achromatic vision. Ann. N.Y. Acad Sci., 74: 388-404.

Tamura, T. and Niwa, H. (1967) Spectral sensitivity and colour vision of fish as indicated by S-potential. Comp. Biochem. Physiol., 22: 745-754.

Tomita, T. (1965) Electrophysiological study of the mechansims subserving colour coding in the fish retina. Cold Spring Harb. Sympos. Quant. Biol., 30: 559-566.

Vaughan, D.K. and Lasater, E.M. (1990) Distribution of F-actin in bipolar and horizontal cells of bass retinas. Am. J. Physiol., 259 C205-C214.

Wagner, H.-J. (1978) Cell types and connectivity patterns in mosaic retinas. Adv. Anat. Emryol., 55: 6-79.

Wagner, H.-J. (1980) Light-dependent plasticity of the morphology of horizontal cell terminals in cone pedicles of fish retinas. J. Neurocytol. 9: 573-591.

Wässle, H., Boycott, B.B. and Rohrenbeck, J. (1989) Horizontal cells in the monkey retina: cone connections and dendritic networks. Eur. J. Neurosci., 1: 421-435.

Weiler, R. and Wagner, H.-J. (1984) Light-dependent change of cone - horizontal cell interactions in carp retina. Brain Res. 298: 1-9.

Wheeler, T.G. (1982) Color vision and retinal chromatic information processing in teleost: a review. Brain Res. Rev., 4: 177-235.

Witkovsky, P. and Powell, C.C. (1981) Synaptic formation and modification between distal retinal neurones in larval and juvenile Xenopus. Proc. R. Soc. Lond. B, 211: 373-389.

Yazulla, S. (1986) GABAergic mechanisms in the retina. Prog. Retinal Res., 5: 1-52.

Yazulla, S. and Kleinschmidt, J. (1983) Carrier mediated release of GABA from retinal horizontal cells. Brain Res., 263: 63-75.

NEW ASPECTS OF CELLULAR AND MOLECULAR MECHANISMS IN LEARNING PROCESSES

Giovanna Traina, Rossana Scuri, Denise Cecchetti
and Marcello Brunelli*

Department of Physiology and Biochemistry
"G.Moruzzi" Via S.Zeno,31, 56127, Pisa, ITALY

INTRODUCTION

The term "Plasticity" of Nervous System was introduced, in the early fifties, by Konorsky (1948) and it was related mainly to all the experience-dependent modifications which underlay learning processes in adult animals. Changes occurr either during the development and the differentiation of neural elements, or during aging, but changes occurr also in behavior and consequently in the networks of adult's neural structure during learning and memory.

In the case of development and aging it should be better to speak about "trophic" influences driving the maturation or protecting nervous system from degenerative processes. More specifically the idea, largely circumstantial, is that neurons compete for survival. For instance we can single out the case of development in the course of which at least three main influences modulate competition between axon terminals:
 1) the availability of specific trophic agents likely supplied by the target cells, to which different classes of axons respond;
 2) the level and temporal pattern of neural activity among competing axons;
 3) the geometrical complexity of target cells.

So since the liver growths, or regenerates, and nobody speaks about "plasticity of the liver" this means that the difference consists in the fact that the capability of Nervous System to be plastic implies that it changes continually throughout life. And this brings about a persistent ability in animals to modify their behavior to environmental changes.
What are the relationships between this plasticity subserving learning and memory and that observed during maturation?
It is therefore so difficult to define the point at which neural development ends (if indeed it ever does), that many investigators have endeavoured to design an unitary theory of the mechanisms of plasticity.

Learning has developed along the evolution in the way that it endows organisms with fantastic adaptative capabilities. It is possible to pinpoint some aspects of learning which can lead to a formal definition:
a) a change in behavior following individual experience;
b) a sustained process and not a brisk and transient response;
c) learning is the process through which it is possible to collect informations, while memory is the storage of the engrams.
Learning and memory can be analysed at different levels of biological organization: in behaving organisms, or in integrated systems, or in neuronal networks both in vertebrate

The Changing Visual System, Edited by P. Bagnoli and
W. Hodos, Plenum Press, New York, 1991

and in invertebrate animals. But, what it is important to clarify, is the common feature which links all the learning processes, in other words, what is the molecular alphabet underlying learning and memory.

In order to elucidate the elementary biochemical and biophysical events subserving learning events a few neurobiologists have been attracted by the idea of studying synaptic modifications in relatively simple invertebrate nervous system following a kind of reductionistic approach.

The reductive step is a shift in analysis from the level of a system as a whole to the level of single cellular and molecular components. It is clear that, for understanding the complexity of learning processes which subserve the modifications of behavior is necessary to extend the cellular studies to different neuronal networks underlying various more or less complicated behavioral acts in order to single out the putative common mechanisms of learning phenomena.

The rationale of this approach seemed indeed appealing.

In invertebrate it is possible to select a single behavior and to identify all the neurons of the network underlying it.

In this system one can study, when the behavior changes, during learning,the sites and the modifications that occur in the cellular network. The best advantage for this project was offered by the sea mollusc "Aplysia" which has a relatively simple nervous system,with cells clustered in to well-defined ganglia. Within each ganglion the cells can be identified and characterized for their distinctive shape and function. Some of the nerve cells of "Aplysia" CNS are among the largest neurons. Kandel and his collaborators have focused their attention to the study of cellular changes underlying elementary forms of learning such as non associative learning of the habituation and sensitization type. The study has been carried out in the abdominal ganglion where are localized the neurons which mediate a simple behavioral act, the withdrawal reflex of the gill and the siphon.

In these conditions the complex phenomenon of learning has been dissected into elementary components in order to facilitate experimental analysis. Habituation and sensitization are considered the most elementary forms of learning; they are defined as "non associative learning processes".

<u>Habituation and sensitization</u>

Habituation consists of a progressive reduction of a response to a stimulus, after repetitive application. It contributes to fitness, enabling adaptation to the "milieu" and the animal learns to ignore stimuli that are ongoing and innocuous. Sensitization is a potentiation of the response to a test stimulus when another, usually strong or noxious, is applied in another site.It increases arousal and attention lowering the threshold of defensive response. Dishabituation is referred to a potentiation that occurs in an habituated response. Kandel and his collaborators have combined many molecular methodologies in an extense interdisciplinary investigation of the cellular and molecular basis of these simple forms of learning in "Aplysia" (Kandel and Schwartz,1982).

NON ASSOCIATIVE LEARNING IN "APLYSIA"

In "Aplysia", an extensive study has been carried out taking as a behavioral model the gill and siphon withdrawal reflex (WR). This reflex has been analysed at cellular level during simple forms of non associative learning,such as habituation and sensitization.Intracellular recordings from all the cells of the WR in the abdominal ganglion have revealed that the monosynaptic connection between sensory and motoneuron changes in efficacy. Habituation were correlated with a progressive decrease in the amplitude of EPSP recorded in the motoneuron whereas dishabituation (or sensitization) exibited a facilitation of this EPSP (Castellucci et al., 1970; Kandel et al., 1973; Castellucci and Kandel, 1974, 1976; Kandel, 1976).

Similar results have been obtained in a simplified system of co-culture "in vitro" of sensory and motoneurons which reconstructs the synaptic array between them. Repetitive stimulation produced a depression of the EPSP recorded on the motoneuron, reproducing homosynaptic depression in absence of other ganglion constituents (Dagan and Levitan, 1981; Schacher and Proshansky, 1983; Rayport and Schacher,1986).

Voltage clamp experiments were employed to analyze the conductance modifications in habituated sensory neurons (Klein et al., 1980). It has been observed that repeated stimulation of the sensory neuron resulted in a decrease in the inward Ca current.The detailed molecular mechanisms for habituation are so far not completely elucidated. Several hypotheses can be taken in consideration for this mechanism of homosynaptic depression :1) inactivation of Ca channels by intracellular Ca^{2+}; 2) activation of second messengers cascade of phospholipid type, initiated by the binding of the released transmitter to autoreceptors onto the presynaptic terminals; 3) in the neural circuitry of WR, inhibitory interneurons and their aminergic and peptidergic transmitters have already been identified. It is possible that they might have a consistent relevance in the habituation acting through an heterosynaptic mechanism. In addition Bailey and Chen (1988) have shown, during habituation, ultrastructural changes in the vesicles of sensory neuron terminals.

The analysis of dishabituation and sensitization of the WR following the same methodological procedure outlined for habituation demonstrated that a facilitation of the sensory to motoneuron synapse occurs. Castellucci and Kandel (1976) have shown that the number of quanta released for each impulse increased, indicating that facilitation is presynaptic.
Brunelli et al. (1976), with a pioneering experiment have demonstrated that serotonin (5HT) was mimicking the facilitatory effect onto the sensory motoneurone synapse. And intracellular injection of cAMP potentiated the monosynaptic EPSP recorded in the motoneurons.

Therefore the molecular model emerging from these experiments is the following: Serotonin activates an adenylate cyclase into the terminals of sensory neurons. This, in turn, increases the level of cAMP, which induces activation of proteinkinases and phosphorylation of preexisting proteins. The phosphoproteins produce the closure of a K channel in the sensory neuron. This K channel is both voltage-dependent and serotonin-regulated channel (Ks).
Ks is active at the resting potential and 5HT decreases the probability to find open the channel. This reduction of K current produces a broadening of spike duration in the sensory neurons which causes an increasing of Ca influx and consequently facilitation of transmitter release (Klein and Kandel, 1980). The direct evidence of this cAMP mediated phosphorylation and the activity of Ks channel emerged from single-channel recordings worked out by membrane patches still attached to the whole cells (Siegelbaum et al., 1982) and later in membrane patches detached from the cell (Shuster et al., 1985). In cell-attached membrane patches,serotonin application or intracellular injection of cAMP caused lasting closure of S channel. In cell-free membrane patches from sensory neurons the catalytic subunit of mammalian Protein kinase A (PKA) produced all-or-none closure of individual Ks channels.

In addition to the S channel closure it has been observed that in voltage clamped sensory neurons long depolarizing steps produced a marked increase of Ca transient after 5HT application. This effect of enhancement of free Ca in the sensory neuron was S channel-independent, since phorbol ester, a PKC activator, induced facilitation without a change in the S current (Hochner et al., 1986). It has clearly demonstrated that 5HT can potentiate the phospholipid-dependent protein kinase PKC in "Aplysia" neurons (Saktor et al., 1986). It was therefore suggested that enlargement of action potential by closure of S channels mediates the sensitization, whereas the S channel-independent mechanism operates during dishabituation (Hochner et al., 1986). This is in accordance with recent experiments (Marcus et al., 1988; Rankin and Carew, 1988) which demonstrated, at behavioral level that dishabituation and sensitization differ at least in three different characteristics: 1) sensitization appears after a delayed onset; 2) sensitization needs stronger stimuli for activation; 3) during ontogeny dishabituation appears before sensitization.In any case this facilitation subserving the behavioral sensitization (or dishabituation) is induced by the formation of phosphoprotein without the synthesis of novel proteins.

NON ASSOCIATIVE LEARNING IN THE LEECH

At the aim of collecting further contributions to the study of mechanisms of short-term learning processes, more recently the analysis has been performed on another invertebrate model, the leech "Hirudo m". The Nervous System of this animal consists of a chain of segmental interconnected ganglia. Several cellular circuitry subserving simple behavioral acts, such as shortening, swimming, etc, have been extensively investigated.

At early stages of the studies the research turned attention to the following items: 1) the mechanisms involved in non associative learning are invariant along the phylogenetic scale?; 2) the neuromodulators and neurotransmitters found out in "Aplysia" play similar roles in short-term changes of different systems?; 3) the molecular mechanism of modulation of Ks channel by phosphoprotein cAMP-dependent subserving short-term sensitization in "Aplysia" is still present in more complex behavioral activity or additional modifications appear to gain relevance in other systems?

A first series of experiments were focused on the shortening reflex of the leech, it has been demonstrated that the potentiation observed during the sensitization is mediated by 5HT, likely through the cAMP increase (Belardetti et al., 1982).

Among the repertoire of behavioral actions, recently the search for learning mechanisms focused on the swimming of the leeches. This complex behavior has already been extensively studied at the cellular level (Stent and Kristan, 1981; Kristan, 1983).

Mechanosensory stimulations brought onto the skin of the body wall produce in each segmental ganglion, the activation of a chain of interconnected neurons starting from the fast oscillatory neurons which trigger pattern generating neurons that, in turn, taking contacts with the dorsal and ventral motoneurons, bring about the rhythmic contraction of the swimming. In animals with a cut between the cephalic and the first segmental ganglion, light tactile or low-threshold electrical stimulation delivered onto body surface of the caudal part produced almost constantly a swim cycle with a predictable latency between the starting of the stimulus and the onset of the response. Repeated tactile or light electrical stimulations applied at very low frequency (1/min) induced a progressive increase in latency (habituation) (Fig.3).

Strong nociceptive stimuli delivered onto various parts of the body wall produced a sudden shortening of the latency, both in habituated (dishabituation) and in non-habituated response (sensitization). The facilitation lasted 30-60 min.

A group of investigations has been planned to characterize such forms of non associative learning utilizing this swim induction in the leech.

The findings can be summarized as follows:

a) Application of 5HT blocking agent, methysergide inhibited the behavioral dishabituation;

b) 5HT injection into the whole animal reduced the latency for swim induction in both habituated and non habituated animals;

c) treatment with neurotoxic agent 5,7 DHT prevented the behavioral dishabituation following noxious stimuli whereas treatment with 6OHDA did not impair the shortening of latency in triggering the swim;

d) dopamine, excitatory and inhibitory aminoacids (GABA, glycine, alanine) failed to produce dishabituation;

e) an adenylate cyclase blocking agent, RMI1233OA (Merrel)

blocked the shortening of the latency in swim induction by 5HT application or by nociceptive stimulation. From all the data taken together two major conclutions emerge; a) that 5HT through the formation of cAMP also in the leech mediates the short-term changes subserving behavioral sensitization; b) the facilitatory effect is mediated by second messengers of cAMP type.

The remarkable analogy with the "Aplysia" model has been pinpointed by these studies; they do share a common framework, but many question arose at this stage.

Are the cellular and molecular mechanisms underlying habituation and dishabituation of swim induction similar to that discovered in "Aplysia", or additional mechanisms with different endurances can set up in this nervous system?
Several experiments have been performed, to find out, at level of the neural circuitry underlying the swim induction, the cascade of molecular events subserving short-term changes of non associative learning type.
At first step the analysis has been carried out onto the first neuronal station of the whole networks represented by the mechanosensory neurons located in each segmental ganglion. A second series of experiments has been focused on the serotonergic neurons, the so called giant or Retzius cells.

MODULATION OF AN ELECTROGENIC PUMP IN THE MECHANOSENSORY NEURON OF THE LEECH

In each segmental ganglion of the leech three types of sensory neurons have been identified: T (touch), P (pressure) and N (nociceptive) (Nicholls and Baylor, 1968).
A burst of action potentials elicited in these neurons produces a lasting afterhyperpolarization (AH) that in T neuron is due to both an electrogenic pump and to an increase in gK whereas in P and in N it is likely due to Ca-dependent K current. One of the major function of AH is to produce a conduction block at the branching points where small axonal processes join the main neurite (Baylor and Nicholls, 1969; Van Essen, 1973).

In a first group of experiments, Belardetti et al.(1984) observed that 5HT application depressed, for a prolonged period of time (3O up to 6O min) the AH amplitude in T neurons (Fig.1). The effect is reversible and is blocked by methysergide. Similar effects have been obtained following the electrical activation of Retzius cells. The effect is not observed in P and in N neurons.
In order to clarify the mechanism underlying this effect of 5HT on T neurons, two series of investigations have been executed (Catarsi and Brunelli, 1991). In the first one the K/Ca dependent channels have been blocked either with $BaCl_2$ or $CdCl_2$. In these experimental conditions 5HT was still capable of further depressing AHP. On the contrary in experiments in which it was possible to get a residual AHP after ouabain treatment 5HT did not further affected the AHP amplitude. In a second series of experiments it has been investigated the effect of 5HT after direct activation of the Na/K electrogenic pump. The activation has been established by three different experiments: 1) Intracellular injection of Na into T sensory neurons produced a ouabain-sensitive hyperpolarization for ATPase stimulation. Perfusion with 5HT generated a depolarization because the ions could not be driven out by the block of the pump. 2) 5HT application brought about a decrease of the repolarization normally obtained with the Na/K pump activator Cs^+ after K free perfusion. 3) 5HT enhanced the depolarization phase during cooling of the ganglia and produced a reduction in the speed of repolarization when the temperature returned to 18°C. Similar effects have been observed with octopamine application. Summing up neurotransmitters, serotonin or octopamine, released by identified neurons , control the functioning of a sensory touch cell through the modulation of an electrogenic pump. This finding represent a completely novel mechanism of the neurotransmitter action (Fig.1).
Changes in the AHP amplitude produce a control of the traffic of impulses travelling along the sensory fibres. When the AHP amplitude decreases, a relief from block in branching point occurs and more action potentials are transported along the neurites and more synapses are invaded by the impulses.
The feature of this scheme is more sophisticated than the "Aplysia" model. In the leech nervous system by controlling specific loci where the fibres are branching it is possible to modulate a synaptic territory below the branching points (Catarsi and Brunelli, 1991). At this stage many questions arose: A) is this mechanism of inhibition by electrogenic pump mediated by second messengers of nucleotide type?
B) Are there substances or physiological situations which activate the electrogenic pump leading to an increase of the AHP? C) Is this effect subserving the elementary forms of non associative learning such as habituation and sensitization?

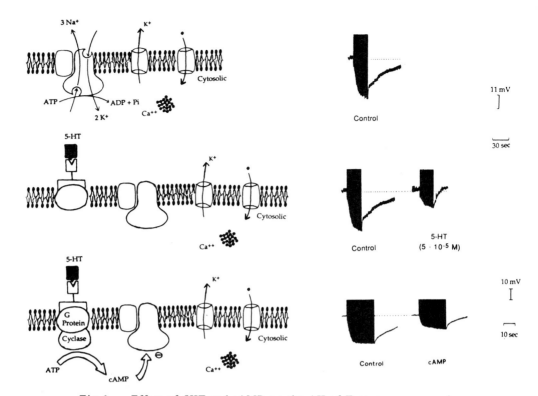

Fig. 1. Effect of 5HT and cAMP on the AH of T sensory neuron in the leech. Top trace- Intracellular stimulation of a T sensory neuron produces a burst of action potentials followed by an afterhyperpolarization (AH).

Middle trace - 5HT application (5x10⁻⁵M) reduces the amplitude of AH. This effect is due (as described in the text) to a block of the electrogenic pump.

Bottom trace - Intracellular iontophoretic injection of cAMP produces a depression of AH amplitude for inhibition of the Na/K electrogenic pump as illustrated in drawing at the left.

A) In order to give an answer to the first question a series of experiments has been planned in which the role of cAMP in mediating the 5HT effects has been studied. It has been clearly established that cAMP increase is the intermediate step which links neurotrasmitter action to the modulation of Na/K electrogenic pump. This emerges also from the recent findings of Catarsi and Brunelli (unpublished results): 1) application of cAMP analogs, 8Br-cAMP and phosphodiesterase inhibitor IBMX, provoked a reversible reduction of the AHP amplitude; 2) intracellular iontophoretic application of cAMP produced a clear cut reduction of the AHP amplitude (Fig.1, lowest trace); 3) intracellular injections of Na ions, activated the pump and generated an hyperpolarization of the resting potential. In presence of 8Br-cAMP and IBMX the hyperpolarizing effect disappeared and a depolarization arose; 4) the physiological relevance of cAMP dependent phosphorylation, triggered by 5HT is further demonstrated by neurochemical experiments in which it has been demonstrated that 5HT raises cAMP levels in the leech CNS and activates cAMP-dependent protein Kinase. A group of protein of 78 kD was phosphorylated in the presence of 5HT, 8 Br-cAMP and phorbol ester, a proteinkinase C activator (Garcia Gil et al., 1989 a,b; Garcia Gil et al., 1991).

B) Experiments still in progress gave evidence that AHP might be increased in amplitude as a result of an excitation of the electrogenic pump. Substances like FMRF-amide applied in the perfusion bath seem to enhance the AHP amplitude.It is still unknown whether this effect might be mediated by second messenger of phospholipid type.

C) Are the described effects really involved in the genesis of the non associative learning and do they play important physiological roles? Some experiments recently performed deserve attention. First of all it has been observed that ouabain injected in the whole animal prevented the dishabituation whereas was ineffective on habituation; in addition 5HT effect of sensitization were blocked by preincubation with RMI (adenylate cyclase inhibitor). These results confirmed, at behavioral level, that 5HT, through the cAMP increase,inhibits the NA/K ATPase in the sensory neuron membrane, reducing the AHP, relieving the block in the branching points and allowing the increase of traffic of action potentials which can potentiate many synaptic fields, facilitating the interconnections between sensory cells and follower neurons. This model would represent the molecular basis subserving dishabituation and/or sensitization. More recently it has been demonstrated, at cellular level, that, low frequency repeated intracellular stimulation of T sensory neurons produced a gradual long lasting increase of AHP amplitude (Fig.2).
This might represent the underlying mechanism of habituation. The increase of AHP induced a block of action potentials in the points where the axons split and get larger. All the synaptic contacts below the block become depressed (habituated). 5HT application or Retzius cells stimulations reduced back the AHP amplitude. The reduction of AHP would potentiate all the synaptic fields and sensitize the contact with the follower cells.

With an elegant experiment made up by a segmental ganglion with the nerve roots left in contact with a patch of body wall skin, it has been shown that, with a micropipette inserted in T neurons it was possible to observe that repetitive tactile stimulation of the skin produced a block of action potentials; in the cell body arrived only small changes in voltage due to the spreading of the electrotonic current. When 5HT was applied or a Retzius cell was stimulated the block was relieved and the action potentials could reach the electrode on the cell body. This represents a clear demonstration of the modulatory role of neurotransmitters on AHP.

NEUROTRANSMITTER MODULATION OF ELECTROTONIC JUNCTION

In an attempt to extende the knowledge about the cellular mechanisms of non associative learning an additional finding emerged by analysing the effect of 5HT on the two Retzius cells. The two giant neurons are usually interconnected trough an electrotonic, non rectifying synapsis (Eckert, 1963; Hagiwara and Morita, 1962).
One cell has been penetrated by two glass microelectrodes whereas one electrode was inserted in the second one.In these conditions it was possible to detect the coupling ratio between the two cells by applying pulse of constant current on one side of the junction. Injection of current into one of the two elements brought about a potential step (V_1) in the cell directly stimulated and a smaller potential shift (V_2) in the other. The attenuation factor (AF) measured by the ratio V_1/V_2, was the parameter usually utilize for quantifying the strength of the electrotonic interaction. This AF depends not only by the junctional membrane resistance, but also by the extrajunctional membrane resistance of the two cells. Application of 5HT and Dopamine (DA) produced a prolonged reduction in the electrotonic coupling between the two Retzius cells. The effect was reversible and was present also with high Mg^{2+} solution, suggesting that the

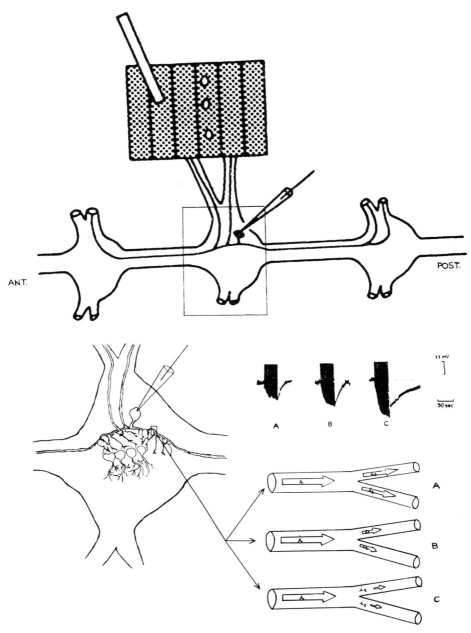

Fig.2.　In the top diagram is presented the experimental arrangement of a semi-intact preparation made up by a skin patch connected to a segmental ganglion of a chain of isolated ganglia. A micropipette is inserted in T neurons. Low frequency repetitive intracellular stimulation of a T sensory cell produces (after 15 trials) a clear increase of the amplitude of the AH. In A (control) the impulses can travel along the fibres, but in B and C, increasing the AH, the block is potentiated and many impulses cannot pass through and are shut out to take contact with follower cells.

monoamine acts directly and not through a synaptic mechanism. Several control experiments excluded that the modification of AF might be associated to a decrease in the cellular input resistance and the decoupling observed account for a direct action of the monoamine on the modulation of the junctional resistance between the two cells.

In order to evaluate whether the effect of neurotransmitter might be controlled by activation of second messengers of nucleotide type,experiments in which the internal cAMP level was handled in different ways were worked out.The decoupling effect was strongly potentiated in the presence of a phosphodiesterase inhibitor IBMX. By means of direct iontophoretical injection of cAMP into one of the Retzius cell in the presence of IBMX a strong reduction in electrotonic strength of the synapsis has been observed. The effect was highly specific because cGMP application did not change the attenuation ratio. In addition intracellular injection of an activator of adenylate cyclase, GTPgammaS (non hydrolisable analog of Guanosine Triphosphate (GTP) which produces a persistent activation of the G subunit of the adenylate cyclase brought about modification in the coupling ratio (Colombaioni and Brunelli, 1988). Perfusion of the ganglia with an agonist for D_1 receptor (SKF) caused a decoupling whereas blocking the D_2 receptor with Clebopride failed to inhibit the uncoupling effect of DA.

All the data converge on the suggestion that neurotransmitters like 5HT or DA modulate, for lasting period of time, the electrical synapses. This effect, mediated by intracellular increase of cAMP appeared to depend upon a real change in junctional pemeability.This was an unexpected phenomenon, that provided evidence that the electrical synapses can be plastic or can undergo to changes in efficacy. Likely 5HT acts through autoreceptors located in the membrane of the giant cells. It is still unknown whether this effect of modulation of gap junction after neurotransmitter application is generalized and widespread or is restricted to specific synapses. We do not know the role of this plastic changes in non associative learning process. Further investigations are needed to elucidate this point.

It is possible that there is no exclusive mechanism of short-term learning, but rather acquisition and retention process might operate in parallel. It is for this reason that we operated an investigation along the phylogenetic scale. The data collected in the leech clearly suggest that might exist a common basic molecular alphabet which can be adapted and modified in different way along the phylogenetic scale.

ENDURING MEMORY: SHORT TO LONG TERM LEARNING PROCESS

All the investigations described suggest that the linkage neurotransmitter-second messenger is critical expecially in acquisition and short-term memory. But is a general knowledge that retention of learned informations has two major components: the so called short-term (S.T.) learning process lasting minutes to hours and long tem (L.T.) learning process in which the engrams remain for days or weeks.
What are the chain of events provoking this passage from S.T. to L.T. one? and which mechanisms are involved in generating enduring memory?
One of the most suggestive idea is represented by the macromolecular synthesis hypothesis. One can assume that in L.T.memory a cluster of newly synthesized protein is set up stabilizing and extending the mechanisms which operate in short-term memory by initiating new type of cellular changes. Many research were oriented to perform experiments in this direction and it has been demonstrated that inhibitor of messenger RNA or protein synthesis may block or disrupt the long term modifications, leaving the short-term unchanged. This occurs when the inhibitors are administered 1 or 2 hours after training (Barondes and Jarvik, 1964; Agranoff et al., 1965; Barondes and Cohen, 1966; Rainbow, 1979).

But in earlier experiments the results were questionable, because the animal models were complicated and it was difficult to keep controlled all the variability of the system and at cellular level was impossible to compare the effects on short-term and long-term modifications. More recently the withdrawal reflex system studied in "Aplysia" has shown powerful experimental advantages. The monosynaptic sensory -motor network of the reflex has been reconstitute in cell culture. In a representative set of investigations, several successive application of 5HT within about 2 hour resulted in a potentiation of the EPSP recorded in the motoneurons for more than 24 hours. This was regarded as long term (Montarolo et al., 1986). Inhibitors of protein synthesis (anysomycin and emetine) and inhibitors of mRNA synthesis (actinomycin D and alfa-amanitine) blocked L.T. sensitization without affecting the short-term ones (Montarolo et al., 1986). There was a critical "time window" for the inhibitory action; the drugs were effective when applied during the serotonin treatment, but not if applied before or after training.This "time window" is present also in various forms of memory in invertebrate and perhaps also in man.

These findings suggest that L.T. sensitization require genic products, depending on translation and trascription processes, whereas the S.T. does not need neoformation of substances, but is set up by changes in preexisting proteins through mechanisms of phosphorylation. In eucariotic cells, many cAMP-inducible genes are activated by protein kinase cAMP-dependent (PK-A) which induces phosphorylation of trascriptional factors which bind a cAMP responsive element (CRE). This, in turn, binds to a protein (CRE binding protein-CREBP) which increases trascription when phosphorilated by kinase A.
Recent experiments (Dash et al., 1990) has been performed in which into the nucleus of sensory neuron (in colture with motoneurons) has been injected a sequence of somatostatin CRE. The rationale of this investigation was the following: if the injected sequence CRE comes in competition with a ligand protein CREBP simil, this protein were inhibited in activating cAMP inducible genes, with a block of long-term potentiation. The data confirmed this hypothesis. The cascade of events which lead to the formation of a L.T. potentiation might be the following:5HT induces activation of protein kinase cAMP dependent (Kinase A), which phosphorylates factors CREBP-like that binds with a cAMP sensitive element(CRE) that activates inducible genes. All the effects described are not present if the motoneurons are absent in the "in vitro" culture. What are the changes triggered by the newly formed proteins? Some suggestions come from two different lines of research.
1) Bailey and Chen (1983, 1988) have found out that during L.T. sensitization three main feature appeared: a) the number of varicosities in the sensory neurons increased up to doubling; b) more varicosities presented an active zone, indicating the increase of synaptic activity; c) it has been detected an increase in the total number of vescicles associated at the releasing pool. All these data suggest that active zone and varicosities are plastic structure that can be modulated during persistent memory enconding.

In addition to these observation are the recent experiments of the same groups which demonstrated that during L.T. sensitization it was present a reduction of adhesion proteins of NCAM type which usually maintain rigid and solid the synaptic contact. This down regulation might induce a decrease of the tight of the synaptic knobs in order to rearrange the synaptic arrays to allow that structural changes important for the plastic modifications. This process appears similar to that operating during development and maturation. During the development the neurons growth and take contacts with target cells generating the synaptic networks with tight ultrastructural contacts. Once reached the maturation those mechanisms are stopped and kept silent. When a learning process arise, through the activation of phosphoprotein, a chain of events in the genoma produces a temporary activation of the factors which worked during the development, likely by means of the block of a repressor which inhibited the development. This theory ehibits undoubtedly a beautiful unity of the cellular process which are functioning both during learning and during growth. In this sense formation of a stable engram of memory might be analogous to what is occurring during developmental process.

It is possible that not all the events undelying L.T. sensitization might be described with this structural model; other changes can be set up at biochemical level, for example a persistent activation of proteinkinase, or some effect on the phosphatases which control the persistance of protein phosphorylation. Further investigations can clarify, at molecular and biophysical level, the question still open.

In "Aplysia" L.T. habituation is impaired by protein synthesis inhibitors and also in this process the Kandel group claims for several ultrastructural changes opposite to that observed in L.T. sensitization. This fascinating hypothesis received strong reinforcement by recent finding collected utilizing the recently developed methodology of low light level video microscopy (Kater and Hadley, 1982; Purves and Hadley, 1985). This technique allows the visualization of a living neuron structure repeatedly over the course of several days. Experiments with fluorescent videomicroscopy have demonstrated that repeated application of 5HT produced an increase in the number of processes or varicosities of sensory neurons. For these changes the presence of the motoneurons was necessary.

From all these studies on the model of "Aplysia" emerges therefore a splendid unitary theory of cellular processes acting either during onthogeny or during plasticity which accompanies learning processes in mature stage of grown up, but a criticism cannot be neglected. Almost all the investigations have been carried out "in vitro", in neuronal networks made up by cells in regeneration or in developing stages. A doubt exists that the structural changes and the synaptic modifications observed might be correlated mostly with the still developing or rearranging processes rather than to the stabilizazion of engrams. For this reason many data deserve confirmation in alternative model.

In order to add more informations to the knowledge of the putative mechanisms responsible of the shift from S.T. into the L.T. processes, several experiments on L.T. sensitization in behavioral model of the swim in the leech have been carried out.
By applying every day a session of stimulation it has been possible to obtain a long term habituation. After 6 days the latency between the stimulus and the onset of the response increased, reached the maximum after 7-9 days and persisted for many weeks. In similar manner, it has been possible to induce L.T. sensitization with the treatment of one session of noxius stimulation daily for 6 days. The experimental group exhibited a shortening of the latency for inducing swim that was markedly lower than that on the control group and than that measured on the first day (Fig.3).This potentiation persisted for several days with slow gradual comeback to normal latency. It has been possible, by applying at regular interval for 24 hours, the same amount of stimuli given over 6 days a kind of " massive potentiation".
Inhibitors of protein synthesis (cychloeximide, puromycin) and mRNA blocking agents (actinomycin D) applied on alternate days blocked significantly the L.T. facilitation of inducing swimming whereas the S.T. modifications were unchanged.
Surprisingly, the L.T. habituation was not affected either by protein synthesis inhibitors, or by mRNA inhibitors.
Summing up: 1) in the behavioral model of the leech, S.T. and L.T. show different mechanisms; 2) L.T. sensitization requires the synthesis of novel proteins.

All these data confirm the framework of the "Aplysia" model, but we have seen that the cellular and molecular mechanisms of the two systems differ substantially. Following the unitary theory of growth and learning,it is only possible to speculate that in this L.T. processes in the leech, one possible explanation can be focused on the neurogenesis. By varying the branching of the neuritic tree,it is possible to enhance or decrease the modulation of the AH exerted by neurotransmitters. But in addition(or in alternative) to this structural dependent modifications some other putative hypothesis can be exploited:
A) For habituation: 1) during the repetitive sessions a peptide or some other substances can build up,exerting its potentiation of AH; 2) phosphorylation of protein can trigger,through cAMP mediation,activation of tubulin and fibrillogenesis which increase the branching points,and therefore the passage of impulses; 3) an increase of autoreceptors binding the neurotransmitters released by the sensory neurons itself.
B) For sensitization: 1) the formation of substances which keep depressed the AH of sensory neuron,or keep inactivated the phosphatase complex; 2) a substance which potentiates the electrical coupling among the sensory cells,in the way that they can work as a whole.

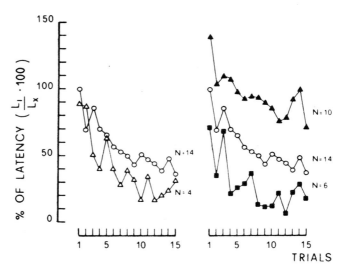

Fig. 3. Long-term sensitization in the swim model.
The animals has a lesion between the cephalic ganglion and the first segmental ganglion. Swimming activity is evoked by electrical stimulation of the tail. The latency between the starting of the stimulus and the onset of the swim cycle is detected by a photocell and recorded. The measurement of the first response is considered as 100% and all the other responses are normalized to the first one. The stimuli are applied at low frequency (1/min). The curves on the left exhibit the habituation of the control group: repetitive stimulation produces a gradual increase in latency (open circle) (the ordinate of the graph represents the reciprocal of this measurements). After seven days without any application of sensitizing stimulation the animals are tested again (open triangles). The two curves have similar slope. The graphs on the right illustrates the results of animals receiving daily sensitizing stimuli. The curve with open circles represents the recordings made on the first day, whereas the curve with black triangles report the recordings made after six days of application of sensitizing stimuli. This curve is statistically higher than that of the control (long-term sensitization). The curve with black square represents the recording made five days after the end of sensitizing stimulation and shows a clear recovery from long-term sensitization.

Only further investigations can give an answer to the knowledge of the real mechanisms. In conclusion, it is clear that in the memory process exists a molecular alphabet represented by the linkage neurotransmitter-chain of second messenger, modification of function of cellular membrane or changes in genomic factors. But the real expression of such mechanisms can vary from different systems in relationship to the specific various adaptative mechanisms that all the species have to set up in the continuous dialogue with the environment and also in consideration of the increasing complexity of the behavioral act of the higher vertebrates.

The reductionistic approach has undoubtedly the merit of discovering the elementary mechanisms of plasticity of neural structures experimented, during the long history of phylogeny, by the different species for their survival.

REFERENCES

Agranoff,B.W.,Davis,R.E.,and Brink,J.J.,1965, Memory fixation in the gold fish, Proc.Natl.Acad.Sci.,54:788-793.

Bailey,C.H.,and Chen,M.,1983,Morpholgical basis of long term habituation and sensitization in "Aplysia",Science,220:91-93.

Bailey,C.H.,and Chen,M., 1988 , Long-term sensitization in "Aplysia" increases the number of presynaptic contacts onto the identified gill motorneuron L7, Proc.Natl.Acad.Sci.,USA, 85: 9356-9359.

Barondes,S.H.,and Jarvik,M.E., 1964 ,The influence of actinomycin D on brain RNA synthesis and on memory, J.Neurochem., 11: 187-195.

Barondes,S.H.,and Cohen,H.D., 1966 , Puromycin effect on successive phases of memory storage, Science, 151: 594-595.

Baylor,D.A.,and Nicholls,J.G., 1969, After-effect of nerve signalling in the central nervous system of the leech, J.Physiol.,Lon., 203: 571-589.

Belardetti,F.,Biondi,C.,Brunelli,M.,Colombaioni,L.,and Trevisani, A., 1982, Role of serotonin and cAMP on facilitation of the fast conducting system activity in the "Hirudo m.", Brain Res., 246:89-103.

Belardetti,F.,Brunelli,M.,Demontis,G.,and Sonetti,D., 1984, Serotonin and Retzius cell depress the hyperpolarization following impulses of the leech touch cell, Brain Res., 300: 91-102.

Brunelli,M.,Castellucci,V.F.,and Kandel,E.R., 1976, Synaptic facilitation and behavioral sensitization in "Aplysia": possible role of serotonin and cAMP, Science,194: 1178-1181.

Castellucci,V.F.,Pinsker,H.,Kupfermann,I.,and Kandel,E.R., 1970, Neuronal mechanisms of habituation and dishabituation of the gill-withdrawal reflex in "Aplysia", Science, 167:1745-1748.

Castellucci,V.F.,and Kandel,E.R., 1974, A quantal analysis of the synaptic depression underlying habituation of the gill withdrawal reflex in "Aplysia", Proc.Natl.Acad.Sci.USA, 71:5004-5008.

Castellucci,V.F., and Kandel,E.R., 1976 , Presynaptic facilitation as a mechanism for behavioral sensitization in "Aplysia", Science, 194 : 1176-1178.

Catarsi,S., and Brunelli,M., 1991 ,Serotonin depresses the after-hyperpolarization through the inhibition of the Na/K electrogenic pump in T sensory neurones of the leech, J.Exp.Bio.,155: 261-273.

Colombaioni,L.,and Brunelli,M., 1988 , Neurotransmitter-induces modulation of an electrotonic synapse in the CNS of "Hirudo m.", Exp.Biol., 47: 139-144.

Dagan,D.,and Levitan,I.B., 1981 , Isolated identified "Aplysia" neurons in cell culture, J.Neurosci.,1:736-740.

Dash P. K., Hochner B., and Kandel, E.R., 1990, Injection of cAMP-responsive element into the nucleus of "Aplysia" sensory neurons blocks long-term facilitation, Nature, 345: 718-721.

Eckert,R., 1963 ,Electrical interaction of paired ganglion cells in the leech, J.Gen.Physiol, 46: 573-587.

Hagiwara,S.,and Morita,H., 1962, Electrotonic transmission between two nerve cells in leech ganglion, J. Neurophysiol., 25: 721-731.

Hochner,B.,Klein,M.,Schacher,S.,and Kandel,E.R., 1986, Additional component in the cellular mechanism of presynaptic facilitation contributes to behavioral dishabituation in "Aplysia", Proc.Natl.Acad.USA,83: 8794-8798.

Kandel,E.R.,Brunelli,M,Byrne,J.,and Castellucci,V.F., 1973, A common presynaptic locus for the synaptic changes underlying short-term habituation and sensitization of the gill withdrawal reflex in "Aplysia", in:"Cold Spring Harbor Symp., Quant.Biol." 48:465-482.

Kandel,E.R,1976,"Cellular basis of behavior" Freeman, S.Francisco.

Kandel,E.R.,and Schwartz,J.H.,1982, Molecular biology of learning:modulation of transmitter release,Science 218: 433-443.

Kater, S.D., and Hadley, R.D., 1982, Intracellular staining combined with videoflorescence microscopy for viewing living neurons. In "Cytochemical methods in neuroanatomy", S. Palay and V. Chan Palay, Alan R. Liss, New York, 441-459.

Klein, M., Shapiro,E.,and Kandel,E.R., 1980 a , Synaptic plasticity and the modulation of the Ca current, J.Exp.Bio.,89:117-157.

Klein,M.,and Kandel,E.R., 1980 b , Mechanism of Calcium current modulation underlying presynaptic facilitation and behavioral sensitization in "Aplysia" , Proc.Natl.Acad.Sci.,USA. 77:6912-6916.

Konorski,J., 1948 ,"Conditioned reflex and neuron organization", Cambridge University Press,Cambridge.

Kristan,W., 1983 , The neurobiology of swimming in the leech,Trend in Neurosci.,6: 84-89.

Marcus,E.A.,Nolen,T.G.,Rankin,C.H.,and Carew,T.J., 1988, Behavioral dissociation of dishabituation,sensitization and inhibition in "Aplysia" ,Science,241:210-213.

Montarolo,P.G.,Goelet,P.,Castellucci,V.F.,Morgan,J.,Kandel,E. and Schacher,S., 1986 , A critical period for macromolecular synthesis in long-term heterosynaptic facilitation in "Aplysia", Science,234: 1249-1254.

Nicholls,J.G.,and Baylor,D.A., 1968 ,Specific modalities and receptive fields of sensory neurons in the CNS of the leech, J.Neurophysiol.,31:740-756.

Purves D., and Hadley, R.D., 1985, Changes in the dendritic branching of adult mammalian neurones revealed by repeated imaging "in situ", Nature, 315: 404-406.

Rainbow,T.C., 1979 ,Role of RNA and protein synthesis in memory formation, Neurochem.Res. 4: 297-312.

Rayport,S.G.,and Schacher,S., 1986 , Synaptic plasticity "in vitro": cell culture of identified "Aplysia" neurons mediating short-term habituation and sensitization, J. Neurosci., 6: 759-763.

Saktor,T.C.,O'Brian,C.A.,Weinstein,I.B.,andSchwartz,J.H., 1986, Translocation from cytosol to membrane of proteinkinase C after stimulation of "Aplysia" neurons with serotonin.Soc.Neurosci.Abstr.,12 :1340.

Schacher,S.,and Proshansky,E., 1983 , Neurite regeneration by "Aplysia" neurons in dissociated cell culture: modulation by "Aplysia" hemolimph and the presence of the initial axonal segment,J.Neurosci.3: 2403-2413.

Shuster,M.J.,Camardo,J.S.,Siegelbaum,S.A.,and Kandel,E.R., 1985, Cyclic AMP-dependent protein kinase closes the serotonin-sensitive K channels of "Aplysia" sensory neurons in cell-free membrane patches, Nature, 313:392-395.

Siegelbaum,S.A., Camardo,J.S.,and Kandel,E.R., 1982 , Serotonin and cAMP close single K channel in "Aplysia" sensory neurons, Nature, 299:413-417.

Stent,G.,and Kristan,W., 1981 , Neural circuits generating rhythmic movements.Neurobiology of the leech. In: "Cold Spring Harbor Laboratory", 52:113-146.

Van Essen,D.C., 1973 , The contribution of membrane hyperpolarization to adaptation and conduction block in sensory neurones of the leech, J.Physiol.,Lond.,230:509- 534.

MATURATION AND PLASTICITY OF NEUROPEPTIDES IN THE VISUAL SYSTEM*

Paola Bagnoli*, Simona Di Gregorio, Margherita Molnar,
Cristina Romei and Gigliola Fontanesi

*Faculty of Science, University of Tuscia, 01100 Viterbo
and Department of Physiology and Biochemistry, University
of Pisa, 56127 Pisa, Italy

INTRODUCTION

A large number of peptides have been recently described within the vertebrate central nervous system. Some of them were previously localized in non-neural vertebrate tissue as well as lower species in which they may serve as primitive elements of intercellular communication (Krieger, 1983).

Neuropeptides are simply small proteins defined as chains of aminoacids held together by peptide bonds. In looking over a list of neuropeptides sets of peptides with similar structures can be identified within a peptide family, suggesting a synthesis from the same precursor. An interesting consequence of peptides being synthetized from a common precursor is cotrasmission within and across peptide families. Cotrasmission also occurs between peptides and "classical" trasmitters (Hokfelt et al., 1980).

Peptide synthesis in neurons is characterized by post-translational proteolitic cleavage of larger precursor molecules, which in themselves have no biological activity. Ribosomial protein synthesis takes place in the endoplasmic reticulum at a considerable

---
*Supported by the CNR Target Project on Biotechnology and Biostrumentation.

distance from the secretory site of the axon terminal. In contrast, classical trasmitters are made by the action of specific enzymes at the synapse.

Although the function of neuropeptides is still not well understood, numerous observations are consistent with a neurotrasmitter/neuromodulator role for neuropeptides in the nervous system. Data obtained so far support a role for peptides in chemical trasmission that is auxiliary to that of classical trasmitters. On the other hand, there is now increasing evidence for a non-trasmitter-like action, expecially trophic effect (Pincus et al, 1990). Considerable evidences do exist on the effects of brain peptides on several homeostatic systems. On the other hand, brain peptides are supposed to exert also a specific role on neural signalling. Electrophysiological results reported so far suggest the possibility that peptides modulate the neuronal excitability (Colmers et al., 1988) either by regulating the release of other trasmitters or by influencing specific ionic currents (Wang et al., 1990).

NEUROPEPTIDES IN THE VISUAL SYSTEM

Over the last years, the vertebrate visual system has been largely used to study the distribution of peptides at the adult stage or during brain maturation. In particular, the value of the vertebrate retina to these studies remains unsurpassed. Less information are available on peptide distribution in central visual regions as well as on the role of retinal afferents in regulating peptide distribution. Moreover, the functional role of peptides in visual processing remains largely to be clarified. The fact that neuropeptides are mostly found in intraretinal neurons and not in the optic nerve implies that they act as solely retinal peptides and do not take part in the direct transmission of visual information through the retina into the optic nerve. Recent experiments with in vitro eye-cup preparations suggest that some peptides do not partecipate in shaping the characteristic receptive field properties of ganglion cells but they rather modulate the excitability of inner retinal neurons (Zalutsky and Miller, 1990). Recent evidences, however, suggest the possibility that retinal ganglion cells use specific peptides in their signalling processes. In particular, numerous evidences indicate that substance P (SP) is localized to ganglion cells in anurans, birds and mammals (Kuljis and Karten, 1986; Tahara et al., 1986; Brecha et al., 1987). The majority of somatostatinergic retinal neurons are classified as wide field amacrine cells with the somata located in the ganglion cell layer and with beaded processes which spread through the nerve fiber and inner plexiform layer (Marshak, 1989). Another somatostatinergic cell type has been recently identified in the cat retina as alpha ganglion cells predominantly of the off-center type (White and Chalupa, 1991). On the other hand, in situ hybridization histochemistry failed to identify somatostatinergic ganglion cells and revealed intraretinal cell bodies expressing mRNA for prosomatostatin (Ferriero et al., 1990). Neuropeoptide Y (NPY) appears to be mainly localized to intraretinal cell groups (Isayama and Eldred, 1988) but recently, NPY localization to the soma and axonal processes of large ganglion cells of the human retina has been also reported (Straznicky and Hiscock, 1988).

THE PIGEON VISUAL SYSTEM AS AN EXPERIMENTAL MODEL

Over the last few years, we used the visual system of the pigeon as a suitable model to study maturative and plastic processes in the brain. Indeed the developmental time-course of the pigeon visual system differs from that of other non-mammalian species. In fact, maturative events that normally occur during incubation "in ovo", take place during the early post-hatching period in pigeons (Bagnoli et al., 1985, 1987; Porciatti et al. 1985). This delayed maturation allows to obtain newborns which are still susceptible to experimental manipulations such as retina removal. Unilateral retinal ablation has marked effects on the organization of the pigeon visual system. If performed immediately after hatching, this procedure results in a drastic shrinkage of the main primary and secondary visual regions contralateral to the removed retina with an associated altered cytoarchitecture which is maintained in the adult. These alterations do not reflect degenerative processes but rather an abnormal maturation induced by removing the retina before ganglion cell axons have completely invaded their targets (Bagnoli et al., 1989a).

We used immunohistochemical methods to study the distribution of NPY, SP and somatostatin (SOM) in central visual regions of normal adults and at different stages during maturation. In addition, adults with one retina removed at different stages after hatching (either before, or after, retinal connections with primary visual regions are established) were also used. The aim of these experiments was to investigate whether the distribution of peptide-immunoreactivity was influenced by retinal afferents either directly or transsynaptically.

The general trend in the variation of peptide-immunoreactivity includes a progressive decrease in the numerical density of immunostained cell bodies and a progressive increase in the density of stained fibers and terminal-like processes. Only if performed immediatly after hatching (i.e. before retinal connections are established), retina removal has marked effects on the distribution of peptide-immunoreactivity in visual structures contralateral to the removed retina.

METHODS

Details of retina removal, fixation procedure and immunochemical methods have been described in Bagnoli et al. (1989 a;b). Rat monoclonal antibodies directed to SP (Sera Lab, MAS 035b Accurate,YMC 1021), rabbit polyclonal antiserum to NPY (Peninsula RAS 7172N) and mouse monoclonal antibody to SOM 8 (generously provided by Allison Buchan) were used in this study.

Quantitative evaluations and statistical analysis of variations in peptide distribution were obtained by a personal system of computerized image processing on coronal sections of the pigeon brain (Bagnoli et al., 1989b). In particular, the number of immunostained cells per cubic millimeter of tissue (numerical density, Nv) was determined by using stereological methods. An analysis of variance showed a significant effect of age on labeled cell numerical density. Variations in Nv of NPY- and SP-positive cell bodies of specific visual regions at the different developmental stages are shown in Fig.1. In addition, Nv of labeled cell bodies in visual structures of adult pigeons with early retina removal is also shown (filled squares in Fig.1).

DISTRIBUTION OF NPY-, SP- AND SOM-IMMUNOREACTIVITY IN THE PIGEON VISUAL SYSTEM: DEVELOPMENTAL CHANGES AND EFFECTS OF RETINA REMOVAL AT HATCHING

Mesencephalon: Optic Tectum and other Mesencephalic Visual Nuclei

NPY-immunoreactivity. In TeO of normal adults no immunoreactive cell bodies can be detected, NPY-positive fibers and terminals show a precise laminar distribution at the level of superficial neuropil with particularly dense processes in retino-recipient tectal layers 3, 5 and 7 (according to the nomenclature of Ramon y Cajal 1891).

This laminar segregation is progressively reached over the first 9 days after hatching when labeled fibers often presenting growth cones are diffusely present. No NPY-immunoreactivity can be detected at any embrional stages. Variations in NPY-positive fibers distribution over age are shown in the photomicrographs of Fig. 2. Early retina removal results in a complete loss of laminar segregation of NPY-immunoreactivity which instead forms a dense band of intensely stained neuropil just below the tectal surface (Fig.2 F). Observed changes likely depend on transsynaptic phenomena especially given the lack of convincing evidence of a retinal NPY contribution. If one excludes the possibility of a contribution of NPY-containing retinal ganglion cells other possible sources of NPY tectal innervation are the thalamic nucleus of the marginal optic tract (nMOT, corresponding to the intergeniculate leaflet of mammals) which projects to the tectal layer 4 and 7 (Hamassaky and Britto, 1990) and the mesencephalic nucleus pretectalis (PT) which projects to tectal layer 5 (Karten et al. 1982).

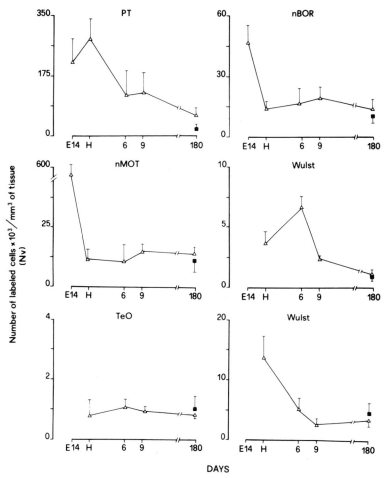

Fig.1 Numerical density, Nv (number of cells per $10^3/mm^3$ of tissue, open triangles) of immunostained cell bodies in visual areas at different stages. Numerical density of NPY-positive cells in the n. pretectalis (PT), the nucleus of the basal optic root (nBOR), the nucleus of the marginal optic tract (nMOT) and the wulst is shown together with the number of SP-positive cells per tissue volume in the optic tectum (TeO) and the wulst. The filled squares refer to Nv of labeled cells in the same visual regions of adult pigeons with one retina removed on the day of hatching.

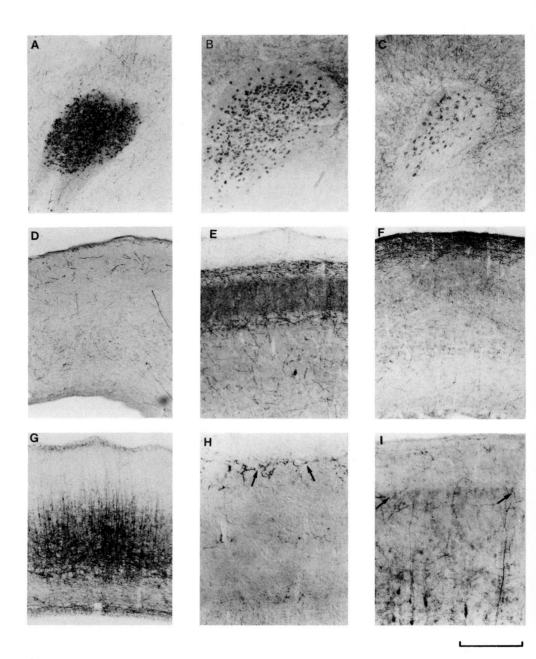

Fig. 2 Photomicrographs to illustrate the distribution of peptide-immunostaining on transverse sections of the pigeon mesencephalon. A-B: NPY-positive cells in the nucleus pretectalis at hatching and 180 days after hatching. C: pattern of immunostaining in the nucleus pretectalis contralateral to the retina removed at hatching. D-E: NPY-stained neuropil in the optic tectum at hatching and in the adult, respectively. F: lamination of NPY-positive fibers and terminals is lost if

In both these nuclei numerous NPY-positive cells can be observed since E14. Their numerical density significantly decreases over time until the adult organization is reached. Early retina removal significantly decreases the density of labeled cells in PT whereas NPY-positive cells of the nMOT are unaffected. Loss of NPY-containing cells in PT likely involves the PT-tectal loop (Karten et al. 1982). In the photomicrographs of Fig. 2 A-C labeled cell bodies of PT are shown at different developmental stages (Fig. 2 A-B) as well as in adults with unilateral retina ablation (Fig. 2 C).

Another primary retinorecipient region in the ventral mesencephalon referred to as the nucleus of the basal optic root (nBOR) of the accessory optic system shows labeled cells, fibers and terminal-like processes in the adult pigeon. Fibers and terminals are likely to derive from NPY-positive somata of the nMOT. From E14 to 9 days after hatching the density of stained neuropil increases whereas the numerical density of stained cells decreases. Retinal removal at hatching does not affect the density of labeled cells whereas the labeled neuropil is reduced to a dense band of labeled fibers superficial to the margin of the ventral mesencephalon.

SP-immunoreactivity. In TeO, the adult pattern is characterized by a laminar distribution of immunoreactivity which is densely present in the dorso-lateral region.

Numerous stained bipolar cells can be observed in the tectal laminae 9-11. They show long apical processes which reach up to layer 2. SP-positive processes are mostly found in laminae 2, 4, 7. Fine granular network with sparse labeled cells can be observed in the ventral tectum. The adult pattern is reached in about 9 days after hatching. No immunoreactivity can be found before the day of hatching. At hatching, intensely stained cells giving off long processes ascending toward the tectal surface can be observed in the central tectal portion. It should be noted that this region is the first to be invaded by retinal axons. Simultaneously to retinal invasion, the progressive lamination of the superficial neuropil occurs (Bagnoli et al., 1987). The possibility of a causal relationship between ingrowing retinal afferents and SP expression by tectal cells can be postulated by the present results. Surprisingly, following retina removal at hatching SP-positive cell bodies can also be detected in the ventral part of the

the retina is removed on the day of hatching. G: SP-stained cells and processes of the lateral tectum at hatching. Cell apical processes reach the superficial tectal laminae. H: SP-positive processes are laminarly distributed in the superficial tectal layers in the adult. I: SP-positive processes of the superficial laminae are drastically reduced in the optic tectum contralateral to the retina removal and apical processes of immunostained cells appear to retract and terminate in layer 8 (arrows). (Scale bar: A-C 340 μm; D-G 310 μm; H-I 100 μm) deafferented tectum. Late retina removal fails to cause such changes suggesting that deafferentation before the establishment of the neural network is a prerequisite for the increased biosynthesis of SP. Other consequences of retina deafferentation are a drastic reduction of SP-positive fibers of the superficial tectal laminae and a retraction of apical processes of SP-positive cells of the dorsal tectum which appear to terminate in layer 8 (rather in layer 2 like in normal adults). In the photomicrographs of Fig. 2 G-I labeled cell bodies and terminal-like processes are shown at different developmental stages as well as in adults with unilateral retina ablation.

Results reported above strongly suggest a role of retinal afferents in regulating the distribution of SP-immunoreactivity in TeO. The almost complete disappareance of labeled processes in the superficial neuropil of the deafferented tectum suggests the possibility of a contribution of SP-positive retinal ganglion cells.

In the rat superior colliculus SP-positive cells and processes are localized mostly at the level of the dorsal half of the stratum griseum superficiale (SGS) and intermedium (SGI). Eye enucleation at birth affects the production of SP by neurons in the ventral part of the SGS and SGI at the deafferented superior colliculus.

The appearance of SP-positive neurons following neonatal eye enucleation may be due at least in part to an increase in SP production at somata induced by possible reorganization of other neuronal systems in the superior colliculus (Hidalgo et al., 1990).

SOM-immunoreactivity. In TeO, the adult pattern includes the presence of: i) labeled fibers and terminals in the tectal layer 2, 8 and 10; iii) numerous labeled terminal-like processes which surround unlabeled cells in layer 8; iv) large weakly stained cells which are diffusely present in layer 12. At E14 rare labeled fibers are present in the superficial neuropil and numerous labeled fibers can be observed in the deep tectal layers. No terminal-like processes are present neither at embrional stages nor at hatching. From hatching to 9 days fiber density progressively increases until to reach the adult-like organization. Retina removal at early stages does not appear to affect immunoreactivity in layers 8, 10 and 12 whereas fibers and terminals of the superficial layers seem to decrease in density.

At the level of the nBOR of the adult pigeon numerous labeled cells can be observed on its dorsal division. This pattern of distribution is reached over the first week after hatching. From E14 to 7-9 days after hatching labeled cells appear diffusely distributed into the nuclear region. Retina removal at hatching induces a significant decrease of SOM-containing cell density.

Diencephalon

NPY-immunoreactivity. Labeled cells and fibers can be observed in the nMOT of the normal adult whereas only numerous fibers can be observed in the nucleus geniculatus lateralis, pars ventralis (GLv). According to the general trend in peptide variation during maturation, cell density significantly decreases whereas fiber density increases over time. Immunoreactive cells in the nMOT can be detected since E14 whereas positive fibers in GLv can first be observed at hatching. Early retina removal does not affect NPY-immunoreactivity in the nMOT whereas the deafferented GLV shows an apparent increase in the staining intensity of the NPY positive band superficial to the lateral margin of the ventral thalamus. If one excludes the possibility of NPY retinal contribution, good candidates to the GLv innervation are NPY-positive cells which are present in a telencephalic region denominated as the visual wulst (telencephalic target of the retino-thalamic visual pathway) .

SP-immunoreactivity. Dense SP innervation is present in the main primary visual thalamic nuclei of the adult pigeon. The adult pattern is reached through a progressive increase in the density of stained fibers. No immunoreactivity can be detected before hatching. The diffuse distribution of SP-positive processes, their varicose appearance and the fact that they are unaffected by retina removal suggest the possibility that SP colocalizes in monoaminergic fibers and terminals. Indeed, the pattern of SP labelling is strikingly similar to that of catecolamine distribution obtained in other studies (Bagnoli and Casini, 1985)

SOM-immunoreactivity. No evident immunoreactivity is present in the visual thalamic regions at any stages.

Telencephalon

NPY-immunoreactivity. In the adult, numerous labeled cells and intensely stained neuropil can be observed in the lateral portion of the anterior wulst. The adult pattern is reached over the first week after hatching through a progressive increase of immunostained cells and processes. No effects can be observed after retina removal.

SP-immunoreactivity. In the adult, SP positive cells and processes show a distinct laminar distribution in the lateral portion of the wulst. This organization is reached over the first 9 days after hatching with a progressive decrease of labeled cells and an increase of stained processes. No changes in SP-immunoreactivity can be observed following retina removal.

SOM-immunoreactivity. Numerous somatostatinergic cell bodies can be observed in the dorsal and lateral telencephalon including the visual wulst and the ectostriatum (the telencephalic target of the retino-tectal visual pathway). Intensely labeled cells are sparsely distributed without an apparent laminar distribution. Numerous moderately stained cells can be observed since E14. In contrast to the diffuse distribution typical of the adult stage, labeled cells appear laminarly organized at early stages in either the wulst or the ectostriatum. Indeed, numerous cells are present in the hyperstriatum accessorium (HA), the nucleus intercalatus hyperstriati accessorii (IHA) and the lamina frontalis superior (LFS) as well as the periectostriatal belt. No effects can be observed following retina removal.

CONCLUSIONS

The wide distribution of neuropeptides in the non-mammalian brain, as well as their early appearance over maturation suggest a rather conservative role of brain peptides during evolution. In addition, the concept of an equivalence among corresponding structures in non-mammalian and mammalian brains is further supported by a comparable distribution of peptidergic systems in the adult or during development.

As shown by the present study, NPY-,SP- and SOM-containing cells and processes of the developing visual system change their distribution over time until to reach the adult-like organization. The adult pattern of distribution shown in this study is in agreement with previous findings either in birds or in corresponding stuctures of the mammalian visual system (Brecha et al., 1987; Nagakawa et al., 1988; Bennet-Clarke et al., 1989; Anderson and Reiner, 1990; Hamassaki and Britto, 1990; Shimizu and Karten, 1990).

In particular, the present findings demonstrate an elaborate laminar pattern of peptide-immunoreactivity at the level of the superficial optic tectum, the main retinorecipient area in the non-mammalian brain. This observation is compatible with the existence of various classes of peptide-containing retinal ganglion cells which contribute at least in part to lamina specific peptidergic arborization in the optic tectum. This possibility is also suggested by the modifications in the pattern of peptide-immunoreactivity induced by early retina deafferentation although transsynaptic phenomena cannot be excluded. Previous studies postulated the existence of peptide-positive retinal ganglion cells and suggested the possibility of their differential functional role strictly related to their differential laminar termination at the mesencephalic level (Kuljis and Karten, 1989).

As shown by our results retinal deafferentation has marked effects on peptidergic systems suggesting an important role of retinal fibers in regulating peptide expression by visual neurons.

Marked effects of retina removal are observed at the level of the optic tectum and related pretectal nuclei. In contrast, the visual thalamus and the visual wulst are almost unaffected by retinal deafferentation. These findings further support the possibility that in non-primates including non-mammals the midbrain pathways (retina to optic tectum/superior colliculus to thalamus, to telencephalon) play an important role for the processing of visual information

Changes in peptide expression over maturation can be attributed to numerous factors including 1) cell death, 2) secondary migration, 3) morphological trasformation, 4) variation in trasmitter level, 5) change in phenotype expression etc.(Huntley et al, 1988).

Generally, the trasmitter status of a neuron represents a dynamic process influenced by multiple factors including genetic program, afferent influences, hormones, efferent innervation etc. Among these factors afferent innervation plays an important role during brain maturation as demostrated here by experiments with early retina ablated pigeons. At the functional level neurons may respond to different factors by altering trasmitter phenotypic expression and, presumably, their functional activity, in terms of signals sent to other neuronal populations. In this respect, modifications in peptidergic systems over brain maturation or following retina ablation are likely to reflect an important role of neuropeptides during the functional development of the visual system.

REFERENCES

Anderson, K. D. and Reiner, A., 1990, Distribution and relative abundance of neurons in the pigeon forebrain containing somatostatin, NPY or both, J. Comp. Neurol., 299:261.

Bagnoli, P. and Casini, G., 1985, Regional distribution of catecholaminergic terminals in the pigeon visual system, Brain Res. 337:277.

Bagnoli, P., Porciatti, V., Lanfranchi, A. and Bedini C., 1985, Developing pigeon retina: light evoked responses and ultrastructure of outer segments and synapses. J.Comp. Neurol. 235:384.

Bagnoli, P., Porciatti, V., Fontanesi, G. and Sebastiani, L., 1987, Morphological and functional changes in the retinotectal system of the pigeon during the early posthatching period, J. Comp. Neurol. 256:400.

Bagnoli, P., Casini, G., Fontanesi, G. and Sebastiani, L. 1989a, Reorganization of visual pathways following posthatching removal of one retina in pigeons, J. Comp. Neurol. 288:512.

Bagnoli, P., Fontanesi, G., Streit, P., Domenici, L. and Alesci, R., 1989b, Changing distribution of GABA-like immunoreactivity in pigeon visual areas during the early posthatching period and effects of retinal removal on tectal GABAergic systems, Visual Neurosci., 3:491.

Bennet-Clarke, C., Mooney, R. D., Chiaia, N. L. and Rhoades, R. W., 1989, A substance P projection from the superior colliculus to the parabigeminal nucleus in the rat and hamster, Brain. Res., 500:1.

Brecha, N., Johnson, D., Bolz, J., Sharma, S., Parnavelas, J. G. and Lieberman, A. R., 1987, Substance P- immunoreactive retinal ganglion cells and their central axon terminals in the rabbit, Nature 327:155.

Colmers, W. F., Lukowiak, K. and Pittman, Q. J., 1988, Neuropeptide Y in the rat hippocampal slice: site and mechanism of presynaptic inhibition, J. Neurosci., 8(10):3827.

Ferriero, D. M., Head, A., Edwards, R. H. and Sagar, S. M., 1990, Somatostatin mRNA and molecular forms during development of the rat retina, Dev. Brain Res., 57:15.

Hamassaki, D. E. and Britto, L. R. G., 1990, Thalamic origin of Neuropeptide Y innervation of the accessory optic nucleus of the pigeon Columba livia, Visual Neurosci., 5:249.

Hidalgo, J. J. M., Senba, E., Takatsuji, K. and Tomyama, M., 1990, Substance P and Enkephalins in the superficial layers of the rat superior colliculus: differential plastic effects of retinal deafferentation, J. Comp. Neurol., 299:389.

Hokfelt, T., Rehfeld J. F., Skirboll, L., Ivernark, B., Goldstein, M. and Markey K., 1980, Evidence for coexistence of dopamine and CCK in meso-limbic neurons, Nature, 285:476.

Huntley, G. W., Hendry, S. H. C., Killacrey, H. P., Chalupa, L. M. and Jones, E.G., 1988, Temporal sequence of neurotransmitter expression by developing neurons of fetal monkey visual cortex, Dev. Brain Res., 43:69.

Isayama, T. and Eldred, W. D., 1988, Neuropeptide Y- immunoreactive amacrine cells in the turtle Pseudemys scripta elegans, J. Comp. Neurol., 271:56.

Karten, H. J., Reiner, A. and Brecha, N., 1982, Laminar organization and origins of neuropeptides in the avian retina and optic tectum, in: "Cytochemical Method in Neuroanatomy", Alan R. Liss. Inc., New York, 189.

Krieger, D. T., 1983, Brain peptides: what, where and why?, Science, 222: 975.

Kuljis, R. O. and Karten, H. J., 1986, Substance-P containing ganglion cells become progressively less detectable during retinotectal development in frog Rana Pipiens, Proc. Natl. Acad. Sci. 83: 5736.

Marshak, D. W., 1989, Peptidergic neurons of the Macaque monkey retina, Neurosci.Res.Suppl., 10:S117.

Nagakawa, S., Hasegawa, Y., Kubozono, T. and Takuni, K., 1988, Substance P-like immunoreactive retinal terminals found in two retino-recipient areas of the Japanese monkey, Neurosci. Lett., 93:32.

Porciatti, V., Bagnoli, P., Lanfranchi A. and Bedini C., (1985) Interaction between photoreceptors and pigment epithelium in developing pigeon retina: an electrophisiological and ultrastructural study, Doc.Opththalmol., 60:413.

Pincus, D. W., DiCicco-Bloom, E. M. and Black, I. B., 1990, Vasoactive intestinal peptide regulates mitosis, differentiation and survival of cultured sympathetic neuroblasts, Nature, 343:564.

Ramon y Cajal, S., 1891, Sur la fine structure du lobe optique des oiseaux et sur l'origine reelle des nerfs optiques, Int. Mschr. Anat. Physiol., 8:337.

Shimizu, T. and Karten, H. J., 1990, Immunohistochemical analysis of the visual Wulst of the pigeon Columba livia, J. Comp. Neurol., 300:346.

Straznicky, C. and Hiscock, J., 1989, Neuropeptide Y-like immunoreactivity in neurons of the human retina, Vision Res., 29(9):1041.

Tahara, Y., Kumoi, Y., Kiyama, H. and Tohyama, M., 1986, Ontogeny of substance-P containing structures in the chicken retina: immunohistochemical anlysis, Dev.Brain Res., 30:37.

Wang, H. L., Reisine, K. and Dichter, M., 1990, Somatostatin-14 and Somatostatin-28 inhibit calcium currents in rat cortical neurons, Neurosci., 38(2): 335.

White, C. A. and Chalupa, L. M., 1991, Subgroup of alpha ganglion cells in the adult cat retina is immunoreactive for Somatostatin., J. Comp. Neurol., 304:1.

Zalutsky, A. and Miller, R. F., 1990, The physiology of Somatostatin in the rabbit retina, J. Neurosci., 10(2):383.

DEVELOPMENT AND PLASTICITY OF THE TECTOFUGAL VISUAL

PATHWAY IN THE ZEBRA FINCH

Hans - Joachim Bischof[1], Kathrin Herrmann[2], and Jürgen Engelage[1]

[1]Universität Bielefeld, Fakultät Biologie, Postfach 8640
4800 Bielefeld 1, F. R. G.
[2]Dept. of Neurobiology, Stanford University
School of Medicine, Stanford, CA 94305, U.S.A.

INTRODUCTION

In the recent years the development of the visual system of mammals and its alterability by environmental influences has been addressed by hundreds of investigations. Detailed knowledge on the development and plasticity of the visual cortex, for example, has been accumulated for a variety of mammals, in particular cats and monkeys (rev. Fregnac and Imbert 1984). In contrast, very few studies were concerned with the development of higher stations of the visual system of other vertebrates. In birds, for example, the retinotectal projection of the chick tectofugal pathway is one of the best investigated paradigms for the development of the specificity of neuronal connections and axonal pathfinding (see Thanos, this volume); however, there were almost no developmental studies of other stations of the tectofugal pathway until recently. In one of the earliest studies Pettigrew and Konishi (1976a,b) showed that the visual wulst has physiological properties very similar to those of the visual cortex in mammals, and that monocular deprivation in these animals induces the same shift in ocular dominance of wulst neurons as it was observed in area 17 of the cat or the monkey.

Owls, however, are not necessarily a representative example of the avian phylum because their eyes are located frontally. Most other species of birds have rather laterally placed eyes. We therefore investigated the development and plasticity of the visual pathway of the zebra finch, a small altricial bird which has recently become a standard laboratory animal because it is easy to keep and has a short reproduction cycle of about 70 days.

Eyes of zebra finches are situated laterally in the head and the optical axes of the eyes are diverging by about 120 degrees (Bischof 1988). As in most birds, the tectofugal pathway, which is equivalent to the visual pathway, leading to the extrastriate cortex in mammals, is much more developed than the thalamofugal projection in the zebra finch. In pigeons, another laterally-eyed bird, the tectofugal pathway plays a prominent role in tasks which are to be said to be a property of the thalamofugal pathway in mammals, as for example the discrimination of patterns or color (Hodos and Karten 1966, Hodos 1969).

Instead of giving a complete overview of our experiments, we intend here to describe the main features of the development of the tectofugal pathway in the zebra finch. Moreover, we want to give some information about the effects of monocular deprivation on the development of this projection, and the existence of a sensitive period during which these effects are most prominent.

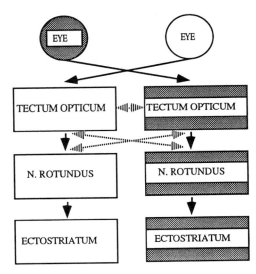

Fig. 1. Simplified diagram of the tectofugal pathway in birds. The cap over one eye symbolizes deprivation. Stippled areas: areas referred to in the text as "deprived eye" or "deprived hemisphere", respectively. Stippled lines: Interhemispheric connections.

VISUAL PATHWAYS IN BIRDS

The avian visual system differs from the mammalian in several aspects. The most important difference is that the avian optic nerve is crossing almost completely to the contralateral hemisphere. From the optic chiasm, two main projections can be traced in birds. The thalamofugal pathway leads from the eye to a variety of thalamic nuclei, commonly called the OPT (opticus principalis thalami) complex and then to a telencephalic target area called visual wulst. This pathway is comparable to the geniculocortical pathway in mammals (Karten 1979, Karten and Shimizu 1989), because the visual wulst has many similarities with the area 17 of the visual cortex in mammals, as was demonstrated by electrophysiological (Pettigrew and Konishi 1976a,b) histochemical (Shimizu and Karten 1990), and tracing studies (Bagnoli et al. 1982).

The second projection, the tectofugal pathway, is the most prominent in most avian species. Retinal ganglion cell fibers project to the mesencephalic optic tectum, the visual information is then transferred to the nucleus rotundus of the thalamus and further to the telencephalic ectostriatum (fig.1). Based on anatomical and physiological data, this pathway has been compared to the mammalian projection to the extrastriate cortex (Karten and Shimizu 1989). Most probably, the ectostriatum is comparable to layer 4 of the extrastriate cortex, whereas the other neocortical layers are represented in birds by other structures of the dorsal ventricular ridge, namely the neostriatum and the archistriatum (Karten and Shimizu 1989).

Due to the almost total crossing of the optic nerve, the visual information of each eye is primarily restricted to the contralateral hemisphere. Interaction of the two hemispheres, however, can be accomplished by a variety of recrossing projections, which have been demonstrated for both the thalamofugal and the tectofugal pathway. Based on experiments in the owl (Bravo and Pettigrew 1981), the thalamofugal pathway has been seen as to processing mainly binocular information from the frontal visual field, whereas the tectofugal pathway has been said to receive input from the lateral visual field. Binocular processing within the tectofugal pathway was considered to be negligible, because the recrossing projections were only small and did not seem to play an important role. Recent experiments, however, showed that this separation of the tasks of the two projections may hold only for birds with frontal vision. In pigeons it was shown that the optic tectum of the tectofugal pathway receives input from all over the retina, whereas the input to the n. opticus principalis thalami (OPT) of the thalamofugal pathway comes mainly from the central

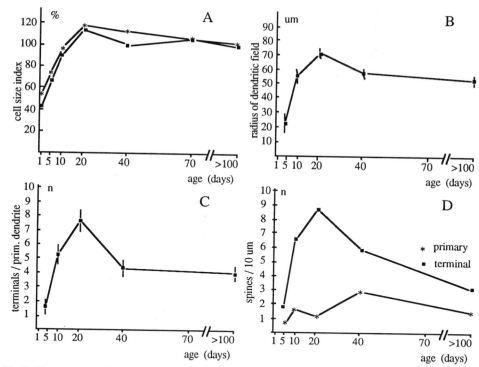

Fig.2. Time course of development of different neuronal elements. a: neuron size in % of the adult values. Stippled line: ectostriatum, full line: n. rotundus. After Herrmann and Bischof (1986a). b-d: ectostriatal measurements. b: average radius of the dendritic field, c: number of terminal segments per primary dendrite, d: number of spines / micrometer for different segments of the dendrite. Primary: segments directly adjacent to the cell body, terminal: end segments of each dendrite. After Herrmann and Bischof (1988b).

retina, which does not contribute to binocular processing in laterally eyed birds because of the large divergence of the eyes (Remy and Güntürkün 1991). Our own studies (Bredenkötter and Bischof 1991) show that the visual wulst in zebra finches receives only minor input from the ipsilateral eye and is accordingly not very likely to be involved intimately in processing of binocular images. We also showed that the recrossing projections within the tectofugal pathway are more prominent than previously believed (Bischof and Niemann 1990), and that a substantial amount of information from the ipsilateral eye is reaching the ectostriatum (Engelage and Bischof 1988, 1989). We therefore propose that in laterally eyed birds information from the binocular part of the visual field is more likely to be processed by the tectofugal pathway.

DEVELOPMENT OF THE TECTOFUGAL PATHWAY

We investigated the development of two of the nuclei of the tectofugal pathway, the nucleus rotundus and the ectostriatum, with light- and electron microscopic methods (Herrmann an 1988a,b, Nixdorf and Bischof 1986,1987). Our data clearly show that the two nuclei seem to develop almost in parallel. Fig. 2. summarizes the data we obtained from light microscopic studies. Fig. 2a (Herrmann and Bischof 1986a) shows the development of neuron size in the nucleus rotundus (solid line) and the ectostriatum (stippled line), as determined by measuring the area of the neurons in Nissl-stained sections with help of a graphics tablet. The next three figures (Herrmann and Bischof 1988b) depict the development of the main type of ectostriatal neurons as revealed by the Golgi method: the radius of the dendritic field measured from the center of the cell body to the most peripheral terminal end of a dendrite (fig.2b), the number of terminals (i.e. free endings) per

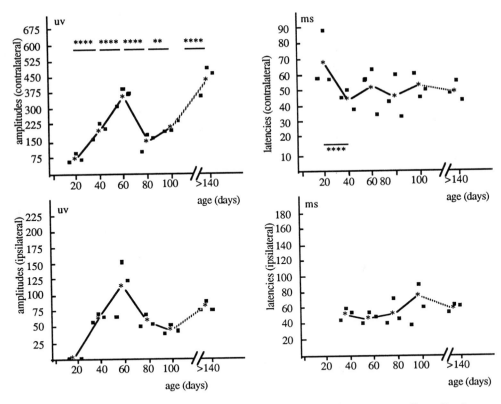

Fig. 3. Time course of development of contralaterally (upper graphs) and ipsilaterally (lower graphs) visually evoked potentials in the ectostriatum of the zebra finch. Left side: amplitudes, right side: latencies. Open circles: means (+- SEM) of individual birds. Closed circles: means (+- SEM) of pooled data from three birds each. Significance levels: ++++ = p<.00001, +++ = p<.0001, ++ = p<.001 (two tailed Student's T-test). No significant difference (p>.05) in all other cases. From Engelage and Bischof (1991).

primary dendrite (fig.2c) and the number of spines/10 μm dendritic length measured at different segments of the dendritic tree (fig.2d).

All light microscopically investigated parameters increase very rapidly from day 5 after hatching to day 20, the increase being most drastically between day 5 and day 10. All measurements show a peak at day 20 and a subsequent significant decrease between day 20 and 40.

In contrast to the data obtained by light-microscopic methods, the patterns obtained by measuring ultrastructural parameters of neurons such as length of the postsynaptic thickening, the size of the presynaptic terminal, and the number of synapses per square unit during development were not as clear-cut. Whereas the synaptic measurements in general showed an increase until day 20, a decline, as observed between day 20 and day 40 in the light microscopic studies, was only very small or even absent in the measurements of ultrastructural features of n. rotundus as well as of ectostriatum neurons (Nixdorf and Bischof 1986, Nixdorf 1990).

Despite of these differences, which will be discussed later, the data allow to conclude that the morphological development of the nucleus rotundus and the ectostriatum is almost complete at about day 40. This does not hold for the physiological development of the ectostriatum. Our measurements of visually evoked responses within this nucleus clearly demonstrate that the

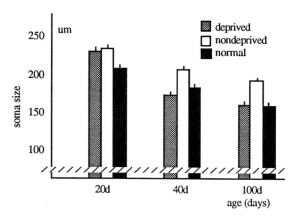

Fig. 4. Effects of different times of monocular deprivation (20, 40, and 100 days from birth) on neuron size of n. rotundus. Deprived, nondeprived: see fig. 1, normal: values from birds raised without deprivation. After Herrmann and Bischof (1988b).

response properties of the ectostriatum are still changing even when the birds are older than 100 days.

As stated earlier, studies from our lab (Engelage and Bischof 1988, 1989) demonstrated that the ectostriatum receives, contrary to earlier prepositions, input from the ipsilateral as well as the contralateral eye. The ectostriatal response evoked by a flashing light (visually evoked potential, VEP) directed to the ipsilateral eye (ipsilateral VEP) is much smaller than that evoked by stimulation of the contralateral eye (contralateral VEP). As can be seen in fig. 3 (Engelage and Bischof 1990), the development of the amplitudes and latencies follows a similar course for either side, but with a delay of about 20 days for the ipsilateral response. The amplitudes of the contralateral VEP's are still very low at day 20 (the earliest developmental stage where stereotaxic access and recording from the ectostriatum was possible) and ipsilateral VEP's are even absent (below noise level). A sharp increase can be observed between day 20 and day 60, followed by a steep decrease until day 80 with contralateral and day 100 with ipsilateral stimulation. Beyond these ages, the amplitudes are rising again, reaching constant levels at about day 140 to day 160.

A shortening of latencies is observed between day 20 and day 40 with stimulation of the contralateral eye, most probably due to myelination of axons, which is adult-like with 40 days (Herrmann and Bischof 1986a). Thereafter, latencies remain at a constant level with contralateral stimulation.

PLASTICITY OF THE TECTOFUGAL PATHWAY

We addressed the question of how the morphological development of the n. rotundus and the ectostriatum is altered by changes of visual experience during development by monocularly depriving the birds for different times starting shortly after hatching, before natural eye opening, and sacrificing them at the end of the deprivation period. Fig. 4 (Herrmann and Bischof 1986c) demonstrates that on neurons of n. rotundus this treatment has different effects according to its duration. After deprivation of 20 days starting shortly after birth there is an increase in cell size of the neurons of both hemispheres, the one driven by the deprived eye as well as that driven by the nondeprived eye, if compared to values obtained in normally reared birds. Deprivation for 40 or 100 days causes a significant hemispheric difference in soma size: neurons of the deprived n. rotundus are 15 % smaller than those of the nondeprived side. This difference is not due to a shrinkage of the neurons on the deprived side, as one would expect, but rather a result of a hypertrophy of the neurons on the nondeprived side, as can be seen by comparison with measurements of normally raised animals of the same ages.

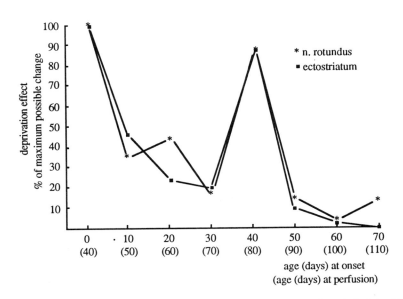

Fig. 5. Sensitive period for the effects of monocular deprivation derived from left-right differences of neuron size in the ectostriatum and n. rotundus of monocularly deprived birds. The difference between the hemispheres of birds deprived for 40 days from birth was set to 100 %. After Herrmann and Bischof 1988a).

Whereas the same effects can be observed in the ectostriatum (Herrmann and Bischof 1986b), no comparable changes of neuronal morphology could be observed in peripheral stations of the visual pathway. Monocular deprivation does not have any significant effect on the size of the retinal ganglion cells, independent of deprivation time. Within the optic tectum, the effects seem to be different for the different layers: No effect could be observed in layer 5 which receives the axons of the retinal ganglion cells. Neurons of layer 13, however, which send their axons to n. rotundus, were smaller in the deprived than in the nondeprived hemisphere. These results clearly show that effects of monocular deprivation become more pronounced in central compared to peripheral areas (Herrmann and Bischof in prep.).

Our results concerning the ultrastructural effects of monocular deprivation on n. rotundus and ectostriatum neurons are less clear-cut (Nixdorf and Bischof 1987, Nixdorf 1990). A finding comparable to our light microscopic studies was that both hemispheres are affected by 20 days of monocular deprivation which started shortly after hatching. However, in contrast to cell size and spine density, measurements of the number of synapses as well as the size of the presynaptic terminal and the length of the postsynaptic density of ectostriatal neurons resemble closely those of normally reared birds if deprivation is maintained for 100 days from birth.

Another study of our lab (Herrmann and Bischof 1988a) demonstrated that the effect of monocular deprivation is critically dependent on the time of the onset of the deprivation period. To determine this, cell size was measured within the right and left n. rotundus and ectostriatum in birds subjected to 40 days of monocular eye closure starting at ages regularly spaced throughout the first 70 days of age. Fig. 5 shows the difference of neuron size between the deprived and the nondeprived hemisphere, respectively, of the different age groups. It demonstrates that monocular deprivation causes marked differences in neuron size in n. rotundus and ectostriatum if the treatment starts at hatching. Starting deprivation between 10 and 80 days of age results in a progressively smaller difference between the two hemispheres with one surprising exception: If deprivation started at day 40, a second sharp increase of hemispheric differences was observed (fig.5).

These data indicate that the sensitivity of both rotundal and ectostriatal neurons for changes of the visual environment is extremely high shortly after birth and a second time at an age between

40 and 80 days, when our morphological measurements indicated that normal development is almost finished.

DISCUSSION

Our light microscopic measurements of the development of the tectofugal visual pathway clearly demonstrate that neurons grow rapidly until day 20. Thereafter, the size of neurons and complexity of neuronal elements such as spines and dendrites decreases until day 40, reaching adult values in most cases. This peak-decline trend (Murphy 1984) can be observed in a variety of animals and for many different neuronal elements (for review see Herrmann and Bischof 1988b). Most theories of brain development argue that this overproduction of neuronal elements is due to the fact that it is not possible for the genetic program to precisely define the structure of the neuronal network for optimal processing of environmental stimuli. Therefore, a redundant network is built which is shaped to its final form by a selection process ("selective stabilization") which favours functionally efficient neuronal connections over those which cannot be driven effectively by the periphery (Hebb 1949, Wiesel 1982, Changeux and Danchin 1976).

Our electron microscopic data do not show the substantial decline after 20 days which was observed for example in the Golgi measures, the values instead remaining on a quite constant level after rising until 20 to 40 days of age. It is conceivable that synaptic features such as the length of the postsynaptic density and the size of the presynaptic terminal should not go down as a consequence of the process of "selective stabilization" since the efficiency of synapses should be positively correlated with the area of the postsynaptic density and the size of the presynaptic bouton. However, the number of synapses should probably show the same decrease as we demonstrated for the density of spines by the Golgi method. This has been shown to be not the case for the ectostriatum. Nixdorf (1990) demonstrated that the proportion of synapses located on spines does not remain constant during development. The percentage of synapses located on dendritic spines is reduced from 40 % in 20 day old birds to 22 % in 100 day old animals. Thus the decrease in spine density reflects, at least partly, a displacement of synapses from spines to dendritic shafts, the total number of synapses remaining constant. Whether this result is a hint against the "selective stabilization" theory, remains open to future research.

Our evoked potential studies clearly demonstrate that the physiological development of the tectofugal pathway has a delay of about 40 days compared to morphological development. This is a conceivable finding because the functioning of the ectostriatal neuronal network should be optimal when the exuberant connections, which lead to a largely random distribution of current flow vectors and a strong cancellation of currents which in turn diminishes the amplitude of the evoked potential (Llinas and Nicholson 1974, Mitzdorf 1985), are fully eliminated and the final network is stabilized.

The most surprising finding of our evoked potential studies was the sharp interruption of the linear increase in the development of the VEP amplitudes after 60 days of age. This dramatic decrease of the visual responsiveness of the ectostriatal neuronal network clearly occurs after the end of neuroanatomically detectable changes. At present, we do not have a fully conclusive interpretation for this decrease. An idea we are following up is that a second wave of progressive events occurs within the ectostriatum. Following the same line of argument already employed in the explanation of the increasing responsiveness of the ectostriatum up to 60 days, the decrease of VEP amplitudes observed at day 80 may be due to a wave of invading fibers which interfere with the originally established patterns of connectivity, leading to desynchronization of the ectostriatal network, and therefore a decrease in the VEP amplitude. This would then be followed by a second period of selective stabilization.

This view is supported by one of our findings in monocularly deprived birds (Herrmann and Bischof 1988a). We have shown that monocular deprivation affects neuronal development not equally at all ages. Instead, the sensitivity to this treatment is high for the first days after birth and, more surprising, a second time when deprivation occurs between 40 and 80 days of age.

The first peak in sensitivity has been observed in a variety of studies concerning monocular deprivation (e.g. Blakemore 1978). Most probably the neuronal tissue is more susceptible to change of input from sense organs until the network is stabilized by selective stabilization. It has been also proposed that myelination of neuronal tissue limits the capability of neurons to undergo alterations (LeVay and Stryker 1979). Myelination is adultlike in the zebra finch visual system with about 40 days of age (Herrmann and Bischof 1986a).

Thus, the drastic effect of monocular deprivation in zebra finches deprived for 40 days from hatching may be due to low myelination and hence more impact of selective stabilization mechanisms during early development. However, with 40 days of age the myelination of ectostriatal neurons is complete; nonetheless, there is a second peak in monocular deprivation effects if deprivation starts at this time. At present we prefer to relate this finding to the electrophysiological results which show a depression of ectostriatal responses after 60 days of age: Both results may indicate a second phase of reorganization of ectostriatal connectivity, probably induced by invasion of new fibers. Experiments to examine this idea are underway.

Finally, we want to discuss another result of our deprivation studies which shows that the effects of monocular deprivation in the tectofugal pathway of birds can clearly be compared to findings concerning the visual cortex of mammals.

In cats as well as in monkeys the most drastic effects of monocular deprivation can be detected on neurons receiving binocular input. The only effect seen in monocularly driven neurons, as for example in the monocular segment of the lateral geniculate nucleus of the cat (Cragg et al.. 1975), was a minor shrinkage of neurons and neuronal elements. When starting our experiments we expected to find only small effects because of the proposed "monocular nature" of the tectofugal pathway. In contrast, our results indicate that the two hemispheres interact in the reaction to monocular deprivation.

In some cases, the nondeprived hemisphere obviously enhances the size of neurons and number of neuronal elements, perhaps in order to compensate for the lack of input of information to one eye by enlarging the stimulus processing capacities of the intact hemisphere. Most probably, the interaction of the two sides implies some sort of competition process between the two visual inputs, as demonstrated for the development of visual cortex neurons in mammals (rev. Fregnac and Imbert 1984). One has to note, however, that the process may not be fully comparable because zebra finches are birds with a very small binocular field. Interestingly, in mammals with laterally placed eyes like rabbits (Chow and Spear 1974) or in the monocular LGN segment of cats (Hickey et al.. 1977) no substantial deprivation effects (except small shrinkage of LGN neurons as a direct consequence of deprivation) could be observed.

The idea that competition mechanisms contribute to the observed effects is supported by our findings (Herrmann and Bischof in prep.) that in retinal ganglion cells and in layer 5 of the optic tectum no effect is observable. Both neuron populations are monocularly driven. The effects found in layer 13 of the optic tectum can already be interpreted as a sign for binocular interaction, because a tecto-tectal projection has been described (Robert and Cuenod 1969).

In addition to the indirect evidence provided by our deprivation studies we have directly demonstrated that areas of the tectofugal systems of both hemispheres are heavily interconnected. Injections of the anterograde tracer 3H-proline into the tectum and of the retrograde tracers RITC and HRP into the n. rotundus revealed that the interhemispheric connection between these two areas are much more massive than previously believed Bischof and Niemann 1990). This was confirmed by an electron microscopic study of lesion- induced degeneration (Bischof and Brinkkötter in prep).

Taken together with our electrophysiological findings which demonstrate that the ectostriatum processes ipsi- as well as contralateral stimuli (Engelage and Bischof 1988,1989), these results suggest that the tectofugal pathway is not, as previously believed, a monocularly driven pathway, but is capable to process binocular information as well. Therefore, our studies support the view that the tectofugal pathway has many characteristics of the geniculocortical pathway of mammals, although the two structures are not homologues.

REFERENCES

Bagnoli, P., Francesconi, W., and Magni, F., 1982, Visual wulst - optic tectum relationships in birds: a comparison with the mammalian corticotectal system. Archives Italienne de Biologie, 120:212-235.

Bischof, H.-J., 1980, The visual field and visually guided behavior in the zebra finch. Journal of Comparative Physiology A, 163:329-337.

Bischof, H.-J., and Niemann, J., 1990, Contralateral projections of the optic tectum in the zebra finch (Taeniopygia guttata castanotis). Cell and Tissue Research, 262:307-313.

Blakemore, C., 1978, Developmental factors in the formation of feature extracting neurons, in: "The Neurosciences: Third Study Program," F.O. Schmitt and F.G. Worden, eds., pp. 105-113, MIT Press, Cambridge, MA.

Bravo, H., and Pettigrew, J.D., 1981, The distribution of neurons projecting from the retina and visual cortex to the thalamus and tectum opticum of the barn owl, Tyto alba, and the burrowing owl, Speotyto cunicularia, Journal of Comparative Neurology, 199:419-441.

Bredenkötter, M., and Bischof, H.-J., 1990, Differences between ipsilaterally and contralaterally evoked potentials in the visual wulst of the zebra finch, Visual Neuroscience, 5:155-163.

Changeux, J.P., and Danchin, A., 1976, Selective stabilization of developing synapses as a mechanism for the specification of neuronal networks, Nature, 264:705-712.

Chow, K.L., and Spear, P.D., 1974, Morphological and functional effects of visual deprivation on the rabbit visual system, Experimental Neurology, 46:429-447.

Cragg, B., Anker, R., and Wan, Y.K., 1975, The effect of age and reversibility of cellular atrophy in the LGN of the cat following monocular deprivation: A test of two hypotheses about cell growth, Journal of Comparative Neurology, 168:345-354.

Engelage, J., and Bischof, H.-J., 1988, Enucleation enhances ipsilateral flash evoked responses in the ectostriatum of the zebra finch (Taeniopygia guttata castanotis, Gould), Experimental Brain Research, 70:79-89.

Engelage, J., and Bischof, H.-J., 1989, Flash evoked potentials in the ectostriatum of the zebra finch: A current source density analysis, Experimental Brain Research, 74:563-572.

Engelage, J. and Bischof, H.-J. (1990) Development of flash evoked responses in the ectostriatum of the zebra finch: An evoked potential and current source density analysis. Visual Neuroscience, 5: 241-248.

Fregnac, Y., and Imbert, M., 1984, Development of neuronal selectivity in primary visual cortex of cat, Physiological Reviews, 64:325-434.

Herrmann, K., and Bischof, H.-J., 1986a, Delayed development of song control nuclei in the zebra finch is related to behavioral development, Journal of Comparative Neurology, 245:167-175.

Herrmann, K., and Bischof, H.-J., 1986b, Monocular deprivation affects neuron size in the ectostriatum of the zebra finch brain, Brain Research, 379:143-146.

Herrmann, K., and Bischof, H.-J., 1986c, Effects of monocular deprivation in the nucleus rotundus of zebra finches: A deoxyglucose and Nissl study, Experimental Brain Research, 64:119-128.

Herrmann, K., and Bischof, H.-J., 1988, The sensitive period for the morphological effects of monocular deprivation in two nuclei of the tectofugal pathway of zebra finches, Brain Research, 451:43-53.

Herrmann, K., and Bischof, H.-J., 1988b, The development of neurons in the ectostriatum of normal and monocularly deprived zebra finches: A quantitative Golgi study, Journal of Comparative Neurology, 277:141-154.

Hickey, T.L., Spear, P.D., and Kratz, K.E., 1977, Quantitative studies of cell size in the cat's dorsal geniculate nucleus following visual deprivation, Journal of Comparative Neurology, 172: 265-282.

Hodos, W., 1969, Color discrimination deficits after lesions of nucleus rotundus in pigeons, Brain, Behavior and Evolution, 2:185-200.

Hodos, W., and Karten, H.J., 1966, Intensity difference thresholds in pigeons after lesions of the tectofugal and thalamofugal pathways, Experimental Brain Research, 2:151-167.

Hubel, D.H., and Wiesel, T.N., 1970, The period of susceptibility to the physiological effects of unilateral eye closure in kittens, Journal of Physiology (London), 208:419-436.

Karten, H.J., 1969, The organization of the avian telencephalon and some speculations on the phylogeny of the amniote telencephalon, Annals of the New York Academy of Sciences, 167:164-179.

Karten, H.J., and Shimizu, T., 1989, The origins of the neocortex: Connections and lamination as distinct events in evolution, Journal of Cognitive Neuroscience, 1: 291-301.

LeVay, S., and Stryker, M.P., 1979, The development of ocular dominance columns in the cat, Society of Neuroscience Symposium, 4:83-98.

Llinas, R., and Nicholson, C., 1974, Analysis of field potentials in the central nervous system, in: "Handbook of EEG and Clinical Neurophysiology," A. Remond, ed.; "Part II: Electrical Activity from the Neuron to the EEG and EMG," O. Creutzfeldt, ed., pp. 62-92, Elsevier, Amsterdam.

Mitzdorf, U., 1985, Current source density method and application in cat cerebral cortex: Investigation of evoked potential and EEG phenomena, Physiological Review, 65:37-100.

Murphy, E.H., 1984, Critical periods and the development of the rabbit visual cortex, in: "Development of Visual Pathways in Mammals," J. Stone, B. Dreher, D.H. Rappaport, eds., pp. 429-462, Allan R. Liss, New York.

Nixdorf, B.E., and H.-J. Bischof, 1986, Posthatching development of synapses in the neuropil of nucleus rotundus of the zebra finch: A quantitative electron microscopic study, Journal of Comparative Neurology, 250:133-139.

Nixdorf, B.E., and H.-J. Bischof, 1987, Ultrastructural effects of monocular deprivation in the neuropil of nucleus rotundus in the zebra finch: A quantitative electron microscopic study, Brain Research, 405:326-336.

Nixdorf, B.E., 1990, Monocular deprivation alters the development of synaptic structure in the ectostriatum of the zebra finch Synapse, 5:224-232.

Pettigrew, J.D., and Konishi, M., 1976a, Neurons selective for orientation and binocular disparity in the visual wulst of the barn owl, Tyto alba, Science, 193:675-678.

Pettigrew, J.D., and Konishi, M., 1976b, Effects of monocular deprivation on binocular neurons in the owl's visual wulst, Nature, 264:753-754.

Remy, M., and Güntürkün, O., 1991, Retinal afferents to the tectum opticum and the nucleus opticus principalis thalami in the pigeon, Journal of Comparative Neurology, 305:57-70.

Robert, F., and Cuenod, M., 1969, Electrophysiology of the intertectal commissures in the pigeon. I. Analysis of the pathways, Experimental Brain Research, 9:116-122.

Shimizu, T., and Karten, H.J., 1990, Immunohistochemical analysis of the visual wulst of the pigeon (Columba livia), Journal of Comparative Neurology, 300:346-369.

Wiesel, T., 1982, Postnatal development of the visual cortex and the influence of the environment, Nature, 299:583-591.

SPATIO-TEMPORAL PROPERTIES OF THE PATTERN ERG AND VEP:

EFFECT OF AGEING

V. Porciatti, D.C. Burr, A. Fiorentini, and C. Morrone

Istituto di Neurofisiologia del CNR
Via S. Zeno 51
Pisa Italy

INTRODUCTION

Several aspects of visual function deteriorate with age, including visual acuity and contrast sensitivity (Morrison and McGrath, 1985; Owsley et al., 1983; Tulunay-Keesey et al., 1988; Elliot et al., 1990; for review see Sekuler and Owsley, 1982; Pitts, 1982). Optical changes (senile miosis, corneal and lens opacification) account for only some of the age-related losses, suggesting that they are at least in part neural (Wheale, 1975; Morrison and McGrath, 1985; Nameda et al, 1989). Neural losses can occur at any stage between the retina and the visual cortex (see for review Wheale, 1986; Ordy et al., 1982), but little is known about the relative contribution of the retina and the post-retinal visual pathway to the age-related dysfunction.

The experiments reported in this chapter were designed to investigate the relative importance of retinal and post-retinal factors in ageing of visual function, by comparing the pattern electro-retinograms (PERGs) and visual evoked potentials (VEPs) of old observers with those of a young control group. The results show that both PERGs and VEPs are affected by age, but the clearest parameter-dependent changes were seen in the VEP. Increased VEP latencies at low temporal frequencies indicate impairment of specific post-retinal mechanisms with ageing.

METHODS

Fourteen older subjects (mean age 72.3 years, SD 7.5) together with twelve young subjects (mean age 21.3 years, SD 6) were investigated. All the older subjects had clear optical media with no ocular or systemic disease, and nine were pseudophakic (i.e. had their cataractous lenses replaced surgically with acrylic lenses of appropriate refractive power inserted into the capsular sac). Refractive errors, when present, were less than +/- 2.0 spherical, +/- 1.5 cylindrical diopters, and were fully corrected. In all subjects the corrected decimal visual acuity was equal to or better than 1.0. Informed consent was obtained after the nature of the technique and the aim of our research were fully explained.

This study was supported in part by a targeted project grant INV.91.4.019 from the Italian CNR.

Stimuli were high contrast (90%) sinusoidal gratings, generated on a Joyce (Cambridge) raster display (200 cd/m^2 mean luminance, 17 deg circular field size within a ganzfeld). The gratings were modulated sinusoidally in counterphase. Both the spatial frequency and temporal frequency were varied throughout this study.

PERGs were recorded by means of skin electrodes placed over the lower eyelid (Fiorentini et al, 1981), and VEPs by electrodes 2cm above the inion with reference to the vertex. Electrical signals were conventionally amplified, filtered and averaged by a PC computer, rejecting single sweeps disturbed by eye blinks or gross eye/body movements. The PC also averaged the signals asynchronously at 1.1 times the temporal frequency of the stimulus to give an estimate of background noise (see figure 1). It performed a discrete Fourier analysis to estimate the amplitude and phase of the 2nd Fourier harmonic (the response component at the reversal rate, and at twice this frequency).

RESULTS

Examples of PERG and VEP responses of an elder observer (83 years-old) are shown in figure 1. The traces were recorded at 7.5 Hz, and show typically strong modulation at twice the frequency of the stimulus (second-harmonic modulation). The dashed lines give an indication of the intrinsic noisiness of the signal, obtained by averaging asynchronously with respect to the pattern reversal, at 1.1 times the stimulus frequency.

Spatial Properties

To investigate spatial dependencies, PERGs and VEPs were measured in young and old observers as a function of the spatial frequency (the inverse of bar size) of the stimulus. The temporal frequency of modulation was fixed at 9 Hz for all measurements, and the contrast at 90% (to ensure a strong PERG response). Figure 2 shows the results. One effect of ageing is that the amplitudes of PERG for the elder observers (open symbols) are systematically lower than those of the younger observers (closed symbols). The effect is quite large, and holds over the entire range of spatial frequencies tested. The average PERG amplitudes for elder observers was about 40% lower than those of the younger group, at all spatial frequencies. The average noise level (not shown) was also lower for the old than for the young observers, suggesting that the lower amplitudes of the elder group does not result from inherent difficulties in registration, but reflects a real change in average amplitude levels.

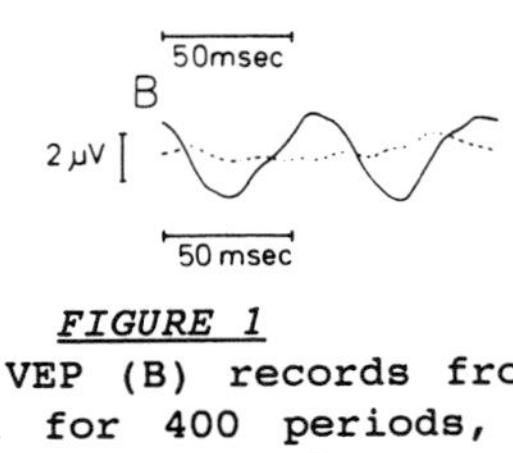

FIGURE 1

Examples of PERG (A) and VEP (B) records from a typical older observer (83 years old), averaged for 400 periods, in synchrony with pattern modulation. The stimulus was a 1.7 c/deg vertical sinusoidal grating of 90% contrast, reversed in contrast sinusoidally at 7.5 Hz. The dotted lines through each record show averages at 1.1 times the frequency of the stimulus, to give an indication of intrinsic noise levels.

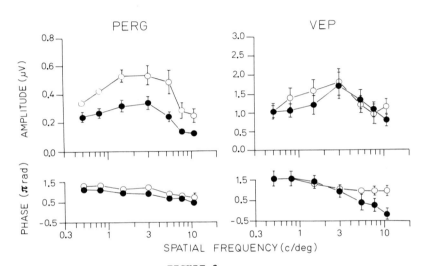

FIGURE 2

Average PERG and VEP second-harmonic amplitude and as a function of spatial frequency, for young (open symbols) and old (filled symbols) observers, with error bars indicating ± 1 SE. The stimuli were vertical sinusoidal gratings of 90% contrast, reversed in contrast sinusoidally at 9 Hz. Spatial frequency is the inverse of the distance between bars of the grating.

The VEP amplitudes did not vary significantly with age at any spatial frequency (at 9 Hz). However, it should be pointed out that the contrast of the stimuli was very high, 90%. This contrast is essential to elicit a clear PERG, but under many conditions may be considered high for VEPs. It is possible that age-related effects might be revealed with less saturating contrasts, and higher spatial frequencies.

The lower curves show the PERG and VEP phase spectra. PERG phases decreased slightly with spatial frequency for both young and old observers, by about 0.6 π radians over the 10 c/deg range. As the temporal frequency of the second harmonic was 18 Hz, this phase change corresponds to a delay of about 17 ms. There was also a slight but systematic tendency for the phase of the older observers to lag behind that the younger observers, by an average of 0.12 π radians (3 ms).

The phases of VEPs showed clearer age-related differences. Phases of old observers decreased with spatial frequency (about 1.9 π radians: 52 ms), whereas those of the young were rather insensitive to spatial frequency. While the phase lag observed in the younger observers may be entirely accounted for by retinal processes (as it was no steeper in the VEP than in the PERG), the steeper phase lag of the older observers implies post-retinal mechanisms.

Temporal Properties

We also examined the temporal properties of PERGs and VEPs, by measuring them as a function of the *temporal frequency* of modulation. For these measurements the spatial frequency of the stimuli was always 1.7 c/deg, and 90% contrast.

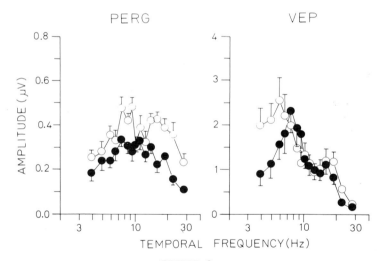

FIGURE 3

Average PERG and VEP second-harmonic amplitude as a function of temporal frequency, for young (open symbols) and old (filled symbols) observers. The stimuli were vertical sinusoidal gratings of 1.7 c/deg and 90% contrast, reversed in contrast sinusoidally.

Figure 3 shows how the PERG and VEP amplitudes varied with temporal frequency. As was observed in figure 2, the PERG amplitude was lower for the elder than the younger observers, at all temporal frequencies. Again the ratio was around 60% at most temporal frequencies (except around 12 Hz, where the data of the younger, but not the older observers showed a systematic dip).

The VEP amplitude curves also reveal age-related effects. Whereas the average amplitudes of young and old observers were similar at high temporal frequencies (as seen in figure 2), below 8 Hz the amplitudes for the elder observers were selectively depressed, by more than a factor-of-two at 4 Hz. The peak amplitude of the young observers was 6 Hz, and that of the older observers 8 Hz.

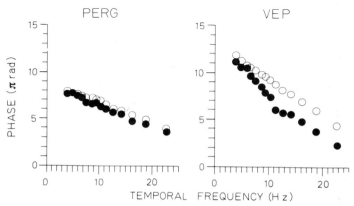

FIGURE 4

Second-harmonic phase as a function of temporal frequency, for young (open symbols) and old (filled symbols) observers. The PERG curves were well fit with a single regression line of slope 58 and 57 ms for old and young respectively. The VEP curves, however, were best fit with two separate regression lines, below and above 10 Hz. The latency estimates from the low temporal frequency limb (of the averaged data) were 153 and 108 ms for old and young respectively, and 94 ms for the high frequency of both young and old.

Figure 4 shows the PERG and VEP phase spectra associated with the amplitude spectra of figure 4. These spectra are particularly interesting, as they provide an indication of response latency. The phases of both PERG and VEPs decrease steadily with temporal frequency at a rate proportional to the "apparent latency" of response at that level. The term "apparent latency" is used to emphasise the fact that the latency does not simply reflect transmission time, but also includes the retinal transduction times, and delays introduced by the filtering properties of retinal and cortical cells (see Regan, 1966).

The PERG curves (on the left) were well fit by linear regression. The average slope estimates were 56 ms for the older group and 55 ms for the younger group (see also figure 5). These estimates are consistent with previous estimates of PERG latency, obtained with both steady-state and transient techniques (Plant *et al.*, 1986; Celesia *et al.*, 1987). The individual data (not displayed) showed the same trend, with very little inter-subject variability either in slope or in absolute values. It is also clear that the temporal sampling was fine enough to be sure of the systematic decrease in phase. These estimates of PERG latency reinforce the previous phase measurements (as a function of spatial frequency) in suggesting that there is little, if any, age-related latency difference in the PERG.

There were, however, large and systematic age-related effects in the latencies of the VEP. The phases of the younger observers were well fit by a single regression line, and the slope of this line yielded average estimates of apparent latency of 102 ms, agreeing with most previous studies (see for example Celesia *et al.*, 1987). However, the phase plots of the older observers were less well fit by a single line, because the curves of most observers tended to change slope around 10 Hz. The fits of both the raw (not displayed) and the averaged data could be greatly improved by allowing a change in slope at 10 Hz. The slopes of the two regression lines were quite different for the older observers, averaging 94 ms for frequencies above 10 Hz, and 153 ms for frequencies below 10 Hz (also see figure 6). The slopes of the curves of the younger observers also tended to change around 10 Hz, but the change was far less: 99 ms for the high frequencies compared with 108 ms for the low.

The PERG and VEP latencies for young and old are summarised in figure 5. PERG latencies, and VEP latencies at high temporal frequencies were similar for young and old, but the low frequency branch of the VEP temporal response curve showed a clear age-related difference. Note that the latency estimates of figure 5 are the average of the individual regressions, while the regression lines of figure 4 were calculated from the averaged data. The latency estimates obtained by these two procedures were in fact very similar.

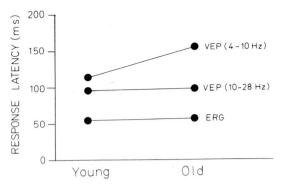

FIGURE 5

Summary of response latencies estimated from PERG and VEP phase responses. The PERG was estimated from the second-harmonic phase response of each observer, over the entire temporal frequency range (4 - 24 Hz). For the VEP, the latency was calculated separately for the lower and upper limbs of the temporal frequency response curves, above and below 10 Hz.

DISCUSSION

To summarise, the major effect observed in this study was that the VEPs of the older group showed a large (40 ms) increase in response latency in the low temporal frequency range, coupled with a reduction in amplitude. This result clearly implies age-related changes in specific neural mechansisms.

The other significant result was an aspecific reduction in PERG amplitude at all spatial frequencies and most temporal frequencies by about 40%. This agrees well with previous studies of ageing of PERG, both with transient (Celesia et al., 1987) and with steady-state (Porciatti et al., 1988) stimuli. Two non-neural possible explanations for the reduction in amplitude could be reduction in pupil diameter in the aged, or reduction in lens transmission. Lens transmission should not play a major role as the majority of our elder subjects were pseudophakic. In our experimental conditions the average decrease in retinal illuminance of old observers due to senile miosis was less than 0.2 log-units. In a control experiment, we have measured PERGs as a function of retinal illuminance, and shown that the 30 decrease in illuminance caused by the smaller pupils has no effect on PERG amplitude. (It could, however, account for the small PERG phase lag in the old. Thus it would seem that the reduced amplitudes reflect a general reduction in average retinal activity in old that could be related to the senile changes reported for both the outer and inner retinal layers (see for review Wheale, 1986).

The largest and most interesting effect reported here is the 40 ms increase in apparent latency of VEPs at low temporal frequencies, together with a decrease in amplitude over this range. These results clearly implicate visual impairment at post-retinal neural sites, and suggest selective ageing of post-retinal mechanisms responsive to low temporal frequencies. The progressive phase lag with spatial frequency in old observers further implies selective ageing of mechanisms responsive to high spatial frequencies.

It is interesting to view these results in the light of recent evidence for anatomically and (to some extent) functionally distinct parallel pathways in primate vision, the so called *magno* and *parvo* pathways (e.g. Derrington and Lennie, 1984; Shapley and Perry, 1986; Shapley, 1990; Kaplan et al., 1990; Merigan and Maunsell, 1990; Livingstone and Hubel, 1988). In the monkey LGN the large, fast-conducting neurones seem to be more sensitive to luminance patterns of low spatial and high temporal frequency. The smaller, slower conducting parvo-cells respond to both luminance and chromatic patterns, but over a higher range of spatial frequencies and a lower range of temporal frequencies. The fact that our older observers exhibited selective deficits at low temporal and high spatial frequencies would seem to imply selective impairment of the parvo-cellular pathway. It would be interesting to have some information from anatomical studies on possible selective deterioration with age of different neural pathways. Although cell losses have been described at all levels in the aged human visual system (see for review Ordy et al., 1982), it is not yet known whether certain pathways may be more vulnerable to cell loss.

As the difference in apparent latency estimates of young and old observers at low temporal frequencies were so clear-cut, we have begun to apply the same technique to investigate patients affected by unilateral optic neuritis. This disease is characterized by an episode of blindness followed by substantial recovery of vision. Preliminary results suggest that these patients, like the aged, show large increases in apparent latencies at low temporal frequencies in VEPs recorded from the affected eye. This may suggest that some structures in the visual pathway are more vulnerable than others, and that optic neuritis may represent a kind of accelerated aging.

REFERENCES

Celesia, G.C., Kaufman, D, & Cone, S. (1987) Effects of age on pattern electroretinograms and visual evoked potentials. *Electroencephalography and clinical Neurophysiology.* 68: 161-171.

Derrington, A.M., & Lennie, P. (1984) Spatial and temporal contrast sensitivities of neurones in lateral geniculate nucleus of macaque. *Journal of Physiology* 357: 219-240.

Elliott D.B., Whitaker, D., & MacVeigh, D. (1990) Neural contribution to spatiotemporal contrast sensitivity decline in healthy ageing eyes. *Vision Research* 30: 541-547.

Fiorentini, A., Maffei, L., Pirchio, M., Spinelli, D., & Porciatti, V. (1981) The ERG in response to alternating gratings in patients with diseases of the peripheral visual pathway. *Investigative Ophthalmology and Visual Science* 21: 490-493.

Kaplan, E., Lee, B., & Shapley, R.M. (1990) New views of primate retinal function. *Progress in retinal Research* 9: 273-336.

Livingstone, M. & Hubel, D.H. (1988) Segregation of form, color, movement and depth: anatomy, physiology and perception. *Science* 240: 740-749.

Merigan, W. H., & Maunsell, J.H.R. (1990) Macaque vision after magnocellular lateral geniculate lesions. *Visual Neuroscience* 5: 347-352.

Morrison, J.D. & McGrath, C. (1985) Assessment of the optical contributions to the age-related deterioration in vision. *Quarterly Journal of experimental Physiology* 70: 249-269.

Nameda, N., Kawara, T., & Ohzu H. (1989) Human visual Spatio-temporal frequency performance as a function of age. *Optometry and Vision Science* 66: 760-765.

Ordy, M.J., Brizzee, K.R., & Johnson, H.A. (1982) Cellular alterations in visual pathways and the limbic system: implications for vision and short-term memory. *In* Aging and Human Visual Functions. eds. Sekuler, R., Kline, D., & Dismukes, K., pp. 79-114. New York: Alan R. Liss.

Owsley, C., Sekuler, R., & Siemsen D. (1983) Contrast sensitivity throughout adulthood. *Vision Research* 23: 689-699.

Pitts, D. (1982) The effects of aging on selected visual functions: dark adaptation, visual acuity, stereopsis, and brightness contrast. *In* Aging and Human Visual Function, eds. Sekuler, R., Kline, D., & Dismukes, K., pp. 131-159. New York: Alan R. Liss.

Plant, G. T., Hess, R.F., & Thomas, S.J. (1986) The pattern evoked electroretinogram in optic neuritis. *Brain* 109: 469-490.

Porciatti, V., Falsini, B., Scalia, G., Fadda, A., & Fontanesi, G. (1988) The pattern electroretinogram by skin electrodes: effect of spatial frequency and age. *Documenta Ophthalmologica* 70: 117-122.

Regan, D. (1966) Some characteristics of average steady-state and transient responses evoked by modulated light. *Electroencephalography and clinical Neurophysiology* 20: 238-248.

Sekuler, R., & Owsley, C. (1982) The spatial vision of older humans. *In* Aging and Human Visual Function, eds. Sekuler, R., Kline, D., & Dismukes, K., pp. 185-202. New York: Alan R. Liss.

Shapley, R. (1990) Visual sensitivity and parallel retinocortical channels. *Annual Review of Psychology* 41: 635-658.

Shapley, R., & Perry, H. (1986) Cat and monkey retinal ganglion cells and their visual functional roles. *Trends in Neurosciences* 5: 229-235.

Tulunay-Keesey U., Ver Hoeve J.N., & Terkla-McGrane C. (1988) Threshold and suprathreshold spatiotemporal response throughout adulthood. *Journal of the optical Society of America* A 5: 2191-2200.

Weale, R.A. (1975) Senile changes in visual acuity. *Transactions of the Ophthalmological Society, UK* 95: 36-38.

Weale, R.A. (1986) Retinal senescence. *Progress in retinal Research* 5: 53-73.

METHODS AND MODELS FOR SPECIFYING SITES AND MECHANISMS OF

SENSITIVITY REGULATION IN THE AGING VISUAL SYSTEM

Joseph F. Sturr and Daniel J. Hannon

Vision Laboratories
Department of Psychology
Syracuse University
456 Huntington Hall
Syracuse, NY 13244-2340

1.0 Introduction

In this paper we will be discussing methods and mathematical models for identifying the loci of sensitivity losses that occur with age. The overall goal is to describe an approach to examining changes in the regulation of sensitivity in the aging visual system within the framework of formal models of adaptation. We will not be reviewing specific results from a wide range of experiments, but rather, we will be describing an approach to the understanding of sensitivity losses in the aging visual system that incorporates psychophysical results within the framework of formal models. This approach has been successful at identifying sites and mechanisms of alterations of sensitivity in retinal disease and may also be useful in analyzing changes that occur during visual development.

One function of the visual system is to maintain sensitivity to small differences in contrast over an enormous range of ambient illuminations. The difference in luminance from moonlight to bright sunlight is a factor of 10^{10}. Although this ability is preserved, to a large extent, over the adult lifespan in persons in good ocular health, measurable declines in visual function have been observed in a number of laboratories. We wish to address three questions. First of all, what are the differences in sensitivity between young and old observers under any given set of luminance conditions? Second, what are the differences between young and old observers under changing luminance conditions? Third, what are the mechanisms underlying the above differences? The regulation of sensitivity, otherwise known as adaptation, has been actively investigated by psychophysicists and physiologists in recent years and much has been learned about the mechanisms that subserve this process. Much of what has been learned by these investigations can now be applied to visual development in general and the aging visual system in particular. The general approach of this paper is to describe psychophysical paradigms which may be used to test alternative hypotheses regarding sites and mechanisms underlying changes in visual sensitivity and sensitivity regulation occurring in the aging visual system. Specifically, we will demonstrate how these models can be applied to test hypotheses about receptoral vs. post-receptoral sites of sensitivity loss and about multiplicative vs. subtractive mechanisms of adaptation in aging.

The Changing Visual System, Edited by P. Bagnoli and
W. Hodos, Plenum Press, New York, 1991

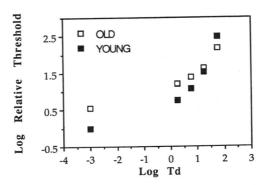

Figure 1. Foveal cone increment thresholds replotted from Sturr et al. (1986). Threshold measured on flashed background (flash-on-flash). Closed circles: young observers, open circles, old observers in good ocular health. +/- 1 standard error of the mean is smaller than symbol size.

1.1 Age-related sensitivity losses

Recent psychophysical evidence exists for an increase in cone and rod absolute thresholds in the aging visual system (Birren et al., 1948; McFarland and Fisher, 1955; Luria, 1960; McFarland et al., 1960; Gunkel and Gouras, 1963; Sturr et al., 1986; Eisner et al., 1987; Werner and Steele,1988; Werner et al., 1990; Sturr et al., 1991). Figure 1 is a replot of foveal cone thresholds from Sturr et al. (1986), measured over a range of background luminance, in young and old observers, in good ocular health. In this experiment the luminance for detecting a test probe presented at the onset of a flashed background field was measured. This is known as the flash-on-flash technique. At low background luminances, the elderly have thresholds that are higher than younger observers. This difference is diminished at the higher background luminance indicated by the convergence of the data points.

Figure 2 is another replot of data taken from Sturr et al. (1986), this time showing foveal cone thresholds measured upon a steadily presented adapting field. Similar to Figure 1, this plot shows differences between old and young observers at low levels of the adapting field. These differences are also diminished at the higher luminance levels of the adapting field.

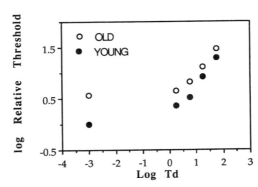

Figure 2. Foveal cone increment thresholds replotted from Sturr et al. (1986). Threshold measured on steady adapting field (steady state). Closed circles: young observers, open circles, old observers in good ocular health. +/- 1 standard error of the mean is smaller than symbol size.

Figure 3 provides a third example of age-related declines in cone sensitivity from Sturr et al. (1991). Thresholds measured following the offset of a bright adapting field are plotted as a function of time following the termination of the background field. This is not the traditional long-term dark adaptation function which usually takes several minutes, but rather is a measure of early-dark-adaptation, or the recovery of visual sensitivity during the first few-hundred milliseconds following the offset of an adapting field. The leftmost data points, marked SS, represent the sensitivity of young and old observers under steady-state light adaptation. The two groups are essentially the same. However, the functions diverge during early dark adaptation, with the elderly having a slower time course of recovery. The rightmost data points, marked RT, illustrate differences in absolute thresholds in the cones for these two age groups.

1.2 Potential sites and mechanisms

What are the possible causes of these sensitivity losses in the aging visual system? We can delineate three broad sites: 1.) preretinal screening of the light reaching the retina, 2.) loss of receptoral function, and 3.) neural loss beyond the receptors.

There are three possible factors at the preretinal level: 1.) increased lens density, 2.) senile miosis, 3.) increase in macular pigmentation. The lens progressively yellows with age causing a greater relative loss in sensitivity to shortwave stimuli. Johnson et al. (1988) and Werner and Steele (1988) have measured the contributions of ocular media density in individual observers and have concluded that 40% or more of the age-related loss in sensitivity of the short-wavelength sensitive cones is attributable to light loss in the ocular media. The remaining losses must be due to receptoral and/or post-receptoral changes.

The second pre-retinal factor is senile miosis, which is a chronic decrease in pupil diameter with age resulting in a progressive decrease in retinal illuminance (Kornzweig, 1954). The third potential pre-retinal factor is an increase in macular pigmentation. Careful psychophysical evidence by Werner et al. (1987) and direct physical measurements by Bone et al. (1988) of extracted macular pigment have shown wide individual variations but no age- related increase in macular pigment density.

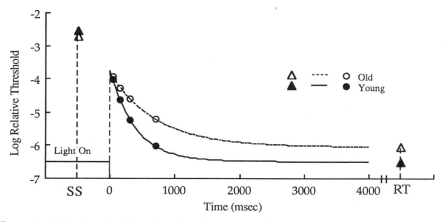

Figure 3. Foveal early dark adaptation in young and old observers in good ocular health, replotted from Sturr et al. (1991). Closed symbols: young, open symbols old observers. SS = increment threshold measured during steady state light adaptation. RT = resting threshold for foveal cones. +/- 1 standard error of the mean is smaller than symbol size.

The second broad site of sensitivity losses with age is at the receptor level. Receptoral factors may include: 1.) a decrease in photopigment density, 2.) misshapen or misaligned receptors, 3.) a loss in number of photoreceptors, 4.) a decrease in amplitude of receptor response, 5.) a decrease in neurotransmitter, 6.) an increase in membrane potential.

Although a decrease in cone pigment density has been reported by some research groups (Kilbride et. al, 1986; Keunen, van Norren, and van Meel, 1987), others report only slight age- related changes in cone pigment density (Elsner et al., 1988). Paradoxically, Liem et al. (1991) have recently reported an increase in rod pigment density in the elderly.

The second receptoral factor is the convolution of the outer segments in aging rods (Marshall et. al., 1979). Rod and cone outer segments continue to grow as new discs are added near the base. The old discs are removed in the pigment epithelium. The convolution of the rods is most likely explained by the fact that the mechanism for clipping the rods is slower in the older eye than the rate of rod growth. The result is an elongated outer segment which may explain the previous paradoxical finding of increased rod photopigment in old age. Evidence also exists for misaligned receptors in old age (Smith et al.,1988). Collectively, these effects reduce the quantum-catching ability of the receptors.

The third receptoral factor is a loss of photoreceptors. A loss of cone photoreceptors has been reported in the aging eye. Cone counts per mm^2 in the foveola by Youdelis & Hendrickson (1986) show a progressive decrease in cell number with age compared to the classic work of Osterberg (1936) . In a more extensive sampling of cone receptors, however, Curcio et al. (1990) have concluded that there is no age- related decrease in foveal receptor density. On the other hand, Curcio et al. (1990) provide persuasive anatomical evidence for significant age- related losses of rod density.

The fourth, fifth and sixth receptoral factors, a decrease in amplitude of response, a decrease in neurotransmitter released, and an increase in membrane potential, have not yet been documented in the aging visual system but could be caused by chronic hypoxia or other age-related metabolic changes. All three of these factors could account for reduced sensitivity in old age.

The third site of sensitivity loss with age may be post-receptoral. There are several possible mechanisms or sites: 1.) a decrease in receptoral pooling, 2.) a decrease in the number of ganglion cells, 3.) a decrease in amplitude of response of post-receptoral cells, 4.) a decrease in neurotransmitter, 5.) a decrease in number of cortical cells, 6.) a decrease in cortical neurotransmitter.

The first factor, a random loss in photoreceptors, will result in a decrease in rod or cone signals sent to the pool. There could also be a change in the temporal or spatial summating properties at the level of the pool which would result in a loss in sensitivity. Second, a decrease in the number of ganglion cells would have an effect on the absolute sensitivity of the system. Third, post-receptoral mechanisms may also experience a reduction in response amplitude apart from a potentially decreased signal from the receptors. For example, a change in center-surround interactive mechanisms at the level of the post-receptoral unit would alter the spatial filtering properties of the system independent of changes at the level of the receptors. The fourth factor, a decrease in neurotransmitter, as well as the fifth and sixth factors, a decrease in the number of cortical cells and a decrease in cortical neurotransmitter, would have similar effects.

In summary, laboratory data from three examples of specific losses of sensitivity and sensitivity regulation with age have been presented and three broadly defined sites of these losses were proposed. Within each site, several possible contributing factors were considered. We now turn our attention to the methods of measurement of these losses of sensitivity and changes of sensitivity regulation with age that will allow us to specify the sites of their activity.

2.0 Psychophysics and Physiology

As illustrated in the first three examples, measuring the changes in absolute threshold associated with aging is clearly insufficient for successful testing of alternative hypotheses regarding sites and mechanisms. We also need to describe how sensitivity is altered under different levels of ambient illumination and how sensitivity changes during the transition from the light adapted state to the dark adapted state and vice versa. In order to characterize sensitivity changes over a wide range of luminance conditions, psychophysicists have measured threshold versus intensity, or t.v.i. functions, that is, the increment in luminance for detection of a flashed test field (I_T) as a function of the luminance of a larger flashed background field (I) and/or a steadily presented adapting field (Aguilar & Stiles, 1954; Wyszecki & Stiles, 1967).

2.1 Psychophysical paradigms

Figure 4 illustrates some of these relationships. Luminance profiles over time are drawn along with accompanying data. As shown in the inset profile 4a on the left, when the flashed background field is used, the onset of the test and background fields are coincident. This is known as the flash-on-flash paradigm. Threshold for detection of a test field as a function of the luminance of a flashed background field is shown in the leftmost curve. As diagramed in the inset profile 4b on the right, when only a test field and a steady adapting field are used, thresholds are determined as a function of the luminance of the steady field. The threshold for detection of a test field is plotted as a function of the luminance of a steady background field in the rightmost curve. The slope of the function measured in the light adapted eye is much shallower than the slope of the function measured in the dark adapted eye.

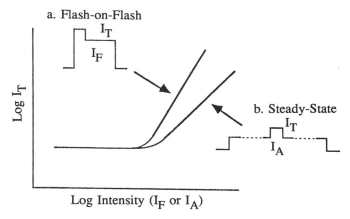

Figure 4. Increment threshold functions measured for the dark adapted eye (left) and the light adapted eye (right), with illustrations of the temporal relationships of the two stimulus conditions (insets a & b). I_T = test probe intensity for threshold. I_F = flashed background intensity, I_A = steady adapting field intensity.

The two flashed fields also can be presented on top of a steady adapting field as illustrated in Figure 5. Detection thresholds are measured as a function of the luminance of the flashed background field. The steady adapting field is presented to control the state of adaptation of the system. Modifications of this paradigm allows for the testing of mechanisms of sensitivity regulation. By varying the time between the onset or offset of the steady field and the presentation of the two flashed fields, changes in sensitivity can be measured as a function of both the luminance of the flashed background and time after the change in the steady field.

2.2 Linking psychophysics and physiology

In order to use the data from these psychophysical procedures to specify sites and mechanisms of sensitivity loss in the aging visual system, it is first necessary to develop a model of the relationship between these methods and the structure of the visual system. Several models of this type have been developed in recent years. Perhaps the most thoroughly developed is the link between the t.v.i. paradigm and visual physiology through the use of the Naka-Rushton equation. In their now classic work, Naka and Rushton (1966) fit the following equation to the intensity response data of retinal neurons:

$$R/R_{max} = I^n/(I^n + \sigma^n) \tag{1}$$

The response R of the cell, normalized to its maximum response, R_{max}, is a function of the stimulus intensity, I, divided by I plus sigma. The semisaturation constant, sigma, is the intensity that gives a response that is one half R_{max}. The exponent n in the equation usually varies between .7 and 1, and for simplicity will be considered to be 1.

As shown in Figure 6a, Log R is plotted as a function of Log I. In this figure, the response in the model first increases with stimulus intensity, but eventually reaches a maximum amplitude, or saturating level. R_{max} is indicated along the ordinate and sigma along the abscissa.

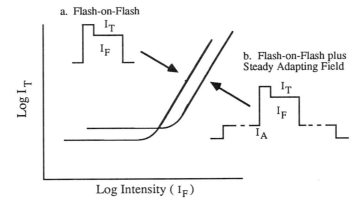

Figure 5. Inset a: illustration of the flash-on-flash paradigm measured in the dark adapted state, as in Figure 4a. Inset b: flash-on-flash paradigm measured in the presence of a third steady adapting field (I_A). See text for details.

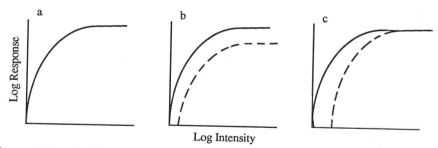

Figure 6. Panel a: Plot of Naka-Rushton function. Panel b: Illustration of the effect of a decrease in R_{max} (dashed line). Panel c: Illustration of the effect of an increase in sigma (dashed line). See text for details.

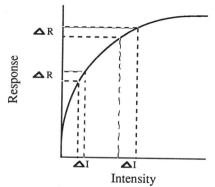

Figure 7. Illustration of the concept of a criterion response in a psychophysical experiment. See text for details. Adapted from Boynton (1979).

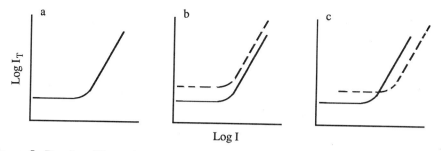

Figure 8. Panel a: Illustration of the t.v.i. function derived from the Naka-Rushton function and the equations described in the text. Panel 8b: The effect of decreasing R_{max} (dashed line). Panel 8c: The effect of increasing sigma (dashed line).

Excluding the exponent, the Naka-Rushton function has two free parameters, sigma and R_{max}. The curve shown in Figure 6a was determined under dark-adapted conditions. Under light-adapted conditions, sigma and R_{max} may increase and decrease respectively. A decrease in R_{max} is illustrated in Figure 6b. The solid curve indicates measurements under dark-adapted conditions, and the dashed curve shows a possible effect of light adaptation upon the intensity-response function.. As can be seen, the dynamic range of the system has decreased with light adaptation . This is known as response compression. If a goal of the visual system is to maintain sensitivity to small contrast differences through adaptation, then response compression, and therefore, a decrease in R_{max}, clearly does not achieve this end.

Figure 6c illustrates an increase in sigma. As before, the response under dark adapted conditions is indicated by the solid function, and the dashed function is obtained under light adapted conditions. It is clear that in this case, the dynamic range has been preserved under light adaptation and the function has simply been shifted to the right along the abscissa. This result is the most common finding among physiological studies of retinal adaptation mechanisms and is known as gain control.

In order to relate the Naka-Rushton function to t.v.i. data we need to make one critical assumption. It is assumed that the incremental threshold in the psychophysical experiment is reached when a criterion increase in response is achieved. Figure 7 illustrates this idea. At very low luminance levels, to achieve the same criterion response, small increments are needed. At higher luminance levels the increment increases in proportion to the background luminance. One can imagine that at the highest levels, an infinitely larger delta I is required.

This relationship is expressed algebraically by:

$$R(I + I_T) - R(I) = \Delta \tag{2}$$

The criterion response, delta, is equal to the response of the system to the background field I plus the increment field I_T minus the response of the system to the background field alone. Substituting I and I_T into equation 1, and then substituting this equation into equation 2 yields:

$$(I + I_T) / [(I + I_T) + \sigma] - I / (I + \sigma) = \Delta \tag{3}$$

Solving for I_T yields:

$$I_T = \Delta (I + \sigma)^2 / k[\sigma - \Delta (I + \sigma)] \tag{4}$$

where k is a constant. This equation describes the generalized psychophysically determined increment threshold function measured in the t.v.i. paradigm.

Just as we have shown the changes in the Naka-Rushton function that come about due to alterations of sigma and R_{max}, we can also do the same for the increment threshold function. Figure 8a shows the standard t.v.i. function. Notice that when R_{max} is decreased, as shown by the dashed function in panel 8b, the t.v.i. curve is shifted vertically. When sigma is increased the t.v.i. curve is shifted along the 45^0 diagonal as indicated by the dashed curve in panel 8c.

Up to now we have shown the relationship between the t.v.i. function and physiology and have demonstrated how changes in the parameters from the original Naka-Rushton function affect the increment threshold curve. We now have a means for analyzing empirically obtained data from the t.v.i paradigm in terms of physiological mechanisms. Differences in the data collected under different conditions can be quantified in terms of the parameter changes necessary to fit the increment threshold function to the data. Once it is recognized that the shape of the function does not vary appreciably between conditions (i.e. n=1) then different experimental conditions or different stages of development reveal themselves in characteristic changes in the values of sigma and/or R_{max}. We thus have an immediately recognizable means for determining the physiological variables that are changing with age.

In summary, psychophysical methods of measuring sensitivity have been introduced, including the t.v.i. and flash-on-flash paradigms. We then presented a model that links psychophysically determined data to underlying physiological processes and have demonstrated how two parameters, sigma and R_{max}, can be used to fit the model to data. Following this we discussed how the t.v.i. paradigm can be used, in principle, to measure sensitivity losses and losses of sensitivity regulation in the aging visual system. We now turn to specific applications of the t.v.i. paradigm and increment threshold model to normal and disease conditions and suggest how these procedures can be modified for the study of development.

3.0 Specific Applications

3.1 R_{max} vs. σ

Perhaps the simplest application of the Naka-Rushton increment threshold model is to fit the model to the data shown in Figure 1. Recall that Log I_T is plotted as a function of Log I of the background field. The "flash-on-flash" paradigm was used with no steady adapting field, i.e. subjects were dark adapted. Filled circles are data from young subjects, and unfilled for the elderly. Since the curves are converging at the higher luminance levels, it appears that there is both a decrease in R_{max} and an increase in sigma. The significance of this finding is that compared to the young, the elderly have a decrease in maximum response in the system and an increase in the semisaturation constant.

We can consider these changes in sigma and R_{max} in terms of the three potential sites of sensitivity loss outlined above as shown in Table 1. Increases in sigma can come about due to prereceptoral contributions such as increased lens density. Both increases in sigma and decreases in R_{max} can occur at the receptoral level. A random loss of receptors, a decrease in photopigment density or misshapen or misaligned receptors would cause an increase in sigma. An increase in membrane potential or a decrease in response amplitude could cause a decrease in R_{max}. Similarly, changes in both parameters can come about due to post-receptoral factors. A loss of ganglion cells, for instance, would produce an increase in sigma, and a decrease in post-receptoral response amplitude would cause a decrease in R_{max}.

Table 1. Sites of sensitivity loss and corresponding changes in R_{max} and σ.

Possible Site	R_{max}	σ
Pre-receptoral	-	↑
Receptoral	↓	↑
Post-receptoral	↓	↑

3.2 Receptoral vs post-receptoral

It is clear from an examination of Table 1 that simply knowing the differences in sigma and R_{max} do not differentiate between potential sites of sensitivity losses with age. What are needed are some additional assumptions about the system that will allow for the identification of specific sites. Recently, Hood (1988) and Hood and Greenstein (1990) developed a model for testing the rod system in disease conditions that incorporated some simplifying assumptions and in turn allowed for the specification of prereceptoral and receptoral versus post-receptoral sites of sensitivity loss. Figure 9 shows a schematic diagram of the model. In the first box, labeled transduction, it is assumed that quantal absorption by the photoreceptors is approximately a linear function of intensity. The second box is the intensity-response function of the rods, which can again be assumed to be a linear function of intensity if the intensity range is restricted to 2.0 log scotopic trolands or less. The output of many rods is pooled, and passes through an adapting mechanism "a". The third box shows the response function at a post-receptoral level. Three potential sites of sensitivity loss are identified as d1, d2, and d3. D1 represents a prereceptoral loss. D2 represents a loss at the receptor level. D3 represents a loss at the postreceptoral level. The data obtained from two different groups of observers, for instance, young and old observers, can be compared in terms of the d1, d2 and d3 parameters.

Figure 10 illustrates the potential differences in the data with losses at d1, d2 and d3. It first should be noted that changes in d1 and d2 cannot be distinguished from each other. Differences between d1 and/or d2 and d3 can be distinguished, however. A pure change in d3, i.e., a loss in sensitivity at the post-receptoral level, will yield a function that is shifted vertically from the comparison function, whereas a d1 or d2 change will be shifted up and to the right. Of course, changes of both kinds are possible as well. It should also be noted that although the curves are shifting in position in ways similar to the analyses with sigma and R_{max} described earlier, a different equation was used to generate these functions, which, along with the simplifying assumptions and differences in experimental procedure, make these two ways of analyzing the data very different from each other. An important distinction in the procedure associated with Hood's model is that the increment threshold be measured under steady-state light adaptation conditions, whereas the previous procedure employed the flash-on-flash paradigm.

Recent work by Hood and Birch (1991) suggests that this model will also hold for cones. We therefore can apply this model to data from our laboratory collected under similar steady-state light adaptation conditions. A re-examination of Figure 2, taken from Sturr et. al. (1986), clearly suggests a difference in d1 and/or d2 between young and old observers, indicating a pre-receptoral and /or receptoral loss in sensitivity.

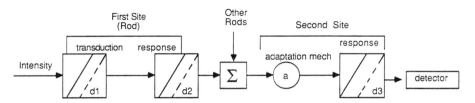

Figure 9. Hood and Greenstein's (1990) model for testing receptoral vs. post-receptoral sites of sensitivity losses in disease or development. Dashed lines labelled D1 and D2 represent losses at receptoral site; dashed lines labelled D3 represents losses at post-receptoral site.

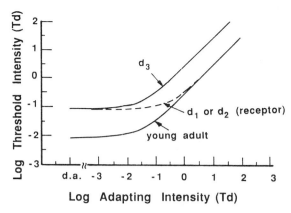

Figure 10. Hypothetical t.v.i. function for young adults compared to elderly observers with either a d1 or d2 loss or a d3 loss. (Adapted from Hood, *J. Opt. Soc. Am.*, *5:*2159, 1988.)

Although this analysis is consistent with a pre-receptoral or receptoral site of sensitivity loss with age, more specific hypotheses regarding mechanisms would have to be tested with other psychophysical paradigms. For instance, these results could be explained on the basis of an increase in lens density with age. Should this analysis not completely account for the differences between young and old, the role of receptoral contributions (i.e., d2 factors) would have to be tested. A decrease of the responsiveness of the receptors is indicated in the model as a change in d2. The hypothesis of a loss in receptor responsiveness could be determined by a follow-up psychophysical experiment. What would be more direct and, therefore, more desirable would be to actually measure receptor responsiveness in an animal model with young and old eyes.

3.3 Mechanisms of sensitivity regulation

Up to this point we have been considering sensitivity measured under dark adapted or steady state light adapted conditions. We are also interested in measuring sensitivity during the transitional periods between these two extremes. As was shown in Figure 3, the time course of recovery during early dark adaptation is slower in the elderly than in the young. What are the mechanisms underlying early light and early dark adaptation and how do they change with age?

Within the past few years techniques have been developed that have allowed for the identification of the functional sensitivity regulating mechanisms. Figure 11 illustrates the adaptation process in cones, taken from Hayhoe et. al. (1987). As in the previous model, the first block represents linear transduction. The final block is a saturating non-linearity. Between these two stages are two components labeled multiplicative process and subtractive process. The multiplicative process is a gain-changing mechanism, set by a steady adapting field, that reduces the response to a test and background flash by a multiplicative constant. The subtractive process acts to remove the signal from the steady adapting field from the signal caused by the test and background flashes that are presented upon the steady field. It is the action of these two processes that results in steady state sensitivity. We wish to measure how these processes change over time and over the adult lifespan.

Several investigators, including Adelson (1982), Geisler (1983), and Hayhoe et. al. (1987), have attempted to measure the time courses of the multiplicative and subtractive processes. The technique involves collecting flash-on-flash increment threshold data as a

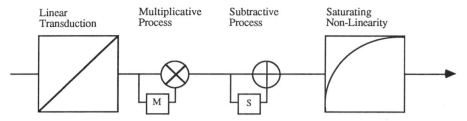

Figure 11. Model of cone adaptation from Hayhoe, Benimoff and Hood (1987). See text for details.

function of time after the onset or offset of a steady adapting field. A family of curves is then plotted showing the change in shape of the t.v.i. curve with time as the parameter. Slight modifications of the Naka-Rushton increment threshold function can be made to incorporate multiplicative and subtractive processes. This model can be fit to the data and the multiplicative and subtractive parameters can be determined as a function of time. The time course of the multiplicative and subtractive processes can then be estimated. However, the specific mechanisms and sites of these processes are only poorly understood at the present time.

The early dark adaptation data from Sturr et. al. (1991), shown in Figure 3, were collected under different stimulus conditions and do not lend themselves to this type of analysis. However, we wish to pursue this technique in the elderly and ask two basic questions. First, how have the time courses of these mechanisms changed with age? Second, have the magnitudes of the processes also changed with age?

4.0 Summary and conclusions

To recap, we have highlighted several different ways of studying sensitivity loss in the aging visual system. We began by illustrating sensitivity loss under three conditions: 1.) at absolute threshold and under different levels of background illumination for the dark-adapted eye, 2.) under different levels of background illumination for the light-adapted eye and, 3.) during the transition from the light-adapted state to the dark-adapted state. We then identified three broad loci of mechanisms that might explain these results: pre-receptoral, receptoral and post-receptoral. Following this, a model was introduced that related the physiology of retinal function to psychophysical data. We showed how this model could be applied to increment threshold data and then presented other models that tested more specific hypotheses. It was shown that with certain assumptions the loci of sensitivity loss can be determined to be at one of the three broad sites just mentioned. Finally, we showed how similar techniques could be used for measuring the time course of multiplicative and subtractive components of sensitivity regulation.

This paper has focused on methods and models and not on specific data from any one experiment. We hope we have convinced psychophysicists of the value of working within the framework of a model and stimulated physiologists to help us take these models one step further. We are not advocating one specific model but rather emphasizing the importance of framing questions within a model. Models allow for quantitative estimates of parameters of visual function and allow for easier communication of results among researchers.

Acknowledgements: This work was supported in part by NEI grant EY07922 provided to JFS and NIA grant T32 AG 00185 provided to DJH.

References

Adelson, E.A., 1982, Saturation and adaptation in the rod system. *Vision Res., 22:* 299.

Aguilar, M. and Stiles, W.S., 1954, Saturation of the rod mechanism of the retina at high levels of stimulation. *Optica Acta, 1:* 59.

Birren, J.E. Bick, M.W. and Fox, C., 1948, Age changes in the light threshold of the dark adapted eye. *J. Gerontol. 3:* 267.

Boynton, R.M., 1979, *Human Color Vision,* Holt, Rinehart and Winston, New York.

Curcio, C.A., Allen, K.A. and Kalina, R.E., 1990, Reorganization of the human photoreceptor mosaic following age-related rod loss. (Abstract), *Invest. Opthalmol. Vis. Sci. Suppl., 31:* 38.

Eisner, A., Fleming, S.A., Klein, J.L., and Mauldin, W.M., 1987, Sensitivities in older eyes with good acuity: Cross-sectional norms. *Invest. Ophthalmol. Vis. Sci. 28:* 1824.

Elsner, A.E., Berk, L., Burns, S.A. and Rosenberg, P. R., 1988, Aging and human cone photopigments. *J. Opt. Soc. Am. A, 5:* 2106.

Geisler, W.S., 1983, Mechanisms of visual sensitivity: Backgrounds and early dark adaptation. *Vision Res. 23:* 1423.

Gunkel, R.D. and Gouras, P., 1963, Changes in scotopic visibility thresholds with age. *Arch. Ophthalmol., 69:* 4.

Hayhoe, M.M., Benimoff, N.I., and Hood, D.C., 1987, The time-course of multiplicative and subtractive adaptation process. *Vision Res. 27:* 1981.

Hood, D.C., 1988, Testing hypotheses about development with electroretinographic and increment-threshold data. *J. Opt. Soc. Am. 5:* 2159.

Hood, D.C. and Greenstein, V.C., 1990, Models of the normal and abnormal rod system. *Vision Res. 30:* 51.

Hood, D.C. and Birch, D.C., 1991, Light adaptation of human cone receptors. (Abstract) *Invest. Ophthalmol. Vis. Sci. Suppl., 32:* 166.

Johnson, C.A., Adams, A.J., Twelker, J.D., and Quigg, J.M., 1988, Age-related changes of the central visual field for short-wavelength sensitive pathways. *J. Opt. Soc. Am. A., 5:* 2131.

Keunen, J.E.E., van Norren, D. and van Meel, G.J., 1987, Density of foveal cone pigments at older age. *Invest. Ophthalmol. Vis. Sci., 28:* 985.

Kilbride, P.E., Hutman, L.P., Fishman, M. and Read, J.S., 1986, Foveal cone pigment density difference in the aging human eye. *Vision Res., 26: 321.*

Kornzweig, A.L., 1954, Physiological effects of age on the visual process. *Sight sav. rev., 24:* 130.

Liem, A.T.A., Keunen, J.E.E., van Norren, D., and van de Kraats, J., 1991, Rod densitometry in the aging human eye. (Abstract). *Invest. Ophthalmol. Vis. Sci. Suppl. 32:* 139.

Luria, S.M., 1960, Absolute visual threshold and age. *J. Opt. Soc. Am. 50,* 86.

Marshall, J., Grindle, C.F., J. Ansell, P.L. and Bowein, B., 1979, Convolutions in human rods: An aging process. *Br. J. Ophthalmol., 63:* 181.

McFarland, R.A. and Fisher, M.B., 1955, Alterations in dark adaptation as a function of age. *J. Gerontol. 10:* 424.

McFarland, R.A., Domey, R.G., Warren, A.G., and Ward, D.C., 1960, Dark adaptation as a function of age: I. A statistical analysis. *J. Gerontol. 15:* 149.

Naka, K.I. and Rushton, W.H.A., 1966, S-potentials from luminosity units in the retina of fish (Cyprinidae). *J. Physiol. 185:* 587.

Osterberg, G., 1935, Topography of the layer of rods and cones in the human retina. *Acta Ophthalmol. Suppl.* (Copenh), *6:* 1.

Smith, V.C., Pokorny, J., and Diddie, K.R., 1988, Color-matching and the Stiles-Crawford effect in observers with early age-related macular changes. *J. Opt. Soc. Am. A., 5:* 2113.

Sturr, J.F., Church, K.L., Nuding, S.C., van Orden, K., and Taub, H.A., 1986, Older observers have attenuated increment thresholds upon transient backgrounds. *J. Gerontol., 41:* 743.

Sturr, J.F., Taub, H.A., and Hall, B.A., 1991, Foveal early dark adaptation in young and older observers in good ocular health. *Clin. Vis. Sci, 6:* 257.

Werner, J.S., and Steele, V.G., 1988, Sensitivity of human foveal color mechanisms throughout the life span. *J. Opt. Soc. Am. A, 5:* 2122.

Werner, J.S., Peterzell, D.H. and Scheetz, A.J., 1990, Light, vision and aging. *Optom. Vision Sci., 67(3):* 214.

Wyszecki, G. and Stiles, W.S., 1967, *Color science.* Wiley, New York.

STRUCTURAL ORGANIZATION AND DEVELOPMENT OF IDENTIFIED PROJECTION NEURONS IN PRIMARY VISUAL CORTEX

Jürgen Bolz, Mark Hübener, Iris Kehrer, and Nino Novak

Friedrich Miescher Labor der Max-Planck Gesellschaft
Spemannstrasse 37-39, 7400 Tübingen, Germany

A characteristic feature of the mammalian cerebral cortex is that each cortical area has outputs to a number of different cortical and subcortical destinations. Cortical neurons projecting to a given target are situated in distinct cortical layers. In the visual cortex for example, cells projecting to the lateral geniculate nucleus (LGN) are located in layer 6, cells projecting to the superior colliculus are located in layer 5, and many cells in layers 2 and 3 project to other cortical areas (for review see Sefton, 1981; Gilbert, 1983). Because cells in different cortical layers differ in their receptive field properties (for review see Bolz et al., 1989), the segregation of projection neurons into layers reflects the specificity of the cortical output. The functional specialization of cortical output neurons was strikingly illustrated in previous studies showing that even cells within a single cortical layer, but with different projection targets, differ in their dendritic morphology and participate in different intrinsic cortical circuits (Katz, 1987; Hübener and Bolz, 1988; Hübener et al., 1990). The proper development of these efferent projections is therefore critical for the correct functioning of the visual system.

In this report we will review our previous studies on the structural organization of projection neurons in primary visual cortex and provide some new data on the development of cortical output neurons. We will first describe the morphological characteristics of two classes of pyramidal neurons, one with cortical and one with subcortical projection targets. Cells within each projection class have a rather stereotypic morphology, but there are distinct differences between the two projection systems. Our developmental studies will then show that this close relationship between pyramidal cell morphology and projection target is not present during early postnatal life. Rather, during postnatal development, the characteristic neuronal phenotypes of these two projection systems are modeled from a common morphological prototype. Finally, we will describe *in vitro* studies that provide some insights into mechanisms generating the specific pattern of cortical outputs during development.

The Changing Visual System, Edited by P. Bagnoli and
W. Hodos, Plenum Press, New York, 1991

Morphological types of cortical projections neurons

Previous retrograde tracing studies demonstrated that in primary visual cortex (area 17), cells in layer 5 project to multiple subcortical targets, including the superior colliculus, the pons, and the lateral posterior nucleus (Kawamura et al., 1974; Gilbert and Kelly, 1975; Albus and Donate-Oliver, 1977; Kawamura and Chiba, 1979). Moreover, double labelling experiments indicated that these neurons innervate more than one subcortical target. Corticotectal cells, for example, often send axon collaterals to the pons or the lateral posterior nucleus (Albus and Donate-Oliver, 1977; Klein et al., 1986; Keizer et al., 1987; Hallman et al., 1988). In addition, cells in layer 5 of area 17 also project to other cortical targets, such as area 18 and 19 in the ipsilateral hemisphere and area 17 in the contralateral hemisphere (Olavarria and Van Sluyters, 1983; Bullier et al., 1984; Ferrer et al., 1988). Again it was shown by double labelling experiments that some cells innervate more than one cortical area (Bullier et al., 1984). However, in all cases examined, very few, if any, double labelled cells were found after tracer injections into cortical and subcortical targets (Weber et al., 1983; Hallman et al., 1988; Hübener and Bolz, 1988). Thus there are two distinct projection systems in layer 5, one projecting to cortical and one to subcortical targets. However, since the transported tracers only labelled cell bodies and the initial portions of primary dendrites, the cellular morphology of these two efferent systems could not be assessed in these studies.

In order to reveal the dendritic morphology and axonal branching patterns of projection neurons in layer 5, we combined retrograde tracing with intracellular staining (Hübener and Bolz, 1988; Hübener et al., 1990). For this, cells were retrogradely labelled from their projection target with fluorescent latex microspheres, and individual projection neurons were subsequently stained intracellularly with the fluorescent dye Lucifer yellow in living brain slices (Katz et al., 1984). This approach is illustrated in Fig. 1, which shows a cell retrogradely labelled with microspheres from the superior colliculus and injected with Lucifer yellow. Both labels can be reliably distinguished by their different fluorescence. Thus this technique allows a complete staining of soma, dendrites, dendritic spines and even very fine axon collaterals of neurons with identified projection targets.

Using this technique, we have been studying the morphology of neurons in layer 5 of rat primary visual cortex projecting to the superior colliculus and the contralateral hemisphere. Fig. 2 shows drawings of Lucifer yellow injected corticotectal cells. Corticotectal cells have the characteristic morphology of pyramidal cells and possess several common morphological features. All cells have a long apical dendrite that runs through all overlaying layers and ends with a large tuft in layer 1. The diameter of the basal dendritic field is smaller than the apical tuft, it is formed by 6-8 primary dendrites. These dendrites are highly branched and form a dense basal dendritic tree. Most basal dendrites are confined to layer 5, and only few dendritic endings reach into upper layer 6.

The morphology of neurons projecting to the contralateral visual cortex is strikingly different from corticotectal cell. As shown in Fig. 2, all callosal cells possess a short

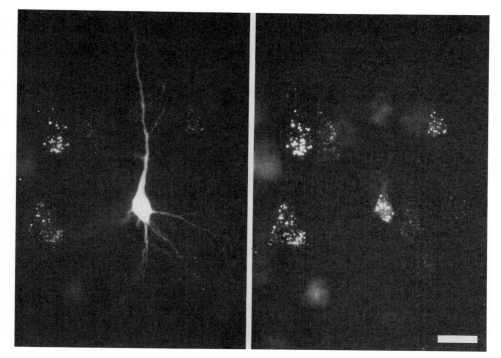

Fig. 1 Combination of intracellular injection in living brain slices after retrograde labelling. Left: high power micrograph of a Lucifer yellow filled neuron. Right: Same field photographed under rhodamine illumination. The cell body of the Lucifer yellow stained cell contains retrogradely transported microspheres, which had been injected into the superior colliculus. Scale bar: 20 μm.

apical dendrite that never reaches higher than the lower part of layer 3. Callosal cells have fewer primary basal dendrites (3-6) than corticotectal cells (6-8). The basal dendrites of callosal cells are less branched. However, compared with corticotectal cells, callosal cells have a larger basal dendritic field and their dendrites usually extend into layer 6 and layer 4. The morphometric data shown in Fig. 5 indicate some of the characteristic differences between callosal and tectal projecting cells.

Development of target specific morphology

The results described in the previous section demonstrated that cortical and subcortical projecting cells in layer 5 of the adult visual cortex have very different morphologies. However, cells within each efferent system possess rather similar patterns of dendrites, suggesting that there is a close relationship between neuronal phenotype and projection target. In order to see how such highly organized and stereotyped efferent connections develop, we examined corticotectal and callosum projecting cells at early postnatal stages. For this we used the technique of neuronal tracing with the fluorescent

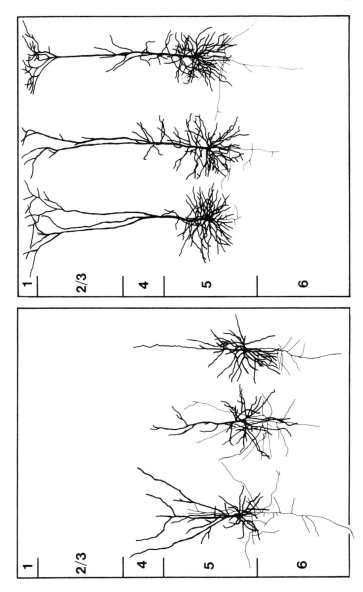

Fig. 2 Drawings of Lucifer yellow injected callosal (left) and corticotectal (right) cells in adult visual cortex. Scale bar: 250 μm.

dye DiI in aldehyde fixed tissue (Godement et al., 1987). In brains of different age-groups, from the day of birth up to 2 weeks after birth, DiI crystals were placed either in the contralateral visual cortex or in the superior colliculus. Since DiI is a lipophilic substance, it diffuses along plasma membranes and, over the period of several months, stains retrogradely the entire dendritic tree of projection neurons via their efferent axon.

In accordance with a previous HRP study (Thong and Dreher, 1986), we detected the first DiI labelled corticotectal cells on postnatal day 3. At this early age, only very few cells were retrogradely labelled from the superior colliculus. All labelled cells were located in layer 5, their appropriate layer, but the morphology of these cells was very immature. The cells had only small apical and basal dendritic fields and many dendrites were tipped with growth cones. Only two days later, on postnatal day 5, many more cells were retrogradely labelled from the superior colliculus, and their morphology appeared more mature (Fig. 3). However, as revealed by our quantitative analysis shown in Fig. 5, in the second postnatal week basal and apical dendrites of corticotectal cells still grow and form new branches.

With DiI injections in the white matter of the contralateral hemisphere, callosal cells can be retrogradely labelled already at the day of birth. During the first postnatal week, the morphology of callosum projecting cells in layer 5 is quite different from the adult morphology (Fig. 4). For example, all cells had an apical dendrite that reached layer 1, where it formed an apical tuft. Thus at this age, both corticotectal and callosum projecting neurons have similar apical dendrites, whereas in adult animals there is a striking difference in the length of the apical dendrite between these two projection classes. Our morphometric analysis revealed that the distinctions in the basal dendritic tree observed in adult animals are also not present during the first postnatal week (Fig. 5). Although there seem to be some more subtle differences, such in the number of apical dendritic endings, overall the dendritic branching patterns of corticotectal and callosal cells are very similar during the first postnatal week. Thus there appears to be an initial common morphological prototype of projection neurons in layer 5, and the characteristic distinctions between the two projection systems are then sculptured during postnatal development.

These observations on the development of projection neurons raise several questions of how these cells have acquired their morphological characteristics. Are there intrinsic differences between these two classes of projection cells ? Are inputs from other cortical or subcortical areas required in defining cell morphology ? Does the target structure influence the neuronal phenotype of projection neurons ? And how, in the first place, do cortical neurons establish their connections with the appropriate target ? Based on observations made in intact animals, it is very difficult to answer such questions. Therefore, in an attempt to get a better understanding of the strategies how efferent connections are established during development, we studied the formation of cortical projections in an *in vitro* system.

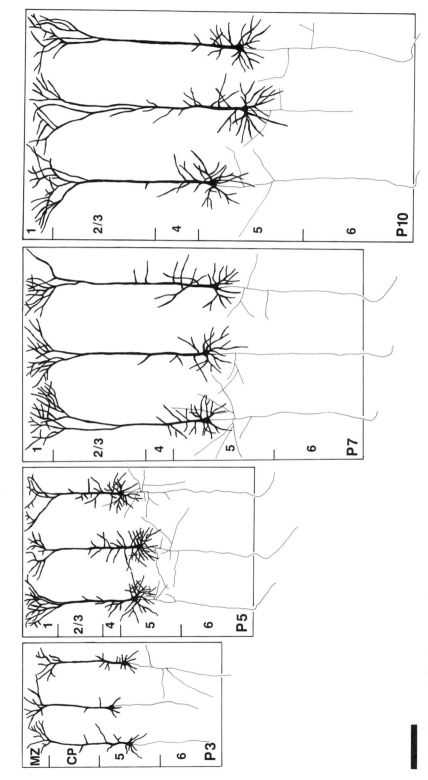

Fig. 3   Postnatal development of corticotectal cells. Drawings of cells retrogradelly labelled with DiI placed in the superior colliculus of fixed brains. Scale bar: 250 μm.

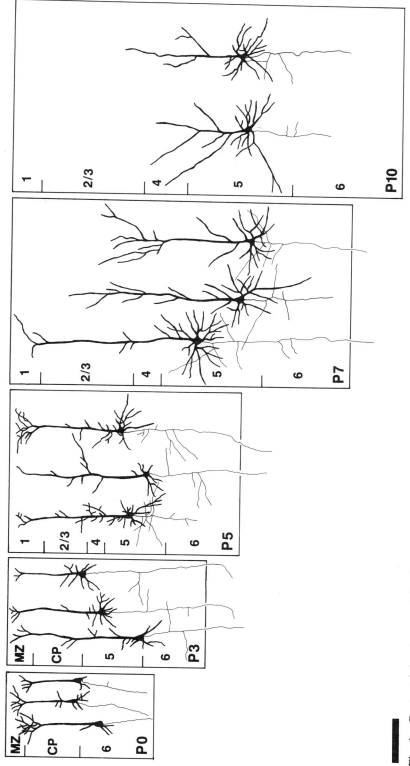

Fig. 4 Postnatal development of callosal projecting cells. Drawings of cells retrogradely labelled with DiI placed in the contralateral hemisphere of fixed brains. Scale bar: 250 μm.

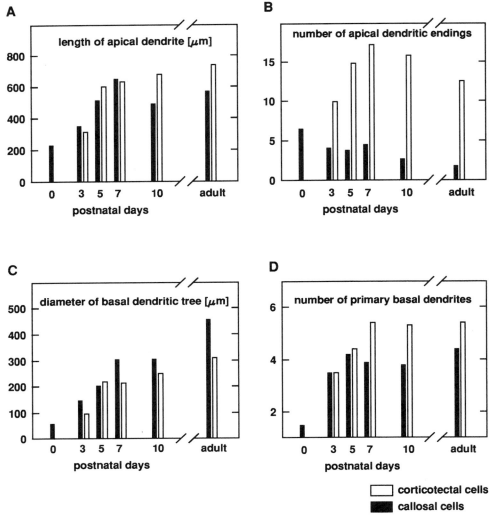

Fig. 5 Quantitative analysis of the morphological differentiation of corticotectal and callosal projecting neurons.

Cortical projections in organotypic slice cultures

For the *in vitro* studies, slice cultures from the visual cortex were prepared using a roller culture technique (Gähwiler, 1981). As we have described previously, cortical slice cultures survive for many weeks and remain organotypically organized. The cytoarchitecture and the cortical layering is preserved in these preparations (Caeser et al., 1989; Bolz et al., 1990; Götz and Bolz, 1990). Cortical slice cultures contain pyramidal cells and different classes of nonpyramidal cells with the typical morphological and neurochemical features of their *in vivo* counterparts (Bolz et al., 1990; Götz and Bolz, 1989). At the electron microscopic level, the pattern of symmetric and asymmetric synaptic connections in slice cultures is similar to that observed in normal cortex (Wolburg and Bolz, 1991). Thus these studies suggest that slice cultures may be a useful *in vitro* model to study mechanisms of cortical development.

In order to examine efferent cortical connections *in vitro*, slices from the visual cortex were cultured next to slices from the superior colliculus. These co-cultures were prepared from animals at the day of birth up to postnatal day 2. As was described above, at this early age the axons of corticotectal cells *in vivo* have not yet reached the superior colliculus. In cultures prepared from such young animals, already after 2 days *in vitro*, many fibers could be seen to leave the cortical and tectal explants. After 9-12 days *in vitro*, many axons of cortical cells had grown into the co-cultured superior colliculus. In contrast, fibers from tectal explants almost never grew into cortical cultures. Thus as in the *in vivo* situation, cortical cells *in vitro* establish connections with the tectum, but there is no back-projection from tectal explants to the co-cultured visual cortex.

To determine the laminar origin and cellular morphology of corticotectal cells *in vitro*, cells in cortical slice cultures were retrogradely labelled by placing DiI in the tectal explant. A micrograph of corticotectal cells *in vitro* is shown in Fig. 6. Almost all cells that established connections with the co-cultured superior colliculus were located in layer 5, precisely were cells projecting to this target are found *in vivo*. Corticotectal cells in slice cultures had the typical morphology of pyramidal cells. They possessed a well developed basal dendritic field and a long apical dendrite that usually reached layer 1, where it formed a large apical tuft. We examined the morphology of these cells using the same quantitative analysis applied for corticotectal cells *in vivo*. As shown in Fig. 7, for the most part corticotectal cells continue their morphological maturation in culture, thus they acquire their target specific pyramidal cell morphology under *in vitro* conditions.

In the experiment shown in Fig. 6, the tectal explant was placed adjacent to the white matter side of the cortical slice culture. Here the axons of the projecting cells first grew through the white matter, their normal route, in order to reach their co-cultured target. However, corticotectal cells also innervated tectal explants placed at ectopic positions. This is illustrated in Fig. 8, where the co-cultured superior colliculus was placed next to the pial surface of the cortical culture. Again, these ectopically positioned targets were innervated from cells in layer 5 with the characteristic morphology of corticotectal cells. In many instances, the target was innervated by axon collaterals that separated from the main axon and grew through the grey matter. Thus the axon collaterals of the projecting cells are not restricted to particular pathways, but rather redirect their growth and head directly towards their target. These experiments therefore suggest that tectal explants attract layer 5 axons by secreting a factor that acts directly on the axons.

In a previous study we showed that cells in cortical slice cultures also establish connections with co-cultured explants from the lateral geniculate nucleus (Bolz et al., 1990). Thalamic explants were innervated by a specific population of projection neurons, no matter whether these explants faced the white matter or the pial side of the cortical

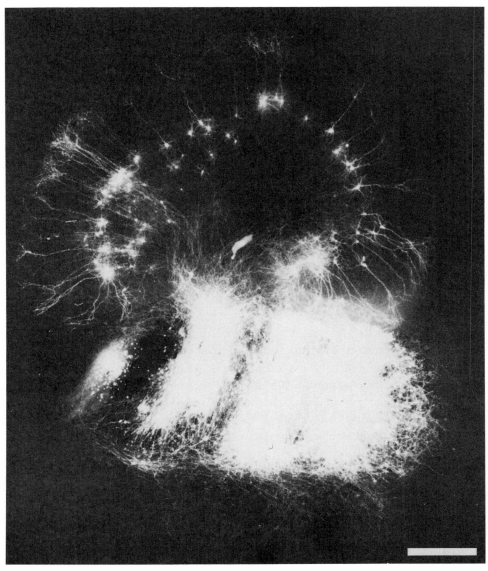

Fig. 6 Micrograph of projection neurons in a cortical slice culture (above) retrogradely labelled with DiI from the co-cultured superior colliculus (below). The pial side is up, the tectal explant faces the white matter zone of the cortical culture. The culture was prepared from a 1 day-old animal and fixed after 12 days *in vitro*. Scale bar: 500 μm.

slice cultures. Almost all corticothalamic cells *in vitro* are located in layer 6 and many of these cells have short apical dendrites. These *in vitro* studies demonstrate that different cortical target areas produce different attractive molecules, and only specific subsets of efferent cortical neurons respond to these molecules. Thus chemotropic guidance may play an important role in the formation of specific connections between cortical neurons and their distant targets.

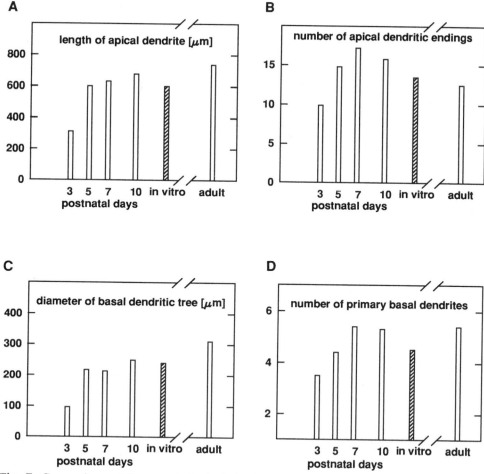

Fig. 7 Comparison of the morphological development of corticotectal cells *in vivo* and in organotypic slice cultures. Co-cultures from visual cortex and superior colliculus were prepared from 0-2 day old animals, and the cellular morphology of cortical cells projecting to the tectal explants was examined after 8-12 days *in vitro*.

Concluding remarks

Here we have considered the sequence of developmental events that lead to the specific pattern of cortical output neurons in the adult visual cortex. We have described two populations of pyramidal cells in layer 5, one with cortical and one with subcortical efferent targets. In adult animals, the neurons that give rise to these two projections show characteristic morphological differences, but cells within each projection class have a stereotyped morphology. This close relationship between neuronal phenotype and projection target is not present during the first postnatal week. At these early stages of development, the morphology of cortical and subcortical projecting neurons in layer 5 is very similar. Thus it appears that the target specific morphological features of cortical

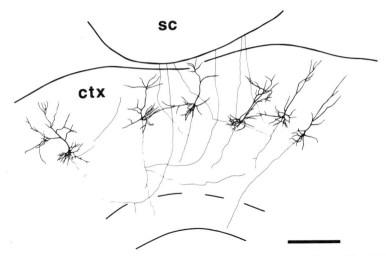

Fig. 8 Drawings of corticotectal cells *in vitro*, retrogradely labelled with DiI from co-cultured superior colliculus positioned close to the pial surface of the cortical slice. The dashed line indicates the border between the grey and white matter. Scale bar: 500 μm.

output neurons are remodeled postnataly from a common morphological prototype. In an attempt to get an insight into the mechanisms underlying the formation of efferent cortical connections, we have also studied cortical projection neurons in an *in vitro* system. These experiments showed that neurons in organotypic cortical cultures establish connections to co-cultured target explants. The morphology of cortical projections neurons *in vitro* was strikingly similar to the morphology of their counterparts *in vivo* at the corresponding age. Thus afferent inputs from extrinsic cortical or subcortical sources are not required for the development of target specific pyramidal cell morphology, since these inputs are eliminated in culture. Furthermore, the axonal trajectories of cortical neurons *in vitro* are always directed towards their appropriate target, and they reorientate their growth if their target is placed at ectopic positions. This suggests that specific subsets of cortical neurons respond to attractive molecules emanating from distant projection targets. Thus there is a significant degree of intrinsic specification in the development of cortical projections.

REFERENCES

Albus, K. and F. Donate-Oliver (1977) Cells of origin of the occipito-pontine projection in the cat: functional properties and intracortical location. Exp.Brain Res. *28*:167-174.

Bolz, J., C.D. Gilbert, and T.N. Wiesel (1989) Pharmacological analysis of cortical circuitry. TINS *12*:292-296.

Bolz, J., N. Novak, M. Götz, and T. Bonhoeffer (1990) Formation of target-specific neuronal projections in organotypic slice cultures from rat visual cortex. Nature *346*:359-362.

Bullier, J., H. Kennedy, and W. Salinger (1984) Branching and laminar origin of projections between visual cortical areas in the cat. J.Comp.Neurol. *228*:329-341.

Caeser, M., T. Bonhoeffer, and J. Bolz (1989) Cellular organization and development of slice cultures from rat visual cortex. Exp.Brain Res. *77*:234-244.

Ferrer, J.M.R., D.J. Price, and C. Blakemore (1988) The organization of corticocortical projections from area 17 to area 18 of the cat's visual cortex. Proc.R.Soc.Lond.B. *233*:77-98.

Gähwiler, B.H. (1981) Organotypic monolayer cultures of nervous tissue. J.Neurosci.Methods *4*:329-342.

Gilbert, C.D. (1983) Microcircuitry of the visual cortex. Ann.Rev.Neurosci. *6*:217-247.

Gilbert, C.D. and J.P. Kelly (1975) The projections of cells in different layers of the cat's visual cortex. J.Comp.Neurol. *163*:81-105.

Godement, P., J. Vanselow, S. Thanos, and F. Bonhoeffer (1987) A study in developing visual systems with a new method of staining neurones and their processes in fixed tissue. Development *101*:697-713.

Götz, M. and J. Bolz (1989) Development of vasoactive intestinal polypeptide (VIP)-containig neurons in organotypic slice cultures from rat visual cortex. Neurosci.Lett. *107*:6-11.

Götz, M. and J. Bolz (1990) Formation of cortical layers in organotypic slice cultures of rat visual cortex. In *Brain - perception - cognition. Proceedings of th 18th Göttingen neurobiology conference* N. Elsner and G. Roth, eds. pp. 282-282, Georg Thieme Verlag, Stuttgart and New York.

Hallman, L.E., B.R. Schofield, and C.-S. Lin (1988) Dendritic morphology and axon collaterals of corticotectal, corticopontine, and callosal neurons in layer 5 of primary visual cortex of the hooded rat. J.Comp.Neurol. *272*:149-160.

Hübener, M. and J. Bolz (1988) Morphology of identified projection neurons in layer 5 of rat visual cortex. Neurosci.Lett. *94*:76-81.

Hübener, M., C. Schwarz, and J. Bolz (1990) Morphological types of projection neurons in layer 5 of cat visual cortex. J.Comp.Neurol. *301*:655-674.

Katz, L.C. (1987) Local circuitry of identified projection neurons in cat visual cortex brain slices. J.Neurosci. *7*:1223-1249.

Katz, L.C., A. Burkhalter, and W.J. Dreyer (1984) Fluorescent latex microspheres as a retrograde neuronal marker for in vivo and in vitro studies of visual cortex. Nature *310*:498-500.

Kawamura, K. and M. Chiba (1979) Cortical neurons projecting to the pontine nuclei of the cat. An experimental study with the horseradish peroxidase technique. Exp.Brain Res. *35*:269-285.

Kawamura, K., J.M. Sprague, and K. Niimi (1974) Corticofugal projections from the visual cortices to the thalamus, pretectum and superior colliculus in the cat. J.Comp.Neurol. *158*:339-362.

Keizer, K., H.G.J.M. Kuypers, and H.K. Ronday (1987) Branching cortical neurons in cat which project to the colliculi and to the pons: a retrograde fluorescent double-labeling study. Exp.Brain Res. *67*:1-15.

Klein, B.G., R.D. Mooney, S.E. Fish, and R.W. Rhoades (1986) The structural and functional characteristics of striate cortical neurons that innervate the superior colliculus and lateral posterior nucleus in hamster. Neurosci. *17*:57-78.

Olavarria, J. and R.C. Van Sluyters (1983) Widespread callosal connections in infragranular visual cortex of the rat. Brain Res. *279*:233-237.

Sefton, A.J. (1981) Cortical projections to visual centres in the rat: an HRP study. Brain Res. *215*:1-13.

Thong, I.G. and B. Dreher (1986) The development of the corticotectal pathway in the albino rat. Dev.Brain Res. *25*:227-238.

Weber, J.T., R.W. Rieck, and H.J. Gould (1983) Interhemispheric and subcortical collaterals of single cortical neurons in the adult cat. Brain Res. *276*:333-338.

Wolburg, H. and J. Bolz (1991) Ultrastructural organization of slice cultures from rat visual cortex. J.Neurocytol. (In Press)

DEVELOPMENTAL STATUS OF INTRINSIC CONNECTIONS

IN VISUAL CORTEX OF NEWBORN HUMANS

Andreas Burkhalter

Departments of Neurosurgery and Anatomy and Neurobiology
Washington University School of Medicine
St. Louis, MO 63110

Although experimental psychological tests of vision in human infants have shown that the visual system is immature at birth (Atkinson, 1984), until recently, neuroanatomical support for these findings was unspecific (Conel, 1939; 1941). This situation has changed with the study of synaptogenesis in the primary visual cortex of humans by Huttenlocher and de Courten (1987), which showed a dramatic increase in synaptic density in the first 10 months after birth. This observation strongly suggests that a large number of neuronal connections are formed postnatally, and that these connections are assembled into functional circuits that may account for much of the sensory maturation seen in psychophysical tests of young infants.

Synaptogenesis in human visual cortex proceeds in phases. In the first 2.5 months after birth there is little change in synaptic density. This slow phase is followed by a phase of rapid proliferation in which synaptic density nearly doubles within a 2 month period. These newly added synapses presumably represent newly established functional connections. This is consistent with the view that cortical circuitry is relatively immature until about 2 months postnatal. Further support for this notion derives from findings that neuronal circuits responsible for cortical functions, such as orientation selectivity and binocular integration, are not functional until 2-3 months of age (Braddick et al., 1983; Braddick et al., 1986). However, the visual system of infants younger than 2 months of age is capable of encoding behaviorally relevant visual information that can initiate visually guided orienting responses. Such reactions can be elicited by static and transient stimuli, but the most effective targets are moving objects in the peripheral visual field (Lewis et al., 1978; Regal, 1981). This capacity together with the presence of saccadic eye movements at birth (Aslin and Salapatek, 1975), was taken to indicate that vision in newborns is controlled primarily or exclusively by subcortical structures, such as the superior colliculus (Bronson, 1974; 1982). But recent studies on the neurophysiological basis of saccadic eye movements have emphasized the contributions of different cortical areas in the generation of saccades (for references see, Andersen and Gnadt, 1989; Goldberg and Segraves, 1989). This may indicate that cortical circuits are functional earlier than previously assumed, and may make it necessary to revise the hypothesis that early infant vision is completely dominated by subcortical structures. To clarify this important issue we need direct information about the developmental status of intracortical connections in newborns. This structural information seems critical for assessing when cortical circuits differentiate into functionally competent circuits.

Until recently, it was impossible to examine the connections of the human brain with experimental neuroanatomical techniques, and the tracing of pathways relied solely on mapping of tissue degeneration patterns in response to neuronal injury produced by experiments of nature (Minkowski, 1920; Putnam, 1926; Van Buren and Borke, 1972; Hitchcock and Hickey, 1980). This has changed with the introduction of the lipid soluble fluorescent dye, diI (Honig and Hume, 1986), and the description of a method for tracing neuronal connections in *postmortem*, aldehyde fixed tissue (Godement et al., 1987). We have recently adapted this approach for tracing connections in the adult human brain (Burkhalter and Bernardo, 1989), and have since made substantial progress in unraveling the development of local circuits in visual cortex of young infants. Before discussing these findings, it seems appropriate to briefly review the functional organization of the visual system in non-human primates and compare it to the organization of the human visual system.

Streams for processing visual information

Anatomical and physiological studies in non-human primates have shown that the information used for visual perception and visually guided behavior is encoded in two principal channels with different but partially overlapping functions (DeYoe and Van Essen, 1988; Felleman and Van Essen, 1991). Neurons of the M (magno) stream have high temporal resolution, high contrast sensitivity, low spatial resolution and show little chromatic opponency. By contrast, cells of the P (parvo) stream have high spatial sensitivity, poor temporal resolution, low contrast sensitivity and are strongly color opponent. The M channel originates from large retinal ganglion cells which project to the magnocellular layers of the lateral geniculate nucleus (LGN). These in turn provide input to layer $4C\alpha$ of primary visual cortex (V1). Cells in layer $4C\alpha$ project to layer 4B which sends inputs to several extrastriate areas, including V2 and MT. Layer 4B is the first stage of the visual pathway in which neurons show direction and disparity selectivity. The circuitry that underlies these receptive field properties is unknown, but it has been suggested that the extensive network of horizontal fibers within layer 4B (Rockland and Lund, 1983; Blasdel et al., 1985) plays an important role for direction selectivity (Lund, 1988). The P channel originates in smaller, P retinal ganglion cells which provide input to the parvocellular layers of the LGN. These in turn project to layer $4C\beta$ of striate cortex. Here, the pathway bifurcates and conveys information via layer 4A to two distinct compartments in superficial layers: the cytochrome oxidase (CO) rich blobs and the CO poor interblobs. Most cells contained within blobs are color selective, are non-oriented and do not respond to binocular disparities. By contrast, only a small fraction of interblob neurons are color selective, but most are orientation sensitive and show disparity selectivity. Similar to layer 4B of the M stream, superficial layers contain an elaborate network of tangential connections that specifically link blobs with blobs and interblobs with interblobs (Livingstone and Hubel, 1984). The function of these lateral connections is uncertain, but their anatomical specificity strongly suggests that they play a role for the intracortical distribution of form and color information and that they may be important for figure/ground discriminations.

Processing streams in human visual cortex

Evidence for functional streams in the human visual system is indirect and, until recently, it was primarily based on the similarity of cytochrome oxidase staining compartments in striate cortex of humans (Horton and Hedley-Whyte, 1984) and monkeys (Horton, 1984). We have now obtained evidence that the secondary visual area (V2) in humans may also have an organization similar to that of non-human primates (Burkhalter and Bernardo, 1989). This notion derives from images such as those in Figure 1. Here, adjacent horizontal sections through V1 and V2 of a 72 old human were stained for cytochrome oxidase activity. Striate cortex shows the familiar array of intensely stained blobs. In V2 a pair of parallel 1-2 mm wide stripes are visible that run perpendicular to the V1/V2 border. This pattern resembles that seen in monkeys (Tootell et al., 1983; Livingstone and Hubel, 1984) in which different sets of thin and thick cytochrome oxidase staining stripes contain non-oriented, color opponent cells and neurons that are direction, orientation and disparity selective, respectively (DeYoe and Van Essen, 1988).

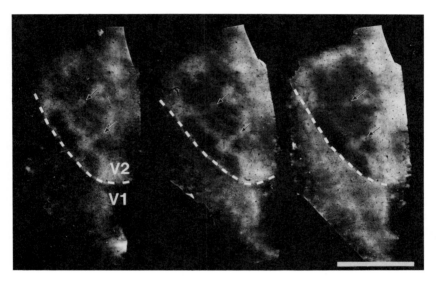

Figure 1. Cytochrome oxidase staining pattern in primary (V1) and secondary (V2) visual cortex of 72 year old human. Photomicrographs of three adjacent horizontal sections. Light areas indicate regions of high cytochrome oxidase activity. Cytochrome oxidase staining blobs are seen in V1. V2 shows a pair of stripes (arrows) that run perpendicular to the V1/V2. Scale bar: 5 mm.

Based on these similarities it seems reasonable to conclude that human visual cortex is parceled into different functional compartments. To further support this view, we examined the connections of blobs and interblobs within striate cortex. The question was whether each functional system is linked through an independent network of local connections, similar to the organization of monkey primary visual cortex (Livingstone and Hubel, 1984). We approached the question by combining axonal tracing with diI and cytochrome oxidase histochemistry in aldehyde fixed blocks of human visual cortex that were obtained at autopsy (Burkhalter and Bernardo, 1989). Small crystals of diI were placed into V1, and the tissue was subsequently stored in phosphate buffer to allow for intramembranous diffusion of the dye along axons. After 1-3 months, sections were cut on a Vibratome and the distribution of diI labeled cell bodies, axons and terminals was examined under the fluorescence microscope. Without exception, the dye spread in highly organized patterns. These were most clearly seen in horizontal sections, in which radial fibers emerged from the injection site and terminated in clusters up to 3 mm from the injection site (Fig. 2A). The clusters contained axon terminals and cell bodies which indicates that these local connections are reciprocal. The size and spacing of the clusters closely matched the dimensions of blob and interblob compartments, and the direct comparison of the diI labeling pattern with the distribution of cytochrome oxidase staining revealed that blobs were connected to blobs and interblobs to interblobs (Burkhalter and Bernardo, 1989). These tangential networks of connections were not confined to superficial layers, but were also seen in layers 4B and 5 (Fig. 2B). The connections within these two layers were indistinguishable from those seen in monkey striate cortex (Blasdel et al., 1985). For the discussion here, it is of particular interest that this resemblance included layer 4B and can, therefore, be assigned to the M stream. In addition it suggests that the connections within layer 4B may also be involved in the generation of direction selectivity. From this comparison of the intrinsic connectivity we conclude that the functional organization of primary visual cortex in humans and monkeys is homologous.

Postnatal development of connections within human primary visual cortex

The cytochrome oxidase staining pattern in primary visual cortex of newborn macaque monkey resembles that of adults (Horton, 1984). We have obtained evidence that this is different in humans. In newborns, high cytochrome oxidase activity was confined to layers 4Cα, 4Cβ and 6. Staining in layer 4B was lighter than in layer 4C, but appeared darker than in adults. The most conspicuous difference, however, was the absence of blobs in newborns. These findings are consistent with the notion that the human visual cortex is immature at birth. In addition, they suggest that the M stream matures in advance of the P stream.

To further support this conclusion, we used neuronal tracing with diI to examine the development of connections within primary visual cortex. Injections were made into striate cortex of humans of different ages: newborns, 2, 4, 7, 15 and 24 months of age. To reveal the complete complement of connections originating from all layers of striate cortex, multiple injections were made throughout the thickness of cortex. This experimental strategy precluded information about the laminar origin of projections. Instead it was focussed on the examination of the developmental status of horizontal and oblique axon collaterals that contribute to the network of connections within layer 4B of the M stream and superficial layers of the P stream. At birth, the connectivity within striate cortex was radically different from that in adults (Figs. 2A, 2B). Horizontal fibers were completely absent from superficial layers and were only seen in layers 4B and 5. At 2 months of age the picture was similar to that in newborns, except that the plexus of fibers in layer 4B was much denser and appeared patchy. Much to our surprise, at 4 months of age, at a time when cytochrome oxidase staining revealed a mature pattern of blobs, superficial layer connections were still absent and even at 7 months of age we were unable to show their existence. To ascertain that this result was not due to methodological

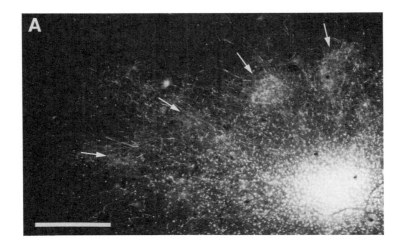

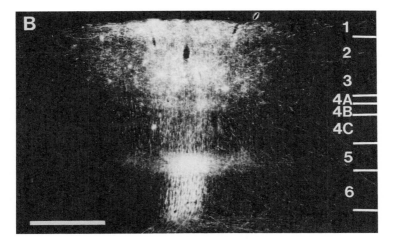

Figure 2. Connections within primary visual cortex of 29 year old human.
A. Fluorescence photomicrograph of horizontal section through primary
visual cortex. DiI injection is seen on lower right side. From the
injection labeled fibers run in all directions and terminate in distinct
clusters (arrows) within a radius of 2-3 mm. Modified from Burkhalter
and Bernardo, 1989. **B**. Fluorescence photomicrograph of transverse
section showing the laminar distribution of dii labeled fibers. The
injection site is located in superficial layers and includes layers 1-4B.
The section is taken ≈ 1 mm outside the margin of the injection site.
The diameter of the injection is 0.5 mm and corresponds to the width of
the vertical fiber bundle in layer 6. Extensive networks of horizontal
fibers extend in Layers 2/3, 4B and 5. These local projections are nonuniform and often show terminal clusters. Scale bars: 1 mm.

problems, we placed diI injections near the V1/V2 border and asked whether neurons in superficial layers of V1 make projections to targets outside striate cortex. This produced asymmetric labeling patterns in superficial layers of striate cortex: a large number of fibers traveled towards the V1/V2 border and penetrated far into V2, but not a single fiber ran in the opposite direction away from the V1/V2 border toward the center of V1. Because diI is a bidirectional tracer it is possible that some of these interareal fibers were feedback fibers from V2 to V1. Injections into V2, however, showed numerous retrogradely labeled cells in V1, which indicates that at least some of the upper layer fibers were axon collaterals of striate cortical neurons. Thus, we are confident that neurons in superficial layers of striate cortex do not develop local axon collaterals until after 7 months postnatal. Thus, connections between blobs and interblobs develop after 7 months of age. So far, we have examined a single case at 15 months of age, which clearly showed horizontal connections within superficial layers. At this age, the labeling pattern was patchy and indistinguishable from adults (Figs. 2A, 2B). It remains to be determined when exactly these connections develop.

Conclusions

Our investigation of the postnatal development of local connections supports earlier conclusions from studies of the cytoarchitecture, myelogenesis, and the formation of synapses and dendrites (Conel, 1939; 1941; Michel and Garey, 1984; Huttenlocher and deCourten 1987) that human primary visual cortex is immature at birth. In addition, our study provides an important extension of this knowledge, by showing that newborns possess an extensive network of connections within layer 4B, while similar connections in superficial layers do not develop until after 7 months postnatal. This indicates that intracortical circuits of the M stream are relatively mature at birth and that components of the M pathway develop several months before intracortical circuits of the P stream. The early presence of intracortical circuits associated with the M stream is interesting and it agrees with observations that newborns show smooth pursuit eye movements (Kremenitzer et al., 1979) which are known to dependent on intracortical circuits (Newsome et al., 1985). It is also consistent with findings that object recognition in infants is more dependent on motion information than on static information (Kellman and Spelke, 1983; Kellman, 1984). Thus, it appears that in newborns cortical circuits of the M stream may be mature enough to assist in visual functions that were previously attributed entirely to subcortical structures. These anatomical results then support the conclusion, drawn by Braddick and Atkinson (1988) from a review of the psychophysical literature, that it is necessary to revise Bronson's (1974) hypothesis of the complete dependence of early vision on subcortical circuits. In fact, our study suggests that cortex may play a more important role in infant vision in the first 2 postnatal months than has previously been recognized.

REFERENCES

Andersen,R.A. and Gnadt,J.W., 1989, Posterior parietal cortex. In: Wurtz and Goldberg (Eds.), The neurobiology of saccadic eye movements, pp. 315-335, Elsevier.

Aslin,R.N. and Salapatek,P., 1975, Saccadic localization of targets by the very young infant. Perception and Psychophysics 17:293-322.

Atkinson,J. 1984, Human visual development over the first 6 months of life. A review and a hypothesis. Human Neurobiol. 3:61-74.

Blasdel,G.G., Lund,J.S., and Fitzpatrick,D., 1985, Intrinsic connections of macaque striate cortex: Axonal projections of cells outside lamina 4C. J.Neurosci. 5:3350-3369.

Braddick,O., Wattam-Bell,J., Day,J., and Aktinson,J., 1983, The onset of binocular function in human infants. Human Neurobiol. 2:65-69.

Braddick,O., Wattam-Bell,J., and Atkinson,J., 1986, Orientation-specific cortical responses develop in early infancy. Nature 320:617-619.

Braddick,O. and Atkinson,J., 1988, Sensory selectivity, attentional control, and cross-channel integration in early visual development. In: A.Yonas (Ed.), Perceptual Development in Infancy. The Minnesota Symposia on Child Psychology, Vol. 20, pp. 105-143.

Bronson,G., 1974, The postnatal growth of visual capacity. Child Development. 45:873-890.

Bronson,G., 1982, Structure, status and characteristics of the nervous system at birth. In: P.Stratton (Ed.), Psychobiology of the Human Newborn. Chichester: Wiley.

Burkhalter,A. and Bernardo,K.L., 1989, Organization of corticocortical connections in human visual cortex. Proc.Natl.Acad.Sci.USA. 86:1071-1075.

Conel,J.L., 1939, The Postnatal Development of the Human Cerebral Cortex, Vol. 1, Cambridge, Harvard Univ. Press.

Conel,J.L. 1941, The Postnatal Development of the Human Cerebral Cortex, Vol. 2, Cambridge, Harvard Univ. Press.

DeYoe,E.A. and Van Essen, D.C., 1988, Concurrent processing streams in monkey visual cortex. Trends in Neurosci. 11:219-226.

Felleman,D.J. and Van Essen, D.C., 1991, Distributed hierarchical processing in the primate cerebral cortex. Cerebral Cortex 1:1047-3211.

Godement,P. Vanselow,J., Thanos,S., and Bonhoeffer,F., 1987, A study in developing visual systems with a new method of staining neurones and their processes in fixed tissue. Development 101:697-713.

Goldberg,M.E. and Segraves,M.A., 1989, The visual and frontal cortices, In: Wurtz and Goldberg (Eds.), The Neurobiology of Saccadic Eye Movements, pp. 283-313, Elsevier.

Hitchcock, P.F. and Hickey,T.L., 1980, Ocular dominance columns: evidence for their presence in humans. Brain Res. 182:176-179.

Honig,M.G. and Hume,R.I., 1986, Fluorescent Carbocyanine dyes allow living neurons of identified origin to be studied in long-term cultures. J.Cell Biol. 103:171-187.

Horton,J.C., 1984, Cytochrome oxidase patches:a new cytoarchitectonic feature of monkey visual cortex. Phil.Trans.R.Soc.Lond.B. 304:199-253.

Horton,J.C. and Hedley-Whyte, T.E., 1984, Mapping of cytochrome oxidase patches and ocular dominance columns in human visual cortex. Phil.Trans.R.Soc.Lond.B. 304:255-272.

Kellman,P.J. and Spelke,E.S., 1983, Perception of partly occluded objects in infancy. Cognitive Psychology 15:483-524.

Kellman,P.J., 1984, Perception of three-dimensional form by human infants. Perception and Psychophysics 36:353-358.

Kremenitzer,J.P., Vaughn,H.G., Kurtzberg,D., and Dowling,K., 1979, Smooth-pursuit eye movements in the newborn infant. Child Development 50:442-448.

Lewis,T.L., Maurer,D., and Kay,D., 1978, Newborns' central vision: Whole or hole ? J.Exp. Child Psychol. 26:193-203.

Livingstone,M.S. and Hubel,D.H., 1984, Specificity of intrinsic connections in primate primary visual cortex. J.Neurosci. 4:2830-2835.

Lund,J.S., 1988, Anatomical organization of macaque monkey striate visual cortex. Annu.Rev.Neurosci. 11:253-288.

Minkowski,M., 1920, Ueber den Verlauf, die Endigung und die zentrale Repräsentation von gekreuzten und ungekreuzten Sehnervenfasern bei einigen Säugetieren und beim Menschen. Schweiz. Arch. Neur. Psychiat. 6:201-252.

Newsome,W.T., Wurtz,R.H., Dürsteler,M.R., and Mikami,A., 1985, Deficits in visual motion processing following ibotenic acid lesions of the middle temporal visual area of the macaque monkey. J.Neurosci. 5:825-840.

Putnam, T.J., 1926, Studies on the central visual connections. Arch. of Neurol. and Psychiat. 16:566-596.

Regal,D., 1981, Development of flicker frequency in human infants. Vis.Res. 21:549-555.

Rockland,K.S. and Lund,J.S., 1983, Intrinsic laminar lattice connections in primate visual cortex. J.Comp.Neurol. 216:303-318.

Tootell,R.B.H., Silverman,M.S., DeValois,R.L., and Jacobs,G.H., 1983, Functional organization of the second cortical visual area in primates. Science 220:737-739.

Van Buren,J.M. and Borke, R.C., 1972, Variations and Connections of the Human Thalamus. Vol. 1, Springer Verlag, Berlin, New York.

DEVELOPMENT OF THE VISUAL CORTEX DEPRIVED PRENATALLY OF RETINAL CUES

Rodrigo O. Kuljis

Department of Neurology
The University of Iowa College of Medicine and
Veterans Affairs Medical Center
Iowa City, Iowa 52242-1053, U.S.A.

INTRODUCTION

The mammalian visual system provides a unique model to analyze some of the factors influencing the development of laminated regions of the brain, especially the visual cortex. This review is focused on the development of the human and nonhuman primate primary visual (striate) cortex under normal and abnormal conditions. Principles of development revealed in this model are contrasted with observations in the visual cortex of other mammals and other sensory cortices, to try to identify rules applicable to the specification of the cerebral cortex in general.

DEVELOPMENT OF THE VISUAL CORTEX IN ANOPHTHALMIC ANIMALS AND HUMANS

Much information has been gathered during the last five decades about the development of the visual cortex in both human anophthalmia and experimental models of this condition. Some of the salient findings are reviewed here, in an attempt to summarize some of the emerging principles of development of the striate cortex deprived of the retinal cues *in utero*.

The visual cortex of anophthalmic rodents

Chase and Chase (1941) described a mutant strain of mice in which 90% of the individulas are eyeless. This trait is primarily due to a failure of the optic vesicle to develop into a normal optic cup about the 10th day of gestation (E10). In normal C57 mice, optic nerve fibers begin to grow out by E13 and reach the diencephalon by E14. According to Chase (1945), the adult ZRDCT congenitally anophthalmic mice (ZRDCT-An) exhibit: (a) a dorsal lateral geniculate body (dLGN) less than half the size of that in the normal; (b) the ventral nucleus of the lateral geniculate body is also small, but over half the size in controls, and (c) the stratum griseum superficiale and stratum opticum of the superior colliculus is markedly reduced in thickness. Except for the visual cortex, these reductions in size are not much greater than those found by Tsang (1937) in rats blinded at birth. Many of the changes observed in adult ZRDCT-An specimens develop postnatally, since both the geniculate nucleus and the superior colliculus appear normal at E18.

Kaiserman-Abramof et al. (1980) found that although the dLGN of ZRDCT-An undergoes a reduction of its neuronal population to 76% of normal, its projection to area 17 exhibits an essentially normal topographic pattern. An interesting additional finding from the latter investigators is that the projection to area 17 from the nucleus lateralis posterior (LP) of the thalamus is considerably greater in congenitally anophthalmic than in normal-eyed mice, which suggests compensatory innervation from LP, perhaps partially substituting reduced dLGN afferents.

The visual cortex of ZRDCT-An, also called "eyeless" (ey; Sidman, Green & Appel, 1965), appears undifferentiated on embryonic day 18 (E18). Layers II/III reportedly become distinct at E19, and layer IV is clearly identifiable at birth. When compared to controls, five to six-month-old eyeless mice were found to have thinner layers II-IV, with a less distinct separation between layers III and IV. Layer V was found to be thicker and layer VI thinner than in controls (Chase, 1945). Unfortunately, precise quantitative determinations of these changes in the visual cortex are not available. This important void of information includes the surface area of the striate cortex, as well as any information about possible associated changes in peristriate cortices.

Interesting additional findings in ZRDCT-An include the formation of cranial nerves III-VI, which are present at birth but disappear or become reduced in the neonatal period and their nuclei become small by six months of age. The only exception is the ophthalmic division of the Vth nerve, which is small at birth but does not change appreciably afterwards.

The visual cortex in human anophthalmia

Anophthalmia in humans has long attracted the attention of clinicians, primarily from the perspective of understanding the mechanisms responsible for the formation of the eye. Relatively little is know, by contrast, about the cortical changes associated with the congenital absence of eyes in humans.

True anophthalmos is a rare clinical entity, the diagnosis of which rests on a careful histological examination of the orbital contents. Such analysis reveals that most cases of presumed anophthalmos are instead the more common condition of microphthalmia in which - contrary to anophthalmia - remnants of the eye, which are sometimes microscopic, can be found embedded among the tissues occupying the orbit (Pritkin, 1980). Given that the scope of this review is limited to instances of complete absence of retinal input to the cerebral cortex, I will address only the pathological findings of true anophthalmia. It should be recognized, nevertheless, that even the restricted category of true anophthalmia comprises a heterogeneous group of conditions. In fact, Mann (1957) subdivided this category into three conditions: (a) primary anophthalmos due to failure of development restricted to the optic vesicles, (b) secondary anophthalmos due to a more generalized maldevelopment of the forebrain, and (c) degenerative (also called consecutive) anophthalmos due to complete regression or involution of the optic vesicles. It should be emphasized that, although by definition there is complete absence of neuroectodermal derivatives in the orbits in all three of these conditions, in practice this can be quite difficult to prove conclusively. For example, cases of extreme microphthalmos can easily be misdiagnosed, and, even when there is no detectable residual eye tissue in the orbits, it is often impossible to establish whether this was primarily due to agenesis or involution. These difficulties are important to keep in mind, since they can contribute to uncertainties in the precise nosological characterization of developmental defects of the orbital contents, which depend critically on the interpretation of histopathological findings.

There are a few well documented cases of anophthalmia in the clinical literature, which will be the basis for this section of the review (Recordon & Griffiths, 1938; Duckworth & Cooper, 1966; Haberland & Perou, 1969; Brunquell et al., 1984). All four cases were characterized by a complete absence of eye tissue, optic nerves, chiasm and tracts. The lateral geniculate nuclei were not found in one case, and were small, nonlaminated and gliotic in three. The calcarine cortex was described as normal in one case, except for the absence of the line of Gennari (Duckworth & Cooper, 1966). The other three cases had abnormalities in the striate cortex which included absence of the line of Gennari in one, a thin line in another, grossly malformed calcarine fissures in another case and a short fissure that did not extend all the way into the occipital pole. The case of Brunquell et al. (1984) had preservation of the basic layering pattern of area 17, although lamination was poor compared with controls and the authors found a general reduction in the density and size of cells throughout this region. This case is the only one in which cytochrome oxidase histochemistry was conducted, which revealed that the continuous laminar pattern of enzymatic activity in layer IVC was present but very weak. The spatially discontinuous cytochrome oxidase puffs in layers II/III could not be visualized. These findings cannot be precisely correlated with those in macaque monkeys subjected to prenatal binocular enucleation (Kuljis & Rakic, 1990), described below, because: (a) precise details about the length of postmortem autolysis and mode of fixation are not available, raising the possibility that technical artifacts such as overfixation in formaldehyde prevented the visualization of the puffs, (b) the patient died at 27 years of age, after suffering significant retardation in psychomotor development and protracted illnesses such as seizure disorder, hypothyroidism and hypoadrenalism, all of which could have had an impact in cortical organization beyond that ascribable solely to the absence of the eyes, and (c) brain weight was low (1,050g), the frontal lobes were small, and there was a right parietal protuberance, all features suggestive of a cerebral maldevelopment extending well beyond the visual cortex, which could have had an additional impact in this region.

Even considering these difficulties in interpretation, the observations in human cases of anophthalmia do seem to indicate that "apparently the visual cortex can still survive, develop, and organize cell layers in the absence of a retinogeniculate pathway" (Brunquell et al., 1984). However, the abnormalities in the stria of Gennari have been interpreted as evidence that intrinsic connections are abnormal.

A primate model of anophthalmia based on prenatal retinal ablation in the macaque monkey

One of the experimental paradigms that has proven helpful in elucidating the role of retinal input in the specification of the visual cortex is the ablation of the retina in the fetal period (Hess, 1958; reviewed in Rakic & Goldman-Rakic, 1985). This model eliminates retinal cues in a manner similar to that discussed previously in human and murine anophthalmia, but potentially in a more tightly timed and controlled manner than the naturally occuring condition. Rakic has recently developed a surgical technique for this purpose in macaque monkeys (Rakic, 1988a,b) that results in a dramatic reduction in the size and cell number in the dLGN, which fails to develop its six characteristic layers. The pattern of gyration in the occipital lobe is altered in animals enucleated prior to mid-gestation, such that abnormal gyri appear where the smooth opercular aspect of the striate cortex is situated in controls. Nevertheless, a variable part of this abnormally gyrated cortex consists of a histologically distinct striate cortex, which is nearly identical in thickness and lamination - as visualized in Nissl-stained sections - to that in normal animals (Rakic, 1988a; Rakic et al., 1991).

Subsequent observations by Dehay et al. (1989) have confirmed the reduction in the surface area of the striate cortex, and found that the cortex surrounding this region has a high density of callosally projecting neurons; a feature characteristic of the prestriate area 18. Taken together with the previous findings by Rakic, these observations have been interpreted by Dehay et al. as indicating that the reduced number of geniculate axons projecting to area 17 results in a reduced areal extent of this cortex. As a result of this, part of the cortical mantle normally destined to become striate cortex - which is deprived of retinal input by the enucleation - becomes area 18 instead, and participates in an expanded callosal projection. In this view - which follows Rakic's (1988a) interpretation - early geniculate input is necessary to specify the portion of occipital cortex that will become striate cortex, which characteristically lacks callosal connections almost completely. Prestriate cortex, by contrast, forms out of occipital cortices that fail to be invaded by axons from the lateral geniculate nucleus and contains substantial callosal connections. The most general hypothesis that can be drawn from these studies is that peripheral input is important among the factors responsible for the parcellation of cortical territories early in ontogenesis (Rakic et al., 1991). Perhaps this input is also important in specifying the differential connectivity among cortical areas.

An interesting finding in prenatally enucleated animals is the presence of cytochrome oxidase-rich regions in layers II/III of the striate cortex, variably called blobs, dots, spots, patches and puffs (Kuljis & Rakic, 1990). The puffs are features unique to the primate striate cortex, which can be used as reliable markers of functionally distinct columns that span the cortical thickness, and that form part of the hypercolumns that make up this region (Horton & Hubel, 1981; Hendrickson et al., 1981; Horton, 1984; Carrol & Wong-Riley, 1984, 1985; Wong-Riley & Carrol, 1984a,b; Livingstone & Hubel, 1982, 1984; Fitzpatrick et al., 1987). In fact, animals subjected to binocular enucleation on the 81st and 120th day of gestation (E81, E120; Term: 165 days) exhibit clearcut puffs in the supragranular layers (Fig. 1) which are of normal size but reduced labeling intensity. As reported by Dehay et al. (1989), the prenatally enucleated animals exhibit also a continous pattern of cytochrome oxidase labeling in layer IV, which is similar to that of normal animals except for a reduced labeling intensity. A recent note by Kennedy et al. (1990) reports an 8% reduction in the space between blobs in an animal enucleated bilaterally on the 68th day of gestation, compared to a normal neonate. This difference was found statistically significant in that it would translate into only a 15% reduction in the surface area of the striate cortex, which differs sharply with the actual finding of more than 70% reduction in animals enucleated at E59-68.

Experiments are in progress in several laboratories to confirm and extend these preliminary quantitative details. What appears conclusive so far is that photoreceptor input is not essential to specify the organization of the hypercolumns in the striate cortex (Kuljis & Rakic, 1990). In fact, retinal ablations at E81 or before take place before the

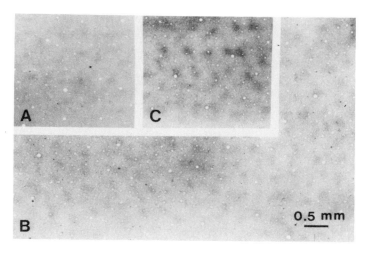

Figure 1. Photomicrographs of cytochrome oxidase-labeled sections through layers II/III of (A) neonate, (B) prenatally enucleated and (C) normal adult macaque monkeys. Note the presence of cytochrome oxidase-rich puffs in this region in all three specimens. Modified from Kuljis & Rakic, 1990.

photoreceptors establish synapses with any type of retinal neuron (Nishimura & Rakic, 1987). Furthermore, the ablation was performed also before thalamic axons invade the *anlage* of the striate cortex, and before layers II/III - where the puffs are situated - were formed (Rakic, 1974). Thus, it would seem that the striate cortex in enucleates formed without any contact-mediated information from photoreceptors. However, an instructive role of the input from retinal ganglion cells to the thalamus cannot be excluded in the cases enucleated at later stages. It is possible, however, that the geniculocortical afferents have a role in the development of the puffs. Although these afferents are reduced in number in prenatal enucleates, Allman and Zucker (1991) have proposed that "the surviving population of neurons in the lateral geniculate nucleus in monkeys with their eyes removed well before birth might be sufficient to provide a tonic drive to the blobs and thus engage their metabolic machinery." So far, however, this hypothesis remains unsubstantiated since information on the physiological activity of the geniculate neurons in prenatal enucleates is not available. Additional factors, such as intrinsic cortical programs that help effect functional and anatomical parcellations within the cortical mantle have not been addressed directly in an experimental fashion so far.

Another interesting aspect of modular parcellation within the striate cortex of prenatally enucleated animals is the distribution of neuropeptide Y (NPY)-containing neurons. These neurons are present throughout major sensory, association, limbic and motor areas of the primate cerebral cortex, and invariably correspond to local circuit neurons (Kuljis & Rakic, 1989a-c). Thus, they are probably not contacted directly by massive numbers of thalamic axons and consequently perhaps not severely affected by the elimination of transsynaptic retinal cues. A distinct spatial distribution of NPY neurons was discovered in the macaque striate cortex: they are situated predominantly outside the cytochrome oxidase puffs (Kuljis & Rakic, 1989a; Fig. 2). This observation appears to indicate that the modules

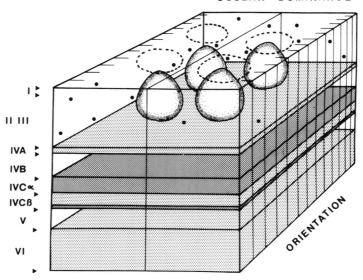

OCULAR DOMINANCE

I

II III

IVA

IVB

IVCα

IVCβ

V

VI

ORIENTATION

<u>Figure 2</u>. Schematic drawing of the organization of the striate cortex
(based on the data from Hubel & Wiesel, 1977; Livingstone & Hubel, 1984,
and Kuljis & Rakic, 1989a). The stippling patterns indicate portions of
the cortex that contain high levels of cytochrome oxidase activity,
where denser stippling represents higher levels of enzymatic activity.
Broken line halos represent the projection of the base of columns of
wavelength-sensitive neurons, which are centered in cytochrome oxidase-
rich puffs (represented by the globular formations in layers II/III).
The dots indicate the position of NPY-containing neurons in these
layers, which are situated predominantly outside the puffs. Thus, NPY-
containing neurons are situated in columns with a high proportion of
cells with orientation-, but not wavelength-selective, binocularly-
driven receptive fields. From Kuljis & Rakic, 1989a, with permission.

that make up the striate cortex are composed of columns that contain
different arrays of local circuit neurons: e.g. columns that do not
contain cytochrome oxidase puffs have a higher proportion of NPY-
containing neurons. This nonuniform distribution of one type of local
circuit neuron among the components of the hypercolumns of the striate
cortex may also indicate that other types of yet unidentified neurons
are distributed inhomogeneously among the columns. If this hypothesis is
correct, their selective distribution among the columns may constitute
another feature of inter-columnar specialization, beyond what is
currently ascribed to differences imposed among columns by their
different thalamic input (i.e. the puffs, but not the interpuffs receive
thalamic input; e.g. Livingstone & Hubel, 1982). An important question
arising from this hypothesis about the distribution of local circuit
neurons among columns is: will their compartmentalization be disturbed
in the absence of input from the periphery? Our findings indicate that,
in the striate cortex, photoreceptor input is not indispensable for the
proper parcellation of NPY neurons in layers II/III (Fig. 3). This
observation suggests that the modular parcellation of local circuit
neurons, like the development of the cytochrome oxidase puffs, occurs

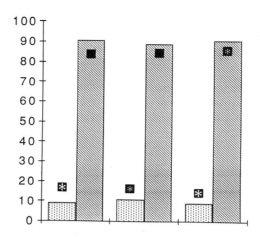

<u>Figure 3</u>. Column chart of the distribution of NPY-containing neurons in layers II/III of a normal 5-day-old infant monkey (n=611 cells; left pair of bars), a prenatally enucleated animal (n=926; middle pair of bars), and six normal adults (n=606; right pair of bars). For each situation, the left bar represents the percentage of labeled neurons found in the puffs plus half the labeled neurons found in the interface with interpuff regions. The right bar indicates the percentage of neurons found in the interpuffs plus half the labeled neurons in the interface with the puffs. Filled squares indicate the percentage of labeled neurons expected on the basis of the volume occupied by puffs and interpuff regions. Asterisks within the squares indicate statistically significant differences (small asterisk, p<0.01; large asterisk, p<0.001) between the number of neurons found in each portion of layers II/III and that expected assuming uniform distribution between puffs and interpuff regions. From Kuljis and Rakic (1990), with permission.

either according to an intrinsic cortical program, and/or is governed by thalamo-cortical interactions that are independent of photoreceptor input.

AN ATTEMPT TO COMPARE THE MODULES IN THE MACAQUE VISUAL CORTEX WITH THE BARRELS IN THE RODENT SOMATOSENSORY CORTEX

Few paradigms in areas other than the visual cortex are available for direct testing of the general validity of the rules of developmental specification that are emerging from the studies reviewed in the preceding sections. Perhaps the most relevant model in this respect is that of the sinus hair representation in the rodent somatosensory cortex. In rats and mice, as well as other species that have mobile mystacial vibrissae, each sinus hair follicle has a unique, anatomically, developmentally and physiologically recognizable representation in the contralateral somatosensory cortex. These representations, which are termed barrels in the mouse cortex, form cytoarchitectonic units that are easily recognizable at low magnification in Nissl stains and subserve a specialization of the somatosensory system capable of detecting form and texture with a degree of sophistication comparable to that of primates using their fingertips (Carvell & Simons, 1990). Since the elegant experiments of Woolsey, Van der Loos and their collaborators (Woolsey & Van der Loos, 1970; Van der Loos & Woolsey, 1973; Van der Loos & Dörfl, 1978; Andrés and Van der Loos, 1985), it is commonly accepted that, in the rodent somatosensory system there is strong evidence that peripheral (vibrissal follicle) receptors have a major role in specifying the modular organization of the barrel cortex. The compelling evidence to that effect rests on at least three major lines of evidence: (1) the failure of barrels to form when their corresponding vibrissal follicles are ablated at or close to the day of birth, (2) the failure of barrels to form after thalamotomy (Wise & Jones, 1978), and (3) the presence of corresponding supernumerary barrels in mutants that have supernumerary vibrissae in the contralateral muzzle (Van der Loos & Dörfl, 1978; Yamakado & Yohro, 1979).

Although these converging lines of evidence are in fact elegant and compelling, there are still several problems with their overall interpretation, with direct comparisons with the primate striate cortex, and with their extrapolation to all cortical areas. First, although the rodent barrel cortex and the macaque striate cortex are among the best characterized models of neocortical modular architecture, they are not comparable to each other but in very general terms, such that several of the differences between them could be very significant in explaining their diverse response to what may superficially appear to be the same experimental manipulation. For example, cytochrome oxidase puffs are situated in layers II/III, are not evident in Nissl sections, and do not receive massive amounts of thalamic axons. By contrast, the barrels are situated in layer IV, are easily recognizable in Nissl stains and their centers (the "hollows") are made up mainly of thalamic afferents. Given the latter characteristics, it is not surprising that barrels fail to form after thalamotomy, since one of their major structural components (i.e. thalamic afferents) is destroyed or at least markedly reduced by this operation.

A second important aspect that bears on the interpretation of lesion studies in the rodent somatosensory system is the timing of the vibrissal ablations, virtually all of which have been performed in the neonatal period. At this time, the somatosensory system has developed to a much larger extent than the visual system of monkeys at the stage that they are subjected to prenatal eye enucleation. For example, cortical histogenesis has been completed in the neonatal mouse (Berry & Eayrs, 1963), and thalamic axons are now known to invade the cortical plate as early as the day after birth (Zhang & Cooper, 1990). Thus, the typical vibrissal ablation takes place in a substantially developed somatosensory cortex - as compared with the paradigm in monkeys - and after the cortex has had abundant opportunities to receive cues from peripheral receptors. Thus, these factors are another major aspect in which the rodent and the primate paradigms not entirely comparable. Therefore, it is not entirely surprising that the response of the two models to different types of manipulation is not identical.

The third major problem with the interpretation of the results after vibrissal follicle ablations is the result of the first two mentioned above, and has been acknowledged in part by Van der Loos and his collaborators (e.g. Van der Loos & Dörfl, 1978; Andrés & Van der Loos, 1985): none of the existing experimental observations rule out the possibility that an interaction between an intrinsic (cortical or thalamo-cortical) program with peripheral input is necessary for the development of the barrels. Taken together, these difficulties in the

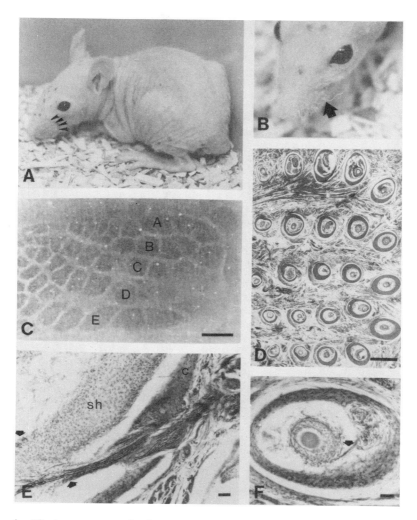

<u>Figure 4</u>. Photomacro- and micrographs of the vibrissaeless (vb) rat, its
somatosensory cortex and muzzle skin. A,B typical mutant animal, which
lacks most pelage hair and vibrissae. However, the elevations in the
muzzle correspond to vibrissal follicles (arrowheads in A), from which
short, tortuous hairs occasionally grow (arrow in B). C. Cytochrome
oxidase histochemistry in tangentially sectioned, flat-mounted
somatosensory cortex demonstrates the presence of cytoarchitectonic
units. Some units appear faint because they are mostly outside of the
plane of the section shown, but they were seen in adjacent sections.
Capital letters designate rows of units according to Woolsey and Van der
Loos' (1970) nomenclature. D. Masson trichrome stained section
from a flat mount of the muzzle skin, which demonstrates a regular
pattern of sinus hair follicles, each of which contains the stump of a
hair. E. Oblique section of a Bielschowsky-impregnated sinus
hair follicle. Branches of axons from the infraorbital nerve (upper
right corner of the panel) enter the capsule (c) of the follicle and
innervate the base of the sinus hair (sh; arrows). F. Transerve
section of another Bielschowsky-impregnated sinus hair follicle.
Bundles of intrafollicular axons (upper left aspect of the capsule)
provide fibers (arrow) that innervate the hair as in panel E.
Calibration bars: C=0.5 mm; D=1 mm; E, F=50 μm.   From Kuljis, 1991a,
with permission.

interpretation of experimental results would suggest great caution in extrapolation of the findings in the rodent somatosensory cortex to the rest of the cerebral cortex.

Recognizing these difficulties I have recently sought new models in the rodent somatosensory system, which offer some advantages to improve our understanding of the factors that regulate the development of this region and, hopefully, offer a basis for a more appropriate comparison with the findings in the striate cortex of anophthalmic primates. These new observations appear to provide additional pieces to the puzzle, but cannot as yet offer a definitive solution to all of the difficulties mentioned in the preceding paragraphs. One model is the rat mutant known as vibrissaeless, which lacks virtually all vibrissae throughout life but has a complete array of sinus hair follicles in the muzzle(Fig.4).This mutant also has a complete array of cytoarchitectonic units in the contralateral somatosensory cortex, indicating that vibrissal stimulation is not indispensable for the development of the barrels (Kuljis, 1991a). In some respects, this paradigm may be comparable to the striate cortex of macaque neonates, who have cytochrome oxidase puffs in layers II/III although they have not had any visual experience (Fig 1A).

It should be emphasized that another mutant without hair in the mouse, called "hairless" (hr), is known to lack mystacial vibrissae but has both vibrissal follicles and barrels (Yamakado & Yohro, 1979). At first glance, it would appear that hr exhibits the same phenomenon discovered recently in vb. This is not the case, however, since hr is known to lose its hair postnatally after barrels have developed (Mann & Straile, 1961), while vb never develops normal vibrissae. Consequently, the vb rat is a far better model of prenatal deprivation of sensory experience than the hr mouse.

Another interesting mutant is the mouse known as Ragged opposum, which has only 3-4 vibrissae in the most posterior aspect of the muzzle (known as "straddlers" in Woolsey & Van der Loos', 1970, terminology). Nevertheless, ragged mice also have a normal set of sinus hair follicles, among which only the most posterior ones produce nearly normal vibrissae. Their somatosensory cortex has a normal array of barrels, but those innervated by the follicles with vibrissae are larger than the rest, suggesting that activity resulting from physiological stimulation of vibrissae is important in determining the amount of cortex devoted to the representation of each vibrissal follicle (Kuljis, 1991b). The latter phenomenon may be comparable in part comparable to the expansion of ocular dominance columns served by the intact eye after unilateral eye enucleation in macaque monkeys (Rakic, 1981), providing another possible analogy among the rodent an primate models. Further experimental observations are nevertheless necessary, before firm and far-reaching conclusions can be drawn. Unfortunately, prenatal ablations of vibrissal follicles before they become innervated by trigeminal afferents about the 16th day of gestation (Tello, 1923) have not been reported so far. This experimental manipulation, is obviously very demanding technically, but may be necessary to make more direct comparisons between the rodent and primate models reviewed here.

CONCLUSIONS

A growing body of evidence indicates that peripheral receptor input can have a role in the specification of certain aspects of the structural and functional specialization of the cerebral cortex. The primary visual (striate) cortex provides a convenient model to address this role, particularly in primate and human paradigms in which retinal cues are absent or can be eliminated early in gestation. It is rather surprising that, even in complete absence of photoreceptor cues, the striate cortex develops with a normal thickness and a seemingly normal lamination as well as a distinct modular organization. This presumably indicates that the latter features of the organization of the striate cortex can be specified in the absence of photoreceptor cues, but perhaps require an intrinsic cortical or thalamo-cortical program that survives the marked shrinkage and cell loss in the lateral geniculate nucleus. Further experiments are needed to understand the reduction in the surface area of the striate cortex that tends to accompany early prenatal binocular enucleation. Nevertheless, existing data are compatible with the notion that the extent of this surface is a function of the number of lateral geniculate axons available to innervate this region.

The elucidation of the extent to which these observations are generally applicable to the entire cerebral cortex, as well as to the extent to which observations in the rodent somatosensory cortex are comparable with seemingly analogous paradigms in the striate cortex necessitate further experimental assessment.

REFERENCES

Allman, J. and Zucker, S.,1991, Cytochrome oxidase and functional coding in primate striate cortex: An hypothesis. In: Cold Spring Harbor Symposium in Quantitative Biology, Vol. 55: The Brain. Cold Spring Harbor Laboratory Press, in press.

Andrés, F.L. and Van der Loos, H., 1985, From sensory periphery to cortex: The architecture of the barrelfield as modified by various early manipulations of the mouse whiskerpad, Anat. Embryol. 172:11-20.

Berry, M. and Eayrs, J.T., 1963, Histogenesis of the cerebral cortex. Nature 197:984-985.

Brunquell, P.J., Papale, J.H., Horton, J.C., Williams, R.S., Zgrabik, Albert, D.M. and Hedley-Whyte, E.T., 1984, Sex-linked hereditary bilateral anophthalmos. Pathologic and radiologic correlation. Arch. Ophthalmol. 102:108-113.

Carroll, E.W. and Wong-Riley, M.T.T., 1984, Quantitative and electron microscope analysis of cytochrome oxidase-rich zones in the striate cortex of the squirrell monkey. J. Comp. Neurol. 222:1-17.

Carroll, E.W. and Wong-Riley, M.T.T., 1985, Correlation between cytochrome oxidase and the uptake and laminar distribution of tritiated aspartate, glutamate, gamma-aminobutyrate and glycine in the striate cortex of the squirrel monkey. Neuroscience 15:959-976.

Carvell, G.E. and Simons, D.J., 1990, Biometric analyses of vibrissal tactile discrimination in the rat. J. Neurosci. 10:2638-2648.

Chase, H.B. and Chase, E.B., 1941, Studies on an anophthalmic strain of mice-I. Embryology of the eye region. J. Morphol. 68:279-301.

Chase, H.B., 1945, Studies on an anophthalmic strain of mice-V. Associated nerves and brain centers. J. Comp. Neurol. 83:121-139.

Cragg, B.G., 1967, Changes in visual cortex on first exposure of rats to light. Nature 215:251-253.

Cullen, M.J. and Kaiserman-Abramof, I.R., 1975, Ultrastructure and quantitative changes in the cellular organization of the dorsal lateral geniculate nucleus in anophtlamic and enucleated mice. Anat. Rec. 181:339-340.

Dehay, C., Horsburgh, G., Berland, M., Killackey, H. and Kennedy, H., 1989, Maturation and connectivity of the visual cortex in monkey is altered by prenatal removal of retinal input. Nature 337:265-267.

Duckworth, T. and Cooper, E.R.A., 1966, A study of anophthalmia in an adult. Acta Anat. 63:509-522.

Fifková, E., 1968, Changes in the visual cortex of rats after unilateral deprivation. Nature 220:379-381.

Fitzpatrick, D., Lund, J.S., Schmechel, D.E. and Towles, A.C., 1987, Distribution of GABAergic neurons and axonal terminals in the macaque striate cortex. J. Comp. Neurol. 264:73-91.

Godement, P., Saillour, P. and Imbert, M., 1977, Etude anatomique des centres visuels de la souris anophthalmique 'Eyeless'. J. Physiol. (Paris) 73:74A.

Haberland, C. and Perou, M., 1969, Primary bilateral anopthalmia. J. Neuropathol. Exp. Neurol. 28:337-351.

Hendrickson, A.E., Hunt, S.P. and Wu, J.-Y., 1981, Immunocytochemical localization of glutamic acid decarboxylase in monkey striate cortex. Nature 292:605-607.

Hess, A., 1958, Optic centers and pathways after eye removal in fetal guinea pigs. J. Comp. Neurol. 109:91-115.

Horton, J.C. and Hubel, D.H., 1981, Regular patchy distribution of cytochrome oxidase staining in primary visual cortex of macaque monkey. Nature 292:762-764.

Horton, J.C., 1984, Cytochrome oxidase patches: a new cytoarchitectonic feature of monkey visual cortex. Phil. Trans. Roy. Soc. Lond. B. 304:199-253.

Hubel, D.H. and Wiesel, T.N. (1977) Functional architecture of macaque visual cortex. Phil. Trans. Roy. Soc. Lond. B. 198:1-59.

Kaiserman-Abramof, I.R., Graybiel, A.M. and Nauta, W.J.H., 1980, The thalamic projection to cortical area 17 in a congenitally anophthalmic mouse strain. Neuroscience 5:41-52.

Kennedy, H., Dehay, C. and Horsburgh, G., 1990, Striate cortex periodicity. Nature 348:494.

Kuljis, R.O. and Rakic, P., 1989a, Neuropeptide Y-containing neurons are situated predominantly outside cytochrome oxidase puffs in macaque visual cortex. Visual Neurosci. 2:57-62.

Kuljis, R.O. and Rakic, P., 1989b, Distribution of neuropeptide Y-containing perikarya ans axons in various neocortical areas in the macaque monkey. J. Comp. Neurol. 280:383-392.

Kuljis, R.O. and Rakic, P., 1989c, Multiple types of neuropeptide Y-containing neurons in primate neocortex. J. Comp. Neurol. 280:393-409.

Kuljis, R.O. and Rakic, P., 1990, Hypercolumns in primate visual cortex can develop in the absence of cues from photoreceptors. Proc. Natl. Acad. Sci. USA 87:5303-5306.

Kuljis, R.O., 1991a, Vibrissaeless mutant rats with a modular representation of innervated sinus hair follicles in the cerebral cortex. Exp. Neurol., in press.

Kuljis, R.O., 1991b, Modifications in the barrel field cortex in ragged mutant mice. Soc. Neurosci. Abstr. 17, in press.

Livingstone, M.S. and Hubel, D.H., 1982, Thalamic inputs to cytochrome oxidase-rich regions in monkey visual cortex. Proc. Natl. Acad. Sci. USA 79:6098-6101.

Livingstone, M.S. and Hubel, D.H., 1984, Anatomy and physiology of a color system in the primate visual cortex. J. Neurosci. 4:309:356.

Mann, I., 1957, Developmental Abnormalities of the Eye, 2nd ed. Harper & Row: Hagerstown, Maryland, pp. 60-66.

Mann, S.J. and Straile, W.E., 1961, New observations on hair loss in the hairless mouse. Anat. Rec. 140: 97:101.

Nishimura, Y. and Rakic, P., 1987, Development of the rhesus monkey retina: II. A three- dimensional analysis of the sequences of synaptic combinations in the inner plexiform layer. J. Comp. Neurol. 262:290-313.

Pritkin, R.I., 1980, The rarity of true congenital bilateral anophthalmos. Metabol. Pediatr. Ophthalmol. 4:165-167.

Rakic, P., 1974, Neurons in rhesus monkey visual cortex: systematic relation between time of origin and eventual disposition. Science 183:425-427.

Rakic, P., 1975, Timing of major ontogenetic events in the visual cortex of the rhesus monkey. In: Brain Mechanisms in Mental Retardation. Academic: New York, pp. 3-40.

Rakic, P., 1977, Prenatal development of the visual system in rhesus monkey. Phil. Trans. R. Soc. Lond. B. 278:245-260.

Rakic, P., 1981, Development of visual centers in the primate brain depends on binocular competition before birth. Science 214:928-931.

Rakic, P., 1988a, Specification of cerebral cortical areas. Science 241:170-176.

Rakic, P., 1988b, Defects of neuronal migration and the pathogenesis of cortical malformations. In: Progress in Brain Research, Vol. 73. Boer, G.J., Feenstra, M.G.P., Mirmiran, M., Swaab, D.F. and Van Haaren, F. (eds.) Elsevier: Amsterdam, pp. 15-37.

Rakic, P. and Goldman-Rakic, P., 1985, Use of fetal neurosurgery for experimental studies of structural and functional brain development in nonhuman primates. In: Perinatal Neurology and Neurosurgery. Thompson, R.A., Green, J.R. and Johnsen, S.D. (eds.) Spectrum: New York, pp. 1-15.

Rakic, P., Suner, I. and Williams, R. W., 1991, A novel cytoarchitectonic area induced experimentally within the primate visual cortex. Proc. Natl. Acad. Sci. USA 88:2083-2087.

Recordon, E. and Griffiths, G.M. (1938) A case of primary bilateral anophthalmia (clinical and histological report). Br. J. Ophthalmol. 22:353-360.

Sidman, R.L., Green, M.C. and Appel, S.H., 1965, Catalog of the Neurological Mutants of the Mouse. Harvard: Cambridge, pp. 21-23.

Tello, J.F., 1923, Genèse des terminaisons motrices et sensitives. II.- Terminaisons dans les poils de la souris blanche. Trav. Lab. Rech. Biol. Univ. Madrid 21:257-384.

Tsang, Y.C., 1937, Visual centers in blinded rats. J. Comp. Neurol. 66:211-261.

Valverde, F., 1967, Apical dendritic spines of the visual cortex and light deprivation in the mouse. Exp. Brain Res. 3:337-352.

Van der Loos, H. and Woolsey, T.A., 1973, Somatosensory cortex: Structural alterations following early injury to sense organs. Science 179:395-398.

Van der Loos, H. and Dörfl, J., 1978, Does the skin tell the somatosensory cortex how to construct a map of the periphery? Neurosci. Lett. 7:23-30.

Wong-Riley, M.T.T. and Carroll, E.W., 1984a, Quantitative and electron microscopic analysis of cytochrome oxidase-rich zones in VII prestriate cortex of the squirrel monkey. J. Comp. Neurol. 222:18-37.

Wong-Riley, M.T.T. and Carroll, E.W., 1984b, Effect of impulse blockage on cytochrome oxidase activity in monkey visual system. Nature 307:262-264.

Woolsey, T.A. and Van der Loos, H., 1970, The structural organization of layer IV in the somatosensory region (SI) of mouse cerebral cortex. The description of a cortical field composed of discrete cytoarchitectonic units. Brain Res. 17:205-242.

Yamakado, M. and Yohro, T., 1979, Subdivision of mouse vibrissae on an embryological basis, with descriptions of variations in the number and arrangement of sinus hairs and cortical barrels in BALB/c (nu/t; nude, nu/nu) and hairless (hr/hr) strains. Am. J. Anat. 155:153-174.

Zhang, L. and Cooper, N.G.F., 1990, Development of layer IV in rat somatosensory cortex. Soc. Neurosci. Abstr. 16:1214 (500.4).

SENSORIAL AND SENSORIMOTOR PHENOMENA IN STRABISMUS

Bruno Bagolini

Dept. of Ophthalmology
Catholic University
Largo A. Gemelli, 8
00168 Rome - Italy

Regardless of its cause, eye misalignment that is present between the time of birth and the seventh or eighth year of life (the plastic age) elicits adaptive sensorial and sensorimotor responses to the problem. These phenomena are considered to be adaptive for several reasons. If, in fact, the angle of strabismus is changed by means of surgery or corrective lenses during this period, the phenomena mentioned above also change to reflect the new type of misalignment. Misalignment that develops in older patients rarely provokes any of the adaptive responses seen in the young child, and the patient consequently experiences diplopia.

BINOCULAR SENSORIAL ANOMALIES (Suppression and anomalous retinal correspondence)

In the past, patients with overt strabismus have been considered almost monocular. It was believed that an important part of the central visual field of the deviated eye was excluded through the phenomenon of suppression in an attempt to avoid diplopia and confusion of images.

The phenomenon of anomalous retinal correspondence (ARC) was and is still, by some, considered to be an abortive attempt to achieve some degree of binocular vision in spite of the deviated eye. Figure 1 illustrates the phenomenon of ARC. On the left side of the drawing (A), the image received by the fixing left eye falls on the fovea (F) while that received by the deviated eye falls on an extrafoveal, nasal area of the retina (X). In children, this second image is not perceived because excitation of the visual field of the deviated eye is suppressed through synaptical inhibition that occurs at some point along the optical pathways.

In some cases, the second image is, at a certain
point in time, no longer suppressed but is perceived
superimposed on the image that falls on the fovea of the
fixing eye. This occurs because there has been a change
in the directional location of the retinal elements of the
deviated eye. The extrafoveal, nasal area (X) of the
retina shown in Figure 1 now corresponds to the fovea of
the non-deviated eye, and the object fixed by the two eyes
is thus perceived as a single image. This phenomenon is
referred to as anomalous retinal correspondence (ARC). It
occurs, however, only during binocular vision. If the
fixing eye is closed, the image falling on the area X of
the deviated eye is, once again, spatially perceived as
peripheral.

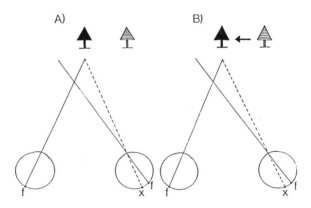

Fig. 1 - Anomalous retinal correspondence

Anomalous retinal correspondence was first observed
in the 19th century. It is a functional condition that is
related to the original ocular misalignment. However,
most investigators found that binocular vision was
impossible with ARC because the phenomenon of suppression
always prevailed. Still, there have been reports of
patients in whom ARC was not completely excluded by
suppression, and an anomalous type of binocular vision was
found to exist. Bielschowsky, for example, reported in
1899 that, when a colored filter was placed in front of
the deviated eye, a small number of strabismus patients
perceived the light as colored. He even found
exceptional cases in which some degree of stereopsis was
observed in the Hearing drop test. Burian (1947) later
confirmed the possibility of color mixing reported by
Bielschowsky and claimed to have also observed fusional
movements in these patients.

Nevertheless, our concepts of the possibility of
attaining some degree of binocularity through ARC began to
change only after the introduction of non-dissociating

tests for binocularity, such as the striated glasses test. Prior to this point, all tests used to determine how much binocular vision there was in a strabismus patient provoked dissociation, i.e. they contained one or more monocular artefacts that allowed the examiner to determine whether one image was being suppressed or whether the two images were being fused in some way. This type of test, however, does not reproduce the condition in which a subject normally sees. And it is only under these conditions, i.e. continual stimulation by the surroundings, that suppression and ARC can develop in a subject with ocular misalignment.

For example, when a colored glass is placed in front of one eye, most strabismus patients react with diplopia. This is obviously an artificial situation which disrupts the sensorial adaptation achieved by the patient who does not see double under normal circumstances. The striated glasses test, which produces only minimal alteration of the subject's habitual vision, is able to show us the actual sensorial status of the patient because its dissociative effect is limited.

The definition we have just given of dissociation is a rather crude one. The elements that disrupt binocularity are those stimuli that introduce retinal rivalry or that alter the image received by one eye with respect to that received by the contralateral eye.

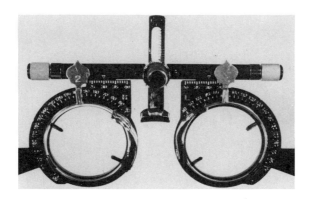

Fig. 2 - Striated glasses

Striated glasses (Fig. 2) are flat lenses that can be inserted into trial frames like any other lens. When a patient is wearing these glasses, his perception of his surroundings is no different than that without the glasses. However, if he fixes a pin-point light, he will see a weakly luminous line passing through the point. This line is caused by invisible striations on the glasses which are perpendicular to the line that is perceived by the patient. These plano lenses are placed inside frames so that the striation axis of one is perpendicular to that of the other. With a left axis oriented to 45 degrees and the right to 135 degrees, a normal subject perceives an X formed by the two luminous lines with the point of light at their intersection.

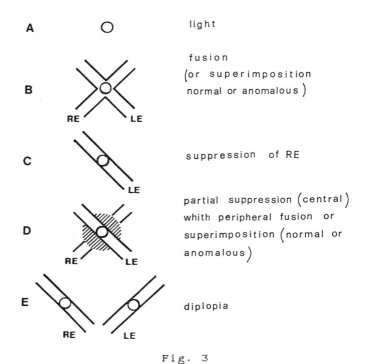

Fig. 3

In the same test, the patient with strabismus may see one of three things. When looking at the pin-point of light (Fig. 3A), he may perceive the same X seen by the normal patient (Fig. 3B), which indicates that he has achieved an anomalous form of binocular vision. He may also see only one arm of the X, that caused by the striations on the lens in front of the non-deviated eye. In this patient, the image received by the deviated is being suppressed (Fig. 3C). Finally, some patients will perceive interruptions in the line seen by the deviated eye. This finding indicates that there are areas of the retina that are being suppressed. Fig. 3D illustrates central suppression. Other findings can also emerge from the striated glasses test, but they are beyond the scope of the present paper.

Extensive suppression of the deviated eye that is demonstrated in the striated glasses test is primarily a function of the angle of deviation. In other tests, the degree of suppression found depended more on the type of dissociation produced by the test itself.

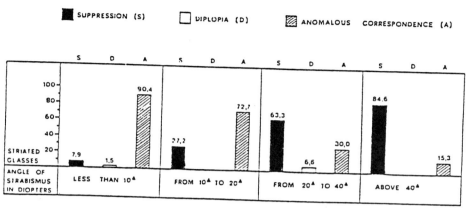

Fig. 4 - A group of 165 patients was divided into 4 groups according to the angle of strabismus in prism diopters (p.d.). The first group includes patients with an angle < 10 p.d., the second between 10 and 20 p.d., the third between 20 and 40 p.d. and the fourth > 40 p.d. The results of the S.G. test suppression (S), diplopia (D) or anomalous correspondence (A).

Figure 4 shows the results of the striated glasses test administered to 165 patients with convergent strabismus. The patients were divided into four sub-groups according to their angle of deviation: < 10△ , 10-20△ , 20-40△ , and > 40△ . In the patients with large-angle deviation, suppression does, indeed, seem to prevail. In these patients, the suppression often involves the entire visual field of the deviated eye. When the angle of deviation was small, however, most patients showed no suppression at all. Diplopia was avoided through ARC and some degree of binocular vision was achieved. This latter category of patients was never observed before the use of the striated glasses test. Now, the concept of ARC as a merely abortive attempt to reinstate binocular vision must be revised. The attempt is abortive only when the angle of deviation is large.

In cases of small-angle deviation, the images of the pin-point light fall on different areas of the retina in the two eyes, but because an anomalous correspondence has developed between these two areas, the image is perceived binocularly. Sometimes, suppression of parts of the visual field of the deviated eye will be observed (Fig. 3D), but in many cases there is no suppression at all. In some cases, the striated glasses test provokes diplopia

(Fig 3E). This is possible because even this test has some dissociative effects although they are far inferior to those of earlier tests for binocularity. When this finding emerges in a patient with small-angle deviation, it indicates that the binocularity achieved through ARC is a very weak phenomenon that is easily disrupted. Most patients with small-angle deviation see binocularly in the striated glasses test just as a normal subject does. The only difference is the lack of stereopsis.

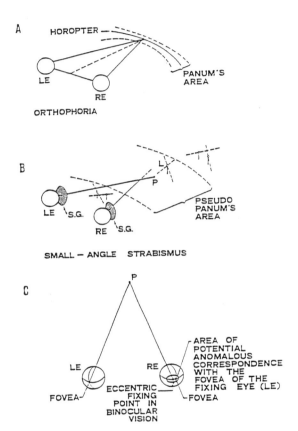

Fig. 5 -
A) Panum's area of binocular vision in an orthophoric subject.
B) Psudo-Panum's area supported by anomalous binocular single vision in small angle stra-bismus. The pseudo-Panum's area is usually larger than Panum's area in normal subjects. This can be demonstrated by modified horopter techniques (Bagolini, 1962/1967).
C) By simple geometrical considerations (Bago-lini, 1976 Part I) a large pseudo-Panum's area implies that a single retinal point in the fixing eye (i.e., the fovea) may correspond to a large retinal area in the deviated eye.

We have used a modified horopter apparatus to determine whether the absence of double vision in these patients was due to suppression or to binocular perception. In patients with small-angle strabismus, we found that the area of binocular vision was usually larger (Fig. 5B) than Panum's area in a normal patient (Fig. 5A). We termed this increased area "Pseudo-Panum's area". In large-angle strabismus, only large areas of suppression were usually found.

As we can see from Fig. 5c, a large pseudo-Panum's area implies through simple geometrical reasoning potential collaboration between a single point in the fixing eye and a large area in the deviated one. The larger the pseudo-Panum's area, the larger is the area of the deviated eye's retina that potentially corresponds to a single point in the retina of the fixing eye.

I first demonstrated this anomalous binocularity with horopter techniques, but it has recently been observed by Campos, Kommerel and Meadorn using campimetry. It involves the superimposition of similar images that fall on anomalously corresponding retinal areas of the two eyes and can occur even in central areas of the binocular visual field.

In many cases, no suppression at all is revealed in either the tridimensional horopter test or in non-dissociating bidimensional campimetric studies. The lack of suppression is confined, however, to those patients who present anomalous binocular vision in the striated glasses test and most of them have small-angle strabismus.

Other investigators are not convinced that suppression can truly be eliminated. Their belief that there is always some degree of suppression in cases of ARC even if the latter permits an anomalous form of binocular vision is, however, based on the results of binocular campimetric techniques that contain dissociating stimuli. Depending on the nature of these stimuli, the patient will react in these tests by suppressing or seeing double. But when the same patient with small-angle deviation is subjected to the non-dissociating striated glasses test, he will, in fact, often see exactly what a normal subject sees.

The fundamental difference between normal and anomalous binocular vision is that the latter lacks stereopsis. It can also be easily disrupted by dissociating tests such as the aploscopic test or red glass test. Under these artificial conditions the patient with anomalous binocular vision will often experience suppression or diplopia. These patients have the potential for suppression though it does not usually occur under normal conditions.

Anomalous binocular vision with very little or no suppression is most commonly seen in the striated glasses test in patients with ARC due to small-angle strabismus. In large-angle patients, the most common finding is that of a large area of suppression. There is, of course, no clear-cut division between the categories of small and large-angle strabismus. Figure 4 gives an idea of the broad areas we are trying to define.

It is interesting from both theoretical and practical points of view to know just how firmly established these two reactions are. A simple method for evaluating the strength of either suppression or ABV is that of gradually introducing more and more dissociation until diplopia occurs. A bar of optical filters of progressive density (Fig. 6) is held in front of the non-dominant eye to avoid altering fixation which may, in itself, provoke diplopia.

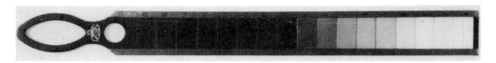

Fig. 6 - Bar of optical filters used with the striated glasses test. The filters are placed in front of the deviated eye. The filter that causes the patient to see a double fixation light gives an index of the intensity of suppression or how deeply rooted a.r.c. is.(Bagolini 1982)

This approach can be used in conjunction with the striated glasses test in order to determine whether the adaptation we are disrupting is ARC or suppression. We use a bar of numbered, red filters in order to identify the eye to which the image belongs. The patient with normal binocular vision will be able to maintain single vision even with filters 15 or 16, whereas those with ABV always experience diplopia with filters 12 or 13 (if not before).

It will obviously be more difficult to convert firmly established ARC to normal retinal correspondence (NRC). Binocular re-education in these patients is almost impossible.

From a theoretical point of view, the strength of the ARC may be a reflection of the number of binocular cells in the cortex that have become capable of stimulation by anomalously corresponding retinal elements. Such cells have been found in the cortex of the cat by Cynader et al. In some of the animals in which unilateral exotropia had been surgically induced, they found receptive fields of binocular neurons in non-corresponding points of the two retinas. The two fields were located in a·manner that allowed the cat to correlate the two images in spite of its divergent strabismus -- exactly what we would expect to find at the cortical level in a patient with ARC.

Campos observed summation of cortical evoked potentials seen in binocular vision in patients that had positive striated glasses tests. The summation disappeared when the anomalous binocularity was interrupted.

Thus, a finding of strong ABV in the filter bar test probably indicates that the binocularly driven cortical cells have become quite numerous.

SENSORI-MOTORIAL ADAPTIVE PHENOMENA

The use of prisms to optically correct strabismus has led to an important observation. Travers and Burian were the first to note that prismatic correction was sometimes associated with an increase in the angle of strabismus. I observed this phenomenon in post-operative patients in which the residual angle had been corrected with prisms.

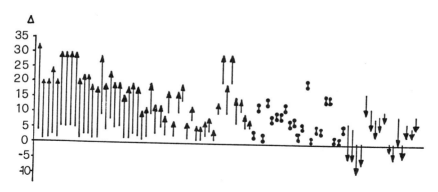

Fig. 7 - Response of 85 esotropic patients to prism correction of residual angle of deviation. Prismatic overcorrection of 20-30 △ caused almost all patients to increase angles of deviation. The length of the arrow indicates, in prism diopters (on the ordinate axis) the variation of the angle of deviation. The cases on the left (arrows pointing up), have completely or partially compensated for prismatic overcorrection by over-convergence.
A few patients did not show any variation of the angle of strabismus, while the cases on the right (arrows pointing down) reacted with divergence (this last possibility occurs more frequently in operated cases). The starting point of the arrow marks the pre-prismatic angle of deviation in prism diopters (△).

Prism compensation takes from a few seconds to several hours to develop fully. The compensatory movements of the eyes are very slow and cannot be perceived with the naked eye, but if the patient is subjected to the cover test, the angle will be found to be increased.

Figure 7 shows the results of 85 patients in which prisms were used to correct strabismus. The patients represented on the left-hand side of the graph were able to compensate for even strong over-correction of their original angle, whereas in those on the right, only a limited amount of prismatic correction could be compensated for. Some of these latter patients actually showed decreases in their original angles under prismatic correction. Adelstein and Cuppers (1970) observed the same response in some post-operative cases.

Jampolsky noted a very important point: prism compensation usually implies that the sensorial status of the patient is anomalous. When it occurs, therefore, we can infer that ARC already exists.

I was interested in knowing how strongly rooted these compensatory reactions were, and therefore devised the very simple progressive prism compensation test. The test is performed as follows: in a patient with an esodeviation of 30Δ, a 10Δ base-out prism that partially corrects the angle is applied and the patient is observed for up to 2 hours. During this time, the cover test is performed at intervals with the patient looking at a distant fixation light. If no compensation has occurred, the cover test will show an angle of about 20Δ. If, on the other hand, compensatory convergent movement has occurred in response to the $10\text{-}\Delta$ prism, the cover test will reveal an angle of 30Δ. The angle of esodeviation has actually increased to about 40Δ. At this point, we add an additional 10 bringing total prism correction to 20Δ, and again we check for compensation with the cover test. Prism correction is thus increased in increments of 10Δ until the patient can no longer compensate for the correction (Bagolini 1976).

The results of the progressive prism compensation test are interesting for two reasons. The results offer objective proof of an anomalous sensorial status which is usually more firmly rooted when the patient is able to compensate for high-diopter prismatic correction. When a patient is able to compensate for even strong over-correction, the probability of poor surgical results is much greater.

THEORETICAL CONSIDERATIONS

Anomalous retinal correspondence is a purely sensorial phenomenon in which the spatial organization of the retina of the deviated eye changes. It occurs in response to eye deviation only in children (from birth to about 8 years of age). Further evidence that this reaction is an adaptive one can be inferred by the fact that it becomes more firmly established in long-standing strabismus. In addition, when the angle of strabismus is corrected by surgery, the ARC changes as well to reflect the new angle of deviation.

Prism compensation, in contrast, is a sensori-motor phenomenon characterized by disjunctive ocular movements. It is quite evident in cases of convergent strabismus. The temporal shift in the retinal image induced by a base-out prism is the sensorial stimulus. In many esotropic patients this stimulus causes a motor reaction mediated by an increase in tone of the medial recti. I believe that the convergent movements that result are fusional in nature and they will, thus, be referred to hereafter as anomalous fusional movements (AFM).

In recent onset esotropia these AFMs are usually absent or weak, suggesting that they represent a sensori-motorial attempt to adapt to the angle of deviation. In addition, they can usually be eliminated by exercises aimed at decreasing the tone of the medial recti. Tsechermak-Seisenegg (quoted by Burian, 1947, p. 646) admits that rudimentary fusional movements may develop in cases of ARC. Bielschowsky proved that there may be fusional movements linked to the anomalous corresponding retinal area. Halden, in a very interesting experimental study, even demonstrated fusional movements in strabismus in spite of anomalous binocularity.

The purpose of these movements is to maintain equal images over anomalously corresponding retinal areas. Their fusional nature was supported by the findings of Campos and Zanasi who found that, in esotropic patients, base-out prisms tend to cause convergent movements while base-in and vertical prisms respectively elicit small, divergent and vertical responses.

There are, however, important differences between normal and anomalous fusional movements. One is related to their velocity. Normal fusional movements are effective within a fraction of a second and can be seen with the naked eye. AFMs may take minutes or hours and can be inferred only by the change in the angle seen in the cover test.

Some investigators have interpreted these movements in other ways. There has been a resurgence of support for the concept of diplopia-phobia first advanced by Van der Hoeve, for example. Jampolsky believes that the convergent movements seen in prism compensation are actually an attempt to avoid diplopia. In the many hundreds of patients I have examined, however, I have rarely heard reports of diplopia in those that compensated for correction or over-correction of their angle. Furthermore, many patients react with compensation and without diplopia even when their angles are only partially corrected by prisms. For these reasons, I am inclined to reject this interpretation.

Gobin explains these movements in yet another way. Like Keiners, he believes that there is a functional superiority of the temporal hemiretina which is enhanced by the suppression of the nasal hemiretina that occurs, in his opinion, in esotropia.

In my view, the weakness of this argument lies in the fact that patients with fairly large angle esotropia may compensate for even partial prism correction. In these cases, even though the image remains in the nasal hemiretina, the tone of the medial recti still increases.

Neither of the above two theories explains the findings of Campos and Zanasi that these patients can react to base-in prisms with divergent movements and to vertical prisms with vertical movements.

In spite of the fact that he admits to having observed vertical fusional movements linked with ARC, Burian interprets the horizontal angle increase seen with corrective prisms as a manifestation of the "horror fusionis" concept introduced by Bielschowsky. According to Burian, the patient with strabismus attempts to "avoid bifoveal stimulation" by turning the eye "until the same distribution of the retinal stimuli is reached which existed prior to the use of prisms". I cannot agree with this opinion because the movements that I believe are fusional in nature occur even if the prism correction does not bring about bifoveal stimulation. On the contrary, when over-correction of the angle is made, the deviated eye may move in a way that initially brings the image toward, rather than away from, the retina. As the eye continues to move, the image will subsequently pass through the fovea on its way to the nasal hemiretina.

In conclusion, the phenomena just discussed are admittedly difficult to interpret and we can still only guess as to their pathophysiological nature. But we can assert the following:

1) Anomalous retinal correspondence is an expression of an alteration in the spatial organization of the retina.
2) Anomalous fusional movements are an expression of an alteration in the motorial value of the retina.
3) Both ARC and AFM are present only when there is binocular vision.
4) Strongly rooted AFMs may interfere with surgical attempts to correct ocular misalignment.

References

Aldestein, F.E., Cüppers, C., 1966, Zum Problem der Echten und der scheinbaren Abducens Lämung (das sogenante) "Blokierungssyndrom").
In:Augenmuskellähmungen,Büch. Augenartz.,46:271.
Bagolini, B., Capobianco, N.M., 1965, Subjective space in comitant squint. Am. J. Ophthalmol. 59:430-432.
Bagolini, B., Part II, 1976, Sensorio-motorial anomalies in strabismus (anomalous movements).
Doc. Ophthalmol. 41:23-41.

Bagolini, B., Campos, E., 1977, Binocular campimetry in small angle of esotropia. Doc. Ophthalmol. Proceeding Series, 14:405.

Bagolini, B., 1982, Usefulness of filters of progressive density as a diagnostic tool for some strabismis problems. In Strabismus II (Isa Asilomar, California, 25 October 1982) p. 561.

Bielschowsky, A., 1899, Untersuchungen über das sehen der Schielenden. Arch. f Ophthalmol. 47:508.

Burian, H.M., 1947, Sensorial retinal relationship in comitant squint. Arch. Ophthalmol. 37:336-68, 504-33, 618-48.

Campos, E., Catellani, T., 1976, Perimetria binoculare nell'esotropia concomitante a piccolo angolo. Boll. di Oculist. 55:205.

Campos, E., Zanasi, M.R., 1978, Die anomalen Fusionsbewegungen: der sensomotorische Aspekt des anomalen Binocularschens. Graefes Arch. Clin. Exp. Ophth. 205:101.

Campos, E., Chiesi, C., 1983, Binocularity in comitant strabismus: objective evaluation with visual evoked responses. Doc. Ophthalmol. 55: 277.

Cynader, M., Gardner, J.C., Mustari, M., 1984, Effects of neonatally induced strabismus on binocular responses in cat area 18. Exp. Brain Res. 53:384-99.

Gobin, M.H., 1968, Sagittalisation of the oblique muscles as possible cause for the A and V and X phenomena. Br. J. Ophthalmol. 52:13.

Haldén, U., 1952, Fusional phenomena in anomalous correspondence. Acta Ophthalmol. 37 (suppl): 1-93.

Jampolsky, A., 1971, A simplified approach to strabismus diagnosis. In: Symposium on strabismus. Trans. New Orleans Acad. Ophthalmol.; 34.

Jampolsky, A., 1984, Discussion of Eisenbaum A.M., Parks, M.M., quoted by Rogers, G.L., Bremer D.L. Surgical treatment of the upshoot and downshoot in Duane's retraction syndrome. Ophthalmol. 91:1380-83.

Kommerel, G., 1986, Das Fixierpunktskotom des scielenden Augen: Ein Artefact. 13:29.

Mehdorn, E., 1989, Suppression scotomas in primary microstrabismus. A perimetric artefact. Doc. Ophthalmol. 71:1.

Travers, T.B., 1936, The comparison between the results obtained by various methods employed for the treatment of comitant strabismus. London: G. Pulman & Sons.

AGE, SEX AND LIGHT DAMAGE IN THE AVIAN RETINA: A MODEL SYSTEM

Katherine V. Fite, Lynn Bengston, and Beth Donaghey

Neuroscience and Behavior Program, Tobin Hall
University of Massachusetts, Amherst, MA 01003, USA

INTRODUCTION

At present, relatively little is known about the senescence of the retina, particularly the outermost layers which are unusually vulnerable to age-related disorders, including the photoreceptors, retinal pigment epithelium (RPE) and its interface with Bruch's membrane and the choriocapillaris. The RPE lies interposed between photoreceptors and the choroidal vascular system and has received increased attention as knowledge of its many regulatory, phagocytotic and reparative processes has advanced. Clearly, any disruption or impairment of the RPE can have progressive, adverse consequences for photoreceptor health, metabolism and functions (Zinn & Marmour, 1979).

RPE cells are particularly interesting for studies of cellular aging in the retina since, like neurons, they do not undergo division after fetal development, except in certain cases of injury or disease when they proliferate in a reparative response. The aging RPE contains several types of pigmented granules: melanin, lipofuscin and melanolipofuscin. Lipofuscin appears to be derived from lipid degradation products associated with incompletely phagocytized outer-segment membranes (Sohol, 1981; Feeney-Burns and Eldred, 1984) which increase over a lifetime of exposure to light and cyclic shedding of outer segments. With aging, both melanosomes and lipofuscin granules are involved in the formation of a third, more complex granule - the melanolipofuscin aggregate - which is the largest inclusion body found in aging RPE cells (Feeney-Burns, et al, 1984).

Human macular RPE cells contain more lipofuscin and melanolipofuscin granules than do peripheral cells (Feeney-Burns, et al., 1984; Weiter, 1986; Dorey, et al., 1989). In nondividing cells, the increased accumulation of indigestible material may ultimately lead to cellular dysfunction and mechanical disruption of intracellular organization with deleterious effects upon photoreceptor functions. Excessive accumulation of lipofuscin may seriously impair RPE cells and lead to a variety of secondary degenerative changes in the outer retina leading to the impairment of crucial interactions

The Changing Visual System, Edited by P. Bagnoli and
W. Hodos, Plenum Press, New York, 1991

between RPE cells and the choriocapillaris, particularly in the macular region.

The increased accumulation of lipofuscin also may result from a loss of phagocytic activity in aging RPE cells. Katz and Robinson (1984) have described a major reduction in the amount of phagocytized outer-segment material in the RPE of aged rats accompanied by an age-related alteration in the morphology of RPE apical microvilli, suggesting that the ability of the RPE to engulf and phagocytize photoreceptor outer-segment tips is impaired. An age-related loss in the number of RPE cells apparently results in an increased ratio of photoreceptors per RPE cell, with increased phagocytic load resulting in higher lipofuscin concentration, all of which may contribute to increased risk of macular disease (Dorey, et al., 1989).

The human fovea seems particularly vulnerable to age-related diseases such as senile or age-related macular degeneration (AMD), the leading cause of blindness in individuals 65 years of age and older in the United States and United Kingdom (Hyman, et al., 1983). The susceptibility of the macula to the effects of aging and its greater vulnerability to age-related diseases may be related to the high density of photoreceptors and the fact that the fovea is the only portion of the human retina without access to an inner retinal circulation. This avascular condition causes photoreceptors, outer nuclear and plexiform layers to be entirely dependent upon the adjacent choriocapillaris for the exchange of nutrients, metabolites and waste products. Thus, any abnormality or impairment in these crucial functions may have severe consequences for the vitality and longevity of foveal photoreceptors.

A major contributing factor to the development of AMD may be the age-related increases in lipofuscin in the macula (Feeney-Burns, et al., 1984; Weiter, et al., 1985; 1986; 1988). A second, potentially harmful factor may be the relatively low concentrations of RPE melanin in the macula compared with other retinal regions (Schmidt and Peisch, 1986). RPE melanin provides several protective functions with respect to ocular light exposure, including absorption of excessive light, particularly short and near-ultraviolet wavelengths (Wolbarsht, et al., 1981) which are especially damaging to photoreceptors. Melanin also scavenges free radicals and excited molecules resulting from photooxidative processes associated with transduction (see Young, 1988, for review). The reduction of RPE melanin that occurs with age appears to be due either to lysosomal digestion of melanosomes through the direct fusion of lysosomes with melanin granules or via extrusions of melanin-containing cytoplasm and its reincorporation by the phagolysosomal system of neighboring RPE cells (Feeney, 1978; Burns and Feeney-Burns, 1980).

A major environmental factor that may contribute both to the increased accumulation of lipofuscin and loss of RPE melanin with aging is light-exposure history. A large body of evidence now indicates that light can have a variety of toxic effects upon photoreceptors and RPE cells. Animals exposed to periods of constant light, or even moderate intensities of

284

cyclic light (depending upon species), show a variety of degenerative changes in the outer retina, including damage to outer segments and loss of photoreceptors (for reviews, see Lanum, 1978; Williams & Baker, 1980; Waxler & Hitchins, 1986). Light mediates the peroxidation of polyunsaturated fatty acids found in photoreceptor outer-segment membranes. The formation of oxygen-free radicals that can oxidize and denature organic lipids are stimulated by excessive light exposure as well (Wiegand, et al., 1982, 1983).

A major need exists for experimental investigations of the systemic and environmental factors influencing both normal and pathological retinal senescence to identify the specific processes that underlie aging in the outer retina. Mammalian species with visual systems most comparable to those of humans (i.e., Rhesus monkeys and domestic cats) are rather inconvenient laboratory residents and are long-lived, making longitudinal studies both impractical and time-consuming. Rodents have been frequently used for studies of retinal aging but are not highly visual animals; their retinae contain few cones and no macular region. Avian species appear to be excellent candidates for investigations of retinal aging, since most birds have excellent vision that may even surpass that of humans in some respects. An attractive feature of the avian retina is the lack of an anterior retinal vasculature and the presence of a highly developed choriocapillaris. Indeed, the avian retina appears to represent a "universal macula", since it has a high density of cones and is avascular over the entire globe (Walls, 1942).

AGE-RELATED CHANGES IN THE JAPANESE QUAIL RETINA

Among graniverous birds, the Japanese quail (Coturnix japonica) is highly precocial, with a lifespan ranging from 1-1.5 years in females and several years for males. A number of characteristics make the Japanese quail an attractive species for studies of aging in the visual system. The quail retina contains two areas of increased cellular density: an afoveate, central, or macular region, and a second, temporally placed area, both of which occur on or near the horizontal meridian (Budnick, et al., 1984). The quail retina is cone-rich, but also contains a significant rod population. The ratio of cones to rods ranges from approximately 2.5:1 in the central retina to 2:1 in the periphery. In addition, an extensive literature exists concerning the genetics, physiology, endocrinology and husbandry of Japanese quail, and an increasing number of laboratories are using this species for studies of aging.

A recent assessment of age-related changes in the outer retina of reproductively active Japanese quail raised on a 12:12 light:dark cycle revealed both age and sex differences in the rate and amount of lipofuscin accumulated in the basal portion of RPE cells (Fite and Bengston, 1989). Female quail showed greater densities of lipofuscin and melanolipofuscin granules and larger-sized granules at 3-months and 1-year of age compared to males. In fact, 1-year old females showed lipofuscin accumulation comparable to that of 3-year old males (Figures 1, 2).

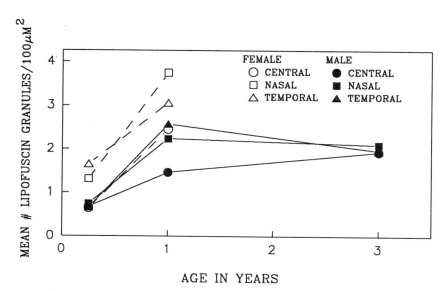

<u>Figure</u> <u>1</u>. Age and sex differences in the mean number of lipofuscin granules occurring in the basal region of the retinal pigment epithelium per 100 uM for central, temporal and nasal areas.

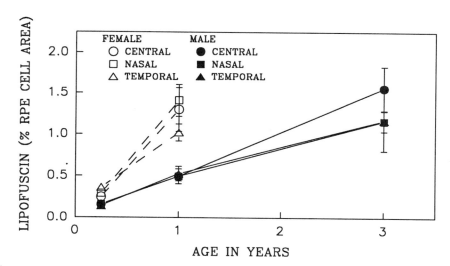

<u>Figure</u> <u>2.</u> Age and sex differences in retinal pigment epithelial (RPE) lipofuscin calculated as percent of average RPE cell area for central, nasal, and temporal regions (bar represents standard error of mean).

A quantitative ultrastructural analysis demonstrated that a substantial (approximately 40%) reduction occurred in the density of melanin granules in males between 4 months and 1-year of age, while females showed no significant change. Both males and females showed a slight decrease in rods at 1-year of age, and a 9-10% reduction in photoreceptor nuclei for the 3 retinal areas sampled (central, temporal, nasal). No loss of RPE cells was observed, but an elongation of RPE cells occurred in both sexes with increased age. Some abnormalities were observed in the RPE basal processes in 3-year old males, including disorientation and loss of processes and deterioration of the basilar membrane. However, no morphological changes were observed in the apical processes or intercellular, RPE- junctional complexes of either sex.

AGE AND LIGHT-DAMAGE EFFECTS IN THE QUAIL RETINA

The inverse relationship observed between RPE melanin and lipofuscin accumulation with aging may increase the vulnerablity of photoreceptors to light exposure. In fact, the effects of aging and those of light-induced damage to the outer retina share a number of similarities; however, the potential linkage of these two factors has not been experimentally investigated in a species with a cone-rich retina. Several studies have indicated that older animals are more susceptible to light damage (O'Steen, et al, 1974; Malik, et al, 1986), but these have been carried out with albino rats which have few cones. Thus, it is difficult to distinguish changes due to aging from those induced by light damage, since in normally pigmented animals, a considerable degree of protection derives from light attenuation by the heavily pigmented iris, RPE and choroid.

Using the Japanese quail, age-related effects following exposure to a single, intense light exposure have been examined in the outer retina using light- and electron-microscopic techniques. Two age groups (6-weeks and 1-year of age), each consisting of six males and six females, were maintained on a 12:12 hour light:dark cycle. Following a single exposure to broad-spectrum, white fluorescent light at 3000-3200 lux, 2mm diameter tissue punches were taken from the central and temporal retinal areas of both eyes of each subject (for detailed procedures, see Fite & Bengston, 1989). Four postexposure (PE) survival times were analyzed: 30 hours, 7 days, 14 days and 42 days. Semi-thin (1 micron) and ultrathin sections were obtained for light-microscopic and ultrastructural analyses, respectively.

Light Microscopic Analyses

Independent histopathology evaluations were made at a magnification of x1000 (oil immersion) by two raters (LB and BD) on 2 sections taken from central and temporal regions from the eye showing the most severe effects of light damage of each animal. These sections were compared with an equal number of sections from control animals (same age and sex). Histopathology ratings were based upon 6 dimensions of morphological abnormality for the outer segments and ONL.

Each histopathology dimension was rated along a 4-point scale: 0 = normal appearance, 3 = most severe condition. The specific dimensions were defined as follows:

Outer Segments- (1) conspicuous separation and disruption of the regular, lamellar arrangement of rod and cone outer segments, (2) outer segments were broken and/or disoriented, (3) outer segments were noticeably truncated and shortened compared to normal.

Outer Nuclear Layer - (1) dark-staining perikarya were present, (2) nuclei were elongated and/or spindle-shaped, (3) nuclei were reduced in density compared to normal. In addition, the width of the ONL was measured at 5, 100-micron sampling intervals in each section evaluated for histopathology.

Numerical ratings were summed separately for outer segments and for the outer nuclear layer. Ratings were then normalized to percentages of the maximum possible value that could have been observed for each layer (i.e., 100% would equal "9").

Results showed that the greatest histopathological effects occurred at the earliest postexposure (PE) time examined, i.e. PE 30 hours. In general, females showed more severe histopathological effects than males with some recovery by PE 42 days. However, the outer segments of males recovered more rapidly as postexposure time increased. Young males (6 weeks of age) showed restoration of normal outer-segment morphology by PE 42 days (light-microscopic analysis, Figures 3, 4).

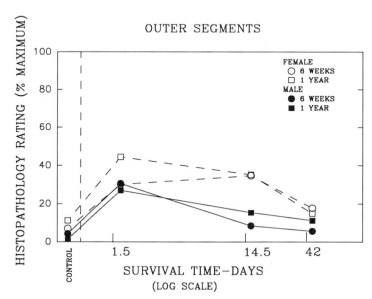

Figure 3. Histopathology ratings for outer segments presented as percentage of maximum possible rating for 6-week old and 1-year old quail at 3 postexposure times.

288

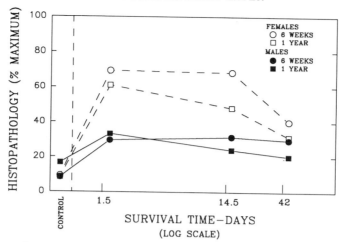

OUTER NUCLEAR LAYER

Figure 4. Histopathology ratings for 6-week old and 1-year old male and female quail at 3 postexposure times after a light-damaging exposure.

The width of the ONL decreased by 18% at PE 42 days in 1-year old males but no change was observed in females. Subsequent counts of rod and cone densities obtained from those sections evaluated for histopathology revealed a decrease in male rod density of 33% ($p \leq .002$), but no change was found in females. Cones showed no significant changes in density in either sex following light damage. This result seems somewhat paradoxical, since females appear to show greater histopathological effects of light damage when compared to males. However, loss of photoreceptors is the ultimate end-point for assessing light damage (Massof, et al., 1976). By this criterion, the rod population in males appears to be more vulnerable to destruction by light damage with increasing age than females. An explanation for this result may lie in the sex differences in lipofuscin accumulation with increasing age (see Figures 1, 2). Since male quail show an age-related loss of RPE melanin and also have substantially less lipofuscin at 1-year of age than females, less overall pigmentation is present in the RPE of males. Thus, the higher levels of RPE melanin and increased accumulation of lipofuscin at 1-year of age may actually provide a protective effect in females.

Ultrastructural Observations

Ultrastructural examination of both rods and cones at PE 30 hours and PE 42 days after the light-damaging exposure revealed that both photoreceptor populations were adversely affected. Both rod and cone outer segments showed morphological abnormalities that included separation of the lamellar array of outer-segment disc membranes, disorientation, convolution, outer segments, vesiculation and fragmentation of portions of outer segments (Figure 5A-D), all of which have been described as characteristics associated with light damage.

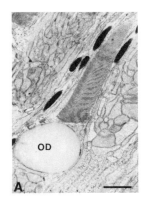
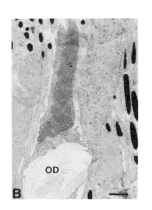
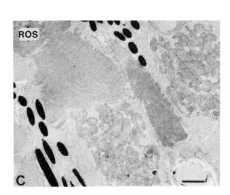
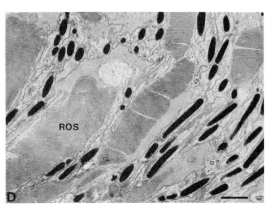
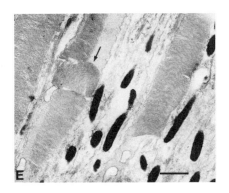

Figure 5. A. Six-week old control female, cone oil droplet (OD) and outer segment; B. six-week old female, 30 hours post-exposure (PE) showing light-damaged cone; C. Six-week old female, 30 hours PE showing light-damaged cone and rod outer segment (ROS); D. One-year old female, 30 hours PE, showing light-damaged cone and rod outer segment (ROS); E. One-year old male showing a convoluted cone outer segment (arrow). Magnification bar = 1 micron.

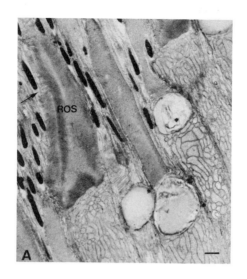

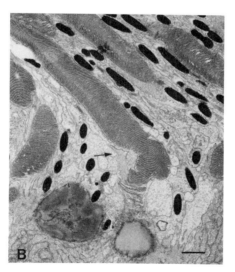

Figure 6. A. Rod and cone outer segments in 1-year-old control
male. Arrow indicates disruption of rod outer segment (ROS).
Magnification bar = 1 micron. B. Cone outer segment in 1-year
old control female. Arrow indicates abnormal region of cone
outer segment. Magnification bar = 1 micron.

With regard to recovery from light damage, at PE 42 days, rods showed a greater restoration of normal morphology than did cones. Young quail (6 weeks of age) of both sexes, showed a nearly complete recovery from light damage by PE 42 days, while 1-year old animals retained some morphological abnormalities from the light-damaging exposure. Many of these morphological alterations resembled those seen less frequently in 1-year old controls (Figure 6 A, B). Presumably, these changes are due to normal aging, perhaps as the result of cumulative light-exposure history (see also, Kuwabara and Gorn, 1968; Marshall, 1978; Marshall, et al. 1979). No abnormalities were observed in the RPE cells, Bruch's membrane or choriocapillaris in young or old animals of either sex.

Although several investigators using species with mixed retinas have concluded that cones are more vulnerable to light damage than rods (Marshall, et al., 1972; Sykes, et al., 1981) our results do not support such a straightforward conclusion. Although the threshold for light damage may be lower for cones (Sykes, et al., 1981), when the end-point criterion of photoreceptor loss is applied (Massof, et al., 1976), rods appear to be at greater risk than cones. Surviving rods may show fewer residual effects due to renewal rates and processes that differ from those of cones [i.e., rod outer segments show a more rapid rate of membrane turnover than cones (Young, 1976)]. The lower levels of lipofuscin and reduced RPE melanin of 1-year old males may be important factors associated with the loss of rods that occurs in older males after light damage. These observations may be relevant to the fact that, in humans, ocular pigmentation provides considerable protection against damage from solar radiation and may also reduce the likelihood of developing AMD (Young, 1988).

Recent studies in our laboratory have provided additional evidence bearing upon the hypothesis that lipofuscin may protect rod photoreceptors against light damage. A dramatic increase has been observed in the amount of RPE lipofuscin, particularly in 1-year old males following a light-damaging exposure (Fite, et al, 1990; manuscript in preparation). An increase in undigested outer-segment debris induced by phototoxicity probably constitutes a major component of the observed increase in RPE lipofuscin.

CONCLUSION

The Japanese quail appears to be an excellent choice of species for experimental investigations of age-related changes in the outer retina in relation to environmental factors such as light-exposure history. Such studies may ultimately lead to the development of strategies for retarding and/or reversing retinal senescence over the life span. The demonstration of sex differences with regard to the accumulation of RPE lipofuscin in the retina of aging Japanese quail may have significant generality for other species with a cone-rich retina including primates and humans.

Both light-exposure history and neuroendocrine factors associated with reproduction appear to have a direct influence on the rate and amount of lipofuscin accumulation in the RPE. Despite the current belief that lipofuscin is deleterious in its effects upon RPE-photoreceptor interrelationships, our results suggest that the higher levels of lipofuscin observed in older females may offer some protection against phototoxicity and partially compensate for the age-related loss of RPE melanin. Ultimately, retinal senescence can only be understood in terms of experimental analyses of the multiple interactions of genetic, environmental and endocrine factors.

ACKNOWLEDGMENTS

The authors thank Julie Gates and Celeste LeBlanc for their valuable technical assistance. This research was supported by NIH Grant EYO-7370.

REFERENCES

Budnick, V., J. Mpodozis, F. J. Varela, and H. Maturana, 1984, Regional specialization of the quail retina: Ganglion cell density and oil droplet distribution. Neurosci. Lett., 51: 145.

Cicerone, C., 1976, Cones survive rods in the light-damaged eye of the albino rat. Science, 194:1183.

Dorey, C. K., G. Wu, D. Ebenstein, A. Garsd, and J. J. Weiter, 1989, Cell loss in the aging retina. Invest. Ophthal. Vis. Sci., 39: 1691.

Feeney, L., Lipofuscin and melanin of human retinal pigment epithelium: Fluorescence, enzyme cytochemical and ultrastructural studies. Invest. Ophthal. Vis. Sci., 17:586.

Feeney-Burns. L. and G. E. Eldred, 1984, The fate of the phagosome: Conversion to "age pigment" and impact in human retinal pigment epithelium. Trans. Ophthal. Soc. 103: 416.

Feeney-Burns, L., E. S. Hilderbrand, and G. E. Eldred, 1984, Aging human RPE: morphometric analysis of macular. equatorial and peripheral cells. Invest. Ophthal. Vis. Sci., 25: 71.

Fite, K. V. and L. Bengston, 1989, Aging and sex-related changes in the outer retina of Japanese quail. Curr. Eye Res., 8: 1039.

Fite, K. V., L. Bengston, and B. Donaghey, 1991, Age, sex and light damage correlates of lipofuscin accumulation in the outer retina of Japanese quail. Invest. Ophthal. Vis. Sci., 32: 1095.

Hyman, L., A. M. Lilienfeld, F. L. Ferris III, and S. L. Fine, 1983, Senile macular degeneration: A case control study. Amer. J. Epidemiol., 118: 213.

Katz, M. and W. G. Robinson, Jr., 1984, Age-related changes in the retinal pigment epithelium of pigmented rats. Exp. Eye Res., 38: 137.

Kuwabara, T. and R. A. Gorn, 1968, Retinal damage by visible light: an electron microscopic study. Arch. Ophthal. 15:64.

Lanum, J. 1978, Review: The damaging effects of light on the retina. Empirical findings, theoretical and practical implications. Surv. Ophthal., 11: 221.

LaVail, M. 1976, Survival of some photoreceptor cells in albino rats following long-term exposure to continuous light. Invest. Ophthal. 15: 64.

Malik, S., D. Cohen, E. Meyer and I. Perlman, 1987, Light damage in the developing retina: an electroretinographic study. _Invest. Ophthal. Vis. Sci._, 27: 164.

Marshall, J., 1978 Aging changes in human cones. In "XXII Concilium Ophthalmologicum, Koyoto," K. Shimizu, and J. A. Oosterhuis, eds., Elsevier, Amsterdam.

Marshall, J., J. Grindle, P. L., Ansell, and B. Borwein. Convolution in human rods: an ageing process. 1979, _Brit. J. Ophthal._ 63: 181.

Marshall, J., J. Mellerio, and D. A. Palmer, 1972, Damage to pigeon retinae by moderate illumination from fluorescent lamps. _Exp. Eye. Res._, 14: 164.

Massof, R. W., S. M. Sykes, L. M. Rapp, W. G. Robinson, Jr., H. Zwick and B. Hochheimer. 1986, In "Optical Radiation and Visual Health," M. Waxler and V. M. Hitchins, eds. CRC Press, Inc., Boca Raton, Fla.

O'Steen, W. K., K. C. Anderson, and C. R. Shear. Photoreceptor degeneration in albino rats: dependency on age. _Invest. Ophthal. Vis. Sci.,_ 13: 334.

Schmidt, S. Y. and Peisch, R. D. 1986, Melanin concentration in normal human retinal pigment epithelium: Regional variation and age-related reduction. _Invest. Ophthal. Vis. Sci._ 27: 1063.

Sohol, R. S. 1981, "Age Pigments", Elsevier/North Holland, Amsterdam.

Sykes, S. M., W. G. Robinson, Dr., M. Waxler and T. Kuwabara, 1981. Damage to the monkey retina by broad-spectrum fluorescent light. _Invest. Ophthal. Vis. Sci._ 20: 425.

Walls, G., 1942, "The Vertebrate Eye and its Adaptive Radiation", Hafner, New York.

Waxler, M. and V. M. Hitchins, (eds), 1986, "Optical Radiation and Visual Health," CRC Press, Inc., Boca Raton, Fla.

THE DAMAGING EFFECTS OF LIGHT ON THE EYE AND IMPLICATIONS

FOR UNDERSTANDING CHANGES IN VISION ACROSS THE LIFE SPAN

John S. Werner

University of Colorado
Boulder, CO 80309-0345 U.S.A.

ABSTRACT

Damage to the lens and retina by photochemical processes upon absorption of light, especially ultraviolet radiation (UVR), has been well documented through laboratory experiments involving short, intense exposures. Throughout life, chronic exposure to less intense light produces the same photochemical effects on molecules contained within cells of the lens and retina, and this absorption may lead to cumulative deterioration in function. Such cumulative damage may explain why lenticular senescence and loss of receptor sensitivity are continuous throughout life. Support for this interpretation was found in patients who had lower short-wave cone sensitivity when chronically exposed to higher, ambient UVR following surgical removal of a cataractous lens and implantation of a prosthetic lens that did not absorb most of the incident UVR.

SOLAR RADIATION AND OCULAR ABSORBING MOLECULES

The extraterrestrial spectrum from the sun is shaped by absorption and scatter of quanta en route to the earth. The dashed curve in Figure 1 illustrates the solar quantum spectrum up to 800 nm that reaches the earth from an angle of 30° from the horizon. The spectrum of sunlight arriving at different regions of the planet may differ from that shown in Figure 1 due to such factors as latitude, altitude, cloud cover, aerosol content, and time of day. Solar UVR having wavelengths from about 285 to 300 nm is only minimally capable of penetrating the stratospheric ozone, but UVR from 300 to 400 nm reaches the surface of the earth. The solar quantum spectrum incident on the cornea will vary with surface reflectances (*e.g.*, snow and sand are better reflectors of UVR than are grass and leaves) and a variety of other factors (*e.g.*, sunglasses and brimmed hats may decrease UVR reaching the cornea).

The energy contained in a quantum is inversely related to its wavelength. Quanta in UVR may contain enough energy to alter molecules in the eye that absorb them. The absorbing molecule may act as a photosensitizer, thereby transferring energy to another molecule, or photochemical damage may ensue through the creation of free radicals which set off oxidative chain reactions that are harmful to biological tissue. Quanta in the visible and infrared contain less energy and have a lower probability of absorption by the ocular media; their absorption may increase the kinetic energy of molecules absorbing them, but this energy is usually not damaging by itself. Excess kinetic energy may, however, combine with energy absorbed at other wavelengths to contribute to threshold for ocular damage. The continuous exposure to light throughout life assures that deterioration will occur in cells containing UVR-absorbing molecules. The life span of these cells would be considerably diminished except for the fact that most visual cells are capable of renewing virtually all of their molecular constituents except DNA (Young, 1976). Nevertheless, molecular renewal is not perfect and can be overwhelmed by excessive radiation. This balance of radiation-induced deterioration and molecular renewal seems to be tipped toward senescence, and both structural and functional changes in the visual pathways occur continuously throughout the life span.

Visible radiation is normally limited to the band between 400 and 700 nm. The limit at long wavelengths is due to the absorption spectrum of the photopigments contained in the rod and cone receptors, while at short wavelengths it is due to the absorption characteristics of the ocular media. The absorbance of components of the ocular media is plotted in Figure 1. These data are transformed from the direct transmittance data of extracted tissue reported by Boettner and Wolter (1962). Quanta with wavelengths below 300 nm are almost completely absorbed by the cornea. Absorption of this radiation can damage the cornea (e.g., actinic keratitis), but long-term effects are rare because the corneal epithelium is capable of rapid molecular renewal. This is probably why the absorption spectrum of the cornea undergoes only small changes with advancing age (Lerman, 1984). Additional attenuation of UVR below 300 nm is provided by the aqueous and vitreous humors. Their absorption spectra change negligibly with age (Boettner & Wolter, 1962) and any damage sustained by absorption of light is likely to be unimportant for senescence because these fluids are rapidly replaced (Young, 1982).

The cornea and aqueous humors transmit UVR from 300 to 400 nm to the crystalline lens where much of it is absorbed. The lens is in a vulnerable position in the eye; only its epithelium and cortex are capable of substantial molecular renewal and it is only the anterior region that has access to antioxidant molecules (Young, 1991). The continual absorption of high-energy photons therefore promotes senescent deterioration in lenticular function and concomitant changes in coloration that lead to dramatic age-related changes in color vision.

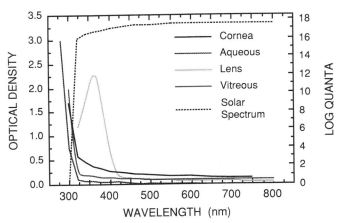

Figure 1. *Optical density (decadic logarithm of the reciprocal of transmittance) of human ocular media is plotted as function of wavelength (left ordinates; from Boettner & Wolter, 1962). Log quanta reaching the surface of the earth from the sun is plotted as a function of wavelength (right ordinates; from Brandhorst, Hickey, Curtis & Ralph, 1975).*

LENTICULAR SENESCENCE AND CATARACTOGENESIS

Molecules that absorb UVR are present in the newborn crystalline lens, but their numbers increase continuosly over the life span. Several studies have shown that the density of the crystalline lens increases with age, leading to a reduction in UVR and short-wavelength visible radiation reaching the retina. Selected data are presented in Figure 2; ocular media density at 400 nm, the peak density in the visible spectrum, is plotted as a function of age. The regression line was fitted only to the points shown as closed symbols. While there are large individual differences at each age, it can be deduced from the regression equation that the average 70-year-old eye transmits about 22 times less light at 400 nm than the eye of the average 1-month-old infant.

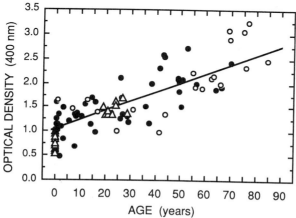

Figure 2. *Optical density of the human ocular media is plotted as a function of age. Filled circles from Werner (1982); unfilled circles from Weale (1988); triangles from Hansen and Fulton (1989).*

The data represented by triangles and filled circles were obtained from comparisons of the rhodopsin absorbance spectrum and log scotopic spectral sensitivity. Ocular media density represented by these symbols thus represents all media of the eye combined, not just the crystalline lens. The unfilled circles show density spectra of extracted human lenses with an upward scaling of 0.48 for comparison with the closed symbols. This difference in the two sets of results is consistent with the combined, average, density of the cornea, aqueous and vitreous humors measured by Boettner and Wolter (1962) but does not factor in possible small age-related changes in corneal absorption.

The linear increase in ocular media density with age shown in Figure 2 may describe most of the life span, but some data suggest that optical density may increase at a faster rate above about age 65 years. A linear increase in optical density would be expected (if the lens pigment were uniformly distributed) because of a linear increase in lens thickness with age. Sample *et al.* (1988) have reported a nonlinear increase in ocular media density with age. The nonlinearity in their data appears to be due to an acceleration in the aging function above about age 65 years, but is largely due to the inclusion of some patients with cataract. While many investigators assiduously avoid inclusion of patients having a cataract, their inclusion is defensible. This "disease" is largely a matter of definition and may represent only an extreme in the continuous process of aging. The change in lens density is continuous throughout life, and when the more extreme changes in density produce measurable interference with visual resolution they are labelled cataractous. In his recent comprehensive monograph on this subject, Young (1991) presents an impressive body of data that lead to the conclusion that: "No discontinuity between senescent and cataractous changes can be detected at the molecular level in the human lens....The most sophisticated techniques of modern biophysical and biochemical analysis have so far failed to uncover any feature of the cataractous lens that suggests cataract is anything more than an advanced stage of normal aging" (p. 56).

To the extent that cataract is only an extreme of normal aging, evidence regarding its formation can be culled to shed light on normal senescence. Considerable experimental and epidemiological evidence has shown that lenticular senescence and cataract is, in part, associated with the absorption of high-energy photons of UVR. For example, *in vivo* studies indicate that the action spectrum for lens opacities rises sharply at about 295 nm (due to corneal absorbance), peaks at about 300 nm and falls sharply with increasing wavelength (Bachem, 1956). This action spectrum is initially and primarily due to photon capture by tryptophan in the lens cortex and nucleus, and by DNA in the posterior subcapsule. The dissipation of this energy can lead to the formation of free radicals and oxygen biproducts which ultimately lead to development of yellow pigments (oxidative degradation products of tryptophan) that further extend the absorption spectrum of the lens into longer UV wavelengths and the visible spectrum. While cataracts can be of several different types (*e.g.*, nuclear, cortical, posterior subcapsular), they all appear to involve UVR-initiated photochemical processes. Weale (1983) has proposed that the specific form of cataract depends on genetic factors, while the common etiology is solar radiation. Young (1991) shares Weale's view that genetic factors may be related to individual differences in the form of cataract, and proposes specific hypotheses about the underlying mechanisms. For example, individuals low in antioxidation defences normally found in lens cortex and epithelium may be more susceptible to cortical cataract, while others having normal antioxidation defences may experience opacities of the nucleus, a part of the lens that has little access to oxidation defences and scavengers of free radicals. Still other individuals may develop subcapsular cataract due to inadequate DNA repair processes. Thus, while radiation contributes to all types of cataract formation, individual variation in the weakest defences may result in variations in the site of lenticular senescence and cataractogenesis.

Epidemiological evidence further buttresses the role of solar radiation in senescent deterioration of the lens. For example, there is a correlation between incidence of cataract and other diseases (*e.g.*, pterygium and skin cancer) clearly associated with exposure to sunlight. If one examines a large number of studies of cataract prevalence, it is found to vary systemically with latitude. The onset of cataract and its incidence in the population increases from the poles to the equator. Young's (1991) summary of this literature indicates a prevalence rate of about 14% for countries above 36°, 22% for mid-latitude (28° to 36°) countries and 28% for low (10° to 26°).latitude countries Such epidemiological studies are complex and open to alternative interpretations because many variables change with latitude. However, UVR may be the only variable that changes with latitude *and* has been shown to play a significant role in aging of the lens.

Based on a wide range of experimental and epidemiological studies, it is evident that senescent changes in the human lens such as those illustrated by Figure 2 are due, at least in part, to exposure to UVR over the life span.

RETINAL SENESCENCE REVEALED BY AGE-RELATED CHANGES IN THE SENSITIVITY OF CONE MECHANISMS

The penetrance of some UVR through the ocular media and its high concentration of oxygen make the retina susceptible to some of the same photochemical and photodynamic effects that accelerate aging in the lens. The retina, however, is more complex than the lens due to its greater variety of cell types, cell functions, nutritional and metabolic requirements, and light-absorbing molecules. Therefore, aging of the retina is likely to be more varied than in the lens and the role of radiation in accelerating aging is likely to be more difficult to unravel.

When the cornea is uniformly illuminated, as in natural viewing, a high concentration of quanta will be imaged onto the fovea. This concentration of light is sufficient to raise the temperature of the retina, but the heat is sufficiently dissipated by the retinal pigment epithelium (RPE) and choroidal vasculature so that it is seldom damaging (Parver et al., 1980). The highest energy photons of the visible spectrum (ca, 400-520 nm) are also attenuated by the macular pigment in the receptor fiber layer and inner plexiform layer. The density of this pigment is highest in the fovea and decreases radially outward so that by about 5° there is virtually no change in density with further eccentricity. Its presence reduces short-wavelength spectral sensitivity and the effects of chromatic aberration. Based on its absorption spectrum, the macular pigment is generally believed to be a carotenoid (3,3' dihydroxy-alpha-carotene) similar to leaf xanthophyll or perhaps a mixture of two carotenoids (Bone et al., 1985). While the presence of melanin provides the retina with an excellent scavenger of free radicals, macular pigment may provide an additional defence for the fovea as carotenoid pigments tend to neutralize photosensitized molecules (Kirschfeld, 1982) and inhibit free radical reactions (Krinsky, 1979).

We (Werner et al., 1987) have measured the density of the macular pigment in the fovea for 50 observers ranging in age from 10 to 90 years using noninvasive procedures. Following Wald (1949), spectral sensitivity was compared for the fovea and parafovea, but an improvement in his method was to use a short wavelength adapting field and a 15 Hz flickering stimulus so that short-wave-sensitive (SWS) cones and rods would not contribute to thresholds. This was necessary because these receptor types are not distributed equally in the fovea and parafovea. Macular pigment measurements under our conditions depended only on a constant ratio of middle-wave-sensitive (MWS) to long-wave-sensitive (LWS) cones from the fovea to the parafovea. The results are presented in Figure 3, which shows mean optical density at 460 nm, the peak of the macular pigment absorption spectrum, as a function of age. Like the lens, there is substantial individual variation; unlike the lens, there is no significant change with age between 10 and 90 years.

These findings have been verified and expanded by direct measurements of extractable macular pigment (Bone et al., 1988). This study shows that macular pigment accumulates over the first two-to-three years of life, after which there is no systematic change in density with further increases in age. Infants' reduced macular pigmentation and more transparent lens imply that they may have considerably weaker defenses against UVR and short-wave visible radiation than do adults.

While the infant eye may differ from the older eye in its preretinal screening pigments, it does not differ (at least after about the fifth postnatal week) from the adult in the types of photopigments contained in the receptors. The presence of all three classes of cone photoreceptors and rods has been demonstrated in early infancy, but detailed functions showing how each class of cone changes between infancy and early adulthood have not been reported. One approach to determining sensitivity of cone mechanisms is to measure two-color increment thresholds (Stiles, 1953; Wald, 1964). An adapting background is chosen to selectively suppress activity of two of the

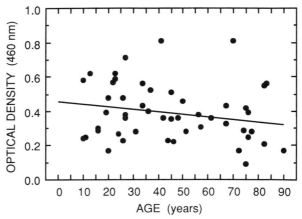

Figure 3. *Optical density of human macular pigment for the central 1° of retina is plotted as function of age (from Werner et al., 1987). The slope of the linear regression equation is not significantly different from zero.*

three classes of cones, leaving the third type to dominate spectral sensitivity to superimposed monochromatic stimuli. For example, an intense yellow adapting background will suppress MWS and LWS cones, rendering the SWS cones relatively more sensitive. This approach has been used by Volbrecht and Werner (1987) to isolate a SWS-cone mechanism in 4-6-week-old infants. Averages of cortically-evoked responses to a series of test flash intensities were measured at a number of short wavelengths, and threshold for each wavelength was defined by a fixed-criterion response interpolated from the response vs. intensity function. The data were consistent with the view that average sensitivity of infant SWS cones is about 1.0 log unit less than in 20-30 year-old adults. A subsequent study demonstrated that adult sensitivities may not be reached by 6-8 years of age (Abramov *et al.*, 1984). Sensitivities of mechanisms dominated by MWS and LWS cones have not yet been systematically measured for infants and young children.

Several studies have attempted to measure age-related changes in the sensitivity of the individual classes of cone receptors and/or cone pathways (Eisner *et al.*, 1987; Johnson *et al.*, 1988; Werner & Steele, 1988). Each of these studies reported age-related decreases in sensitivity of SWS cones. In our laboratory, sensitivity of all three cone mechanisms was measured for the same 76 individuals sampled evenly over the range of about 10 to 80 years. We found continuous change in all three cone types from about 10 years of age throughout the life span. Figure 4 summarizes these results. Each panel represents average sensitivity across the wavelengths in which one cone type dominated sensitivity; SWS (440, 460, 500 nm); MWS and LWS (500, 530, 560, 590, 620 nm). The decline in sensitivity with advancing age is statistically significant for each of the three cone classes. Indeed, the slopes of the regression lines shown in the figure were similar for all three cone types and imply a decline of 0.13 ± 0.01 log unit, per decade. That is, cones sustain a sensitivity loss of about 26% per decade over most of the life span.

The results in Figure 4 refer to sensitivity specified at the cornea and so some of the loss must be attributable to a reduction in the retinal illuminance arising from age-related increases in ocular media density. Correction of sensitivity for losses in ocular media density implies that the SWS cones decline at 440 nm by about 0.08 log unit per decade, which is in agreement with results of Johnson *et al.* (1988), who

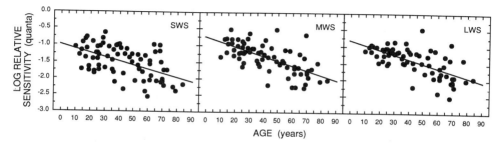

Figure 4. *Log relative sensitivity (on a quantal basis) of mechanisms dominated by short-wave sensitive (SWS), middle-wave sensitive (MWS) or long-wave sensitive (LWS) cones is plotted as a function of age (from Werner and Steele, 1988).*

report an age-correlated decline in short-wave-cone sensitivity of 0.15 log unit per decade at the cornea, and a decline of 0.09 log unit per decade after corrections for ocular media absorption. Thus, in these investigations, 30-40% of the age-correlated loss in sensitivity of the SWS cones (defined in terms of light delivered to the cornea) is attributable to light-losses in the ocular media, with the remaining loss ascribable to receptoral and/or postreceptoral changes. The data presented in Figure 4 show losses in sensitivity of MWS and LWS cones that are nearly the same as for SWS cones. However, since the age-related changes in ocular media reduce sensitivity to short wavelengths more than to long wavelengths, the loss in sensitivity of SWS cones specified at the retina is relatively less. It is conceivable that the increased density of the aging lens protects the SWS cones from more rapid aging than might otherwise occur as a result of constant bombardment by UVR and short-wave visible radiation. This may explain why a positive correlation has been reported between ocular media density and sensitivity of a SWS-cone mechanism (Johnson *et al.*, 1988). In addition, age-related declines in the sensitivity of SWS cones are greater outside the fovea where macular pigment absorption is reduced, a result consistent with the hypothesis that the yellow macular pigment may protect the fovea against cumulative light damage over the life span (Haegerstrom-Portnoy, 1988). Further evidence consistent with this hypothesis is presented in the final section of this paper.

A DIGRESSION:
TEST OF PARALLEL CHANGES IN CONE SENSITIVITIES WITH AGE

If the three classes of photoreceptor lose sensitivity at essentially the same rate with advancing age, as indicated by Figure 4, one might expect that postreceptoral-opponent processes that combine the cone inputs in a linear fashion should not change with age, as their inputs depend on the balance of activity of the three cone types. For example, Jameson and Hurvich (1968) have expressed the relation between the response of the red-green opponent channel and its receptor inputs as follows:

$$(r,g)_\lambda = k_1 S_\lambda - k_2 M_\lambda + k_3 L_\lambda. \tag{1}$$

Here (r,g) is the response of the red-green channel, S_λ, M_λ, and L_λ are the respective rates of quantal absorption that take place in the SWS, MWS, and LWS cones when stimulated by a light of wavelength λ, and the constants k_1, k_2, k_3 are weighting coefficients used to fit empirical data sets. These coefficients are thought to embody such physiological factors as neural processing of cone signals and the relative numbers of SWS, MWS and LWS cones within an individual. Results from a number of psychophysical investigations indicate that equation 1 is an adequate representation of how the three cone types pool their signals to produce a neural pathway that mediates perception of redness and greenness.

Color theorists have long recognized the existence of four elemental chromatic sensations: blue, green, yellow, and red. These chromatic sensations are said to be perceptually "pure" or "unique" because they contain no traces of any other hue. Unique hues are significant in opponent-colors theory because they represent a class of stimuli that elicit a null response in one of the two postulated chromatically-opponent processes, either the red-green or blue-yellow channel. For example, a spectral unique yellow, a hue that contains neither traces of red nor green, corresponds to a monochromatic test light that gives rise to a yellow response in the yellow-blue opponent channel and a null response in the red-green opponent channel. Stimuli that produce a null response in one of the two color-opponent channels are called equilibrium hues. Thus, the wavelengths corresponding to unique blue and unique yellow define equilibrium points for the red-green channel. The wavelength corresponding to unique green defines an equilibrium point for the yellow-blue channel, but the complications of this nonlinear system will not be further considered here.

We (Schefrin & Werner, 1990) measured the wavelengths of unique blue and unique yellow for 50 observers ranging in age from 13 to 74 years. Each unique hue was measured at three luminance levels (0.5 log unit steps). These data (means for the three luminance levels) are shown in Figure 5 as closed symbols; open symbols represent an unpublished replication with 50 subjects tested in a Maxwellian-view optical system so that retinal illuminance would be unaffected by pupil size. Both sets of data indicate that the spectral locations of red-green equilibrium hues (unique blue and unique yellow) do not significantly change with age.

Now consider what these results imply in terms of the hypothesis that the sensitivity of the three cone types changes in parallel over the age range tested. In the spectral region encompassing unique yellow, SWS cones are relatively insensitive and consequently the red-green channel essentially receives input only from MWS and LWS cones. Thus, unique yellow can be modelled as a red-green equilibrium state in which:

$$0 = -k_2 M_\lambda + k_3 L_\lambda \qquad [2]$$

The observation that the wavelength of unique yellow does not change with age, as illustrated by Figure 5, is consistent with parallel changes in the sensitivities of MWS and LWS cones as a function of age. Individual variation in the unique yellow locus may be attributable to individual differences in the ratios of MWS to LWS cones.

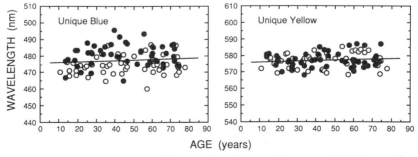

Figure 5. *Wavelengths of unique blue and unique yellow are plotted as a function of age (closed symbols from Schefrin & Werner, 1990).*

In the short wavelength region of the spectrum all three cone types are believed to contribute signals to the red-green channel. As such, the locus of unique blue depends on the rates of quantal absorption in all three classes of cones. It follows from the parallel age-correlated declines in MWS and LWS cones (implied by constancy of unique yellow) and from the nonsignificant age-correlated changes in the locus of unique blue, that the SWS cone contribution to the red-green process declines at the same rate as the contributions from the other two cone types. To wit: all three cone types must decline at similar rates with advancing age, at least in terms of their contribution to a red-green chromatic process.

SITES OF SENESCENT SENSITIVITY LOSS OF A SWS-CONE PATHWAY

Senescent changes in cone sensitivity are partially attributable to age-related changes in ocular media density. Under some conditions, an age-related decrease in the diameter of the pupil will also lead to loss in sensitivity by virtue of reducing retinal illuminance (Weale, 1963). This factor is not likely to have contributed significantly to the data presented in Figure 4 because the adapting backgrounds were sufficiently intense to place the measurements on the approximately linear portion of the log threshold vs. log intensity function. This implies that a smaller pupil for elderly individuals would have affected the test and background approximately equally and hence the same sensitivity would be obtained regardless of pupil area.

Factors affecting the ability of cones to capture quanta almost certainly contribute to some of the observed sensitivity losses of cone mechanisms. For example, fundus reflection densitometry has been used to estimate age-related changes in the density of bleachable photopigment in the central 2° of retina for 19 subjects ranging in age from 22 to 70 years (Kilbride et al., 1986). The density change in the fundus reflectance at 560 nm was quantified in this study, and it can confidently be attributed to combined photopigment density of MWS and LWS cones. The results indicate a linear change in photopigment density as a function of age, with a reduction of 0.03 per decade. There are at least three plausible interpretations for these age-related changes in photopigment density. They could be due to: (1) reduction in the length of the cone outer segments, (2) a change in the alignment of photopigment chromophores that reduces their ability to absorb light, and/or (3) a reduction in photoreceptor numbers. Kilbride et al. favor the last interpretation. This interpretation is consistent with the color-matching results of Elsner et al. (1988) who report no significant age-related change in optical density, inferred from the difference between high and low illuminance color matches for 52 subjects, 13-69 years of age. Color-matching is not affected by number of receptors, but only by the optical density of pigment within individual receptors. At first glance, this summary may seem complicated by a study of van Norren and van Meel (1985) of cone pigment density of 77 observers (age 13-50 years) determined with the Utrecht densitometer. No significant correlation between photopigment density and age was found; however, in a subsequent study, this group did find a decrease in density after age 60 (Keunen, van Norren & van Meel, 1987). This suggests a biphasic relation between photopigment density and age, but when all the data from the Utrecht densitometer were fitted by a single regression equation, a significant linear relation was found ($r^2 = 0.45$, $p < 0.01$), with an overall reduction in optical density of 0.02 per decade. This density is close to the nearly 0.03 reduction reported by Kilbride et al. (1986) using a linear regression analysis. In sum, evidence suggests that reductions in photopigment density are partly responsible for age-related declines in the sensitivity of MWS and LWS cones. Comparable data are not available for SWS cones.

Several types of age-related change in the human retina have been reported on the basis of postmortem light microscopy. Most changes, such as migration of cell nuclei from the outer nuclear layer to the outer plexiform layer, are only rarely observed in early life, become more frequent after the third or fourth decade, and become common after the fifth decade (Gartner & Henkind, 1981)   While these nuclear displacements are rare in the fovea, they are common outside the macula. Gartner and Henkind also noted shrunken and deformed rods and cones in older retinae and a reduction in photoreceptor numbers in the macular zone. It is not clear whether these losses are secondary to the many other retinal changes in the aging eye involving the retinal pigment epithelium, Bruch's membrane and choroidal vasculature. It should be noted that these results are strictly qualitative; quantitative studies show linear changes in numbers of some cell types over the life span (see Werner *et al.*, 1990, Figure 1). For example, losses in cell density at the levels of the optic nerve (Balazsi *et al.*, 1984) and visual cortex (Devaney & Johnson, 1980) are consistent with continuous aging processes. These changes provide a basis for speculating on age-related sensitivity losses of cone pathways. As Weale (1982) has pointed out, however, decrements in specific visual functions do not necessarily have to accompany losses in cell numbers.

The literature thus contains many candidate mechanisms that may contribute to age-related sensitivity losses of cone pathways. This evidence is most pertinent to MWS- and LWS-cone mechanisms; it is less clear what factors contribute to the sensitivity losses of a SWS-cone mechanism. To address this issue, we (Schefrin *et al.*, 1991) measured threshold vs. radiance functions (t.v.r.) for five young (mean age = 24 years) and six older (mean age = 70 years) subjects. Stimulus conditions were chosen to isolate a SWS-cone mechanism; measurements were obtained for a 250 ms, 1° diameter, 440 nm, foveally-viewed test light presented on 470 nm adapting fields and a 570 nm auxiliary field.   Increment thresholds were measured using a temporal, two-alternative, forced-choice method. In addition, ocular media densities were determined for each subject following the method of van Norren and Vos (1974). The resultant t.v.r. functions revealed intensity-dependent sensitivity losses in a SWS-cone pathway of the older group. This can be seen in Figure 6 for one subject's data (open symbols), compared to an average function for the young subjects (solid curve.)

To examine possible causes of the age-related differences in threshold, we modified a model of the π_1 pathway (Pugh & Mollon, 1979) and applied it to individual sets of t.v.r. data. According to this model, output from SWS cones

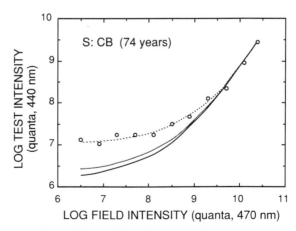

Figure 6.   *Increment threshold function for one observer (open symbols) compared to average function of young observers (solid curve). The middle curve shows the average curve of young subjects adjusted according to the ocular media density of C.B. The top (dashed) curve shows a theoretical function based on age-related changes in photon capture by SWS cones.*

detecting the test light passes through two serial gain sites. The first site is located at the level of the SWS cones (g_1), while the second site represents a stage of cone opponency (g_2). Reductions in gain at either site may be responsible for elevating test thresholds. Gain reductions at the first site are related to increased rates of photon absorption, and gain reductions at the opponent site occur when there is an imbalance between inputs from SWS cones versus MWS and LWS cones. This model can be expressed quantitatively by:

$$\log T_{440} = \log To_{440} - \log \zeta_1 (KoS) - \log \zeta_2 \mid (K_1S) - K_2(M+L) \mid \qquad [3]$$

$$\text{and } K_1 = K_2(M_\mu + L_\mu) / S_\mu.$$

In this equation, $\log T_{440}$ is the intensity of a 440 nm test light at threshold on a 470 nm adapting field and a 570 nm auxiliary field; $\log To_{440}$ is the intensity of the 440 nm test light corresponding to the absolute threshold of an S-cone mechanism; S, M and L are the normalized rates of quantal absorption of the three classes of cones; ζ_1 and ζ_2 are the gain functions at the two adaptation sites which follow Stiles tabulated increment threshold function; and, μ = the wavelength at which the second site is in equilibrium (wavelength of unique green). When this model was applied to the data of observer C.B. in Figure 6, it was found that all of his sensitivity loss could be ascribed to losses in photon capture; that is, he differed from the younger subjects only because of more dense ocular media and lower sensitivity of his SWS cones. When these parameters were inserted into the model for the younger subjects, it produced the theoretical function shown by the dashed curve. Not all subjects' data could be explained in this way. Indeed, an opponent-site loss (second site) had to be assumed in accounting for the data of four of the six older subjects. However, on average, 69% of the age-related sensitivity losses could be attributed to relative reductions in the rate of photon absorption by the cones.

SENESCENCE OF CONE MECHANISMS ACCELERATED BY LIGHT

Senescence of the human lens and receptor mechanisms have been shown to occur *continuously* across the life span. Age-related changes in ocular media transmission are at least partly due to exposure to light itself. One possible advantage of increased lenticular density with advancing age may be to protect the retina from potentially harmful radiation -- radiation which may damage the retina directly at high exposure levels, but which at low levels may have cumulative photochemical effects leading to disease (Young, 1988) and/or aging. Marshall (1978), for example, reported a striking resemblance in the vesicular degeneration of cone outer segments that had sustained damage from intense light exposure and presumably normal receptors of elderly humans. Along the same lines, Fite *et al.* (1991) reported that the age-related increase in lipofuscin in the RPE, presumably due to accumulated outer segment debris, is accelerated in Japanese quail following chronic exposure to light. These pieces of evidence are consistent with the hypothesis that light exposure contributes to what we call normal aging.

In our study of sensitivities of the cone mechanisms, we found linear declines beginning at age 10 years (Werner & Steele, 1988). From a quantitative analysis of t.v.r. functions, we have also shown that a substantial portion of the loss is due to changes in photon capture (Schefrin *et al.*, 1991). It seems likely based on previous literature that some of the loss associated with ocular media changes could be due to light exposure, but it was not clear whether any of the receptor sensitivity loss in this sample was associated with individual light histories. Informal interviews of participants in our studies indicate that individual differences in sensitivity of SWS cones may be related to individual differences in sunlight exposure. For example, participants who worked in outdoor occupations (*e.g.*, ski instructor, power line repairman) and who did not wear sunglasses were often found to have lower short-wave cone sensitivity than others of the same age. Conversely, patients who indicated that they regularly wore sunglasses typically had SWS cones with high sensitivity for their age. It was not possible to verify these self-reports, but the results are consistent with the hypothesis that retinal aging, like lenticular aging, is accelerated by light exposure.

If light contributes to aging, what wavelengths and which class of photoreceptor would most likely be involved? Ham *et al.* (1982) measured the threshold for a funduscopically visible lesion of the monkey retina induced by various wavelengths of light. Damage was usually not apparent until 48 hours after light exposure, indicating that it was due to photochemical processes rather than a thermal burn. The upper 3.0 log units of a function fitted to all of their results (and converted to quanta) is presented as a dashed curve in Figure 7. The graph shows that any wavelength of light may be damaging to the retina, but sensitivity (reciprocal of threshold) for damage by UVR is substantially higher than for visible or infrared wavelengths. Within the visible spectrum, sensitivity was higher for short wavelengths than middle or long wavelengths. Related experiments have used functional criteria to identify the cone types that are most susceptible to photochemical damage. For example, Harwerth and Sperling (1975) have shown that the SWS cones of the monkey retina are less likely to recover from light damage associated with chronic exposure to visible light than are MWS and LWS cones. Thus, if light contributes to normal aging in humans, it seems likely that UVR would be particularly hazardous, and the SWS cones may be most vulnerable.

The relevance of these laboratory experiments to natural situations likely to involve chronic, less intense, exposure to light over the life span is based partly on evidence that retinal damage by photochemical processes is additive over time and intensity (Kremers & van Norren, 1989). This additivity is not complete, though, because rods and cones are capable of molecular renewal (Young, 1976). Thus, rods can replace approximately 30-100 discs per outer segment each day -- and the entire length of the outer segment is replaced every two weeks. As new discs are formed, older discs are pushed into the RPE where they are phagocytized. Renewal of cone outer segments involves piecemeal replacement of molecular constituents and is considerably slower than molecular renewal in rods. Cones may, therefore, be less resilient in their recovery following actinic insult.

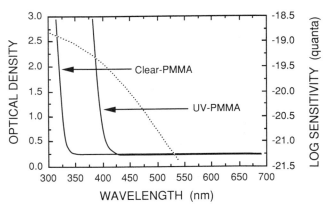

Figure 7. Log quantal sensitivity of the retina to funduscopically-visible damage (dashed curve; right ordinates) is plotted as a function of wavelength (from Ham et al., 1982). Optical density of UV-absorbing and non-UV-absorbing intraocular lenses (solid curves; left ordinates) are plotted as a function of wavelength (from Werner et al., 1989).

We (Werner *et al.*, 1989) reported a novel test of whether UVR exposure can be damaging to the human retina. Eight patients were tested following bilateral cataract surgery and implantation of intra-ocular lenses (IOLs). The IOLs implanted were manufactured from polymethyl methacrylate (PMMA), but one contained UVR-absorbing chromophores while the other did not. Hence, the latter lens did not prevent UVR (between 320 and 400 nm) from reaching the retina. The density spectra for these two IOLs are shown in Figure 7. One lens transmitted about 86% of solar UVR and the other only about 1%. Both IOLs had received approval for implantation by the U.S. Food and Drug Administration and have not been shown to be unsafe (Werner & Spillmann, 1989), but because the UVR-absorbing lens was new, the surgeon elected to use it in only one eye. Patients were included in the study only if they had clear ocular media, normal fundi, and normal intraocular pressure. Snellen acuities were 6/6 for both eyes. It is conceivable that requiring patients to meet these rigid criteria provides a lower-bound estimate of the deleterious effects of UVR, but it was necessary to use these criteria to avoid confounding with other age-related changes in vision or retinal disease.

On average, the clear IOLs were implanted 5 years before testing. The UVR-absorbing IOLs were implanted 2.3 years before testing, but since these IOLs have similar UVR-filtering properties to the natural lens it can be stated that the two eyes differed in their UVR exposure by about 86-to-1 for a period of five years. It should perhaps also be noted that all patients lived near Boulder, CO, where the average daily UVR is about 37% higher than at comparable latitudes on the east coast of the U.S and about 10% higher than comparable latitudes on the west coast of the U.S. Because photochemical damage is cumulative, the results are likely to be applicable to geographical locations that differ in average solar UVR.

Using the same methods to isolate the three classes of cones that were used in our studies of normal aging (Werner & Steele, 1988), it was found that there was a statistically significant loss in sensitivity of the SWS cones for the eyes receiving greater exposure to UVR. On average, the SWS cones were 1.7 times less sensitive in the eye receiving higher UVR exposure. No significant difference between the eyes was found for MWS and LWS cones. These results clearly establish that elevated exposure to UVR is associated with a loss in sensitivity of the photoreceptors, although it is not clear whether these results are mediated by the same processes that mediate age-related losses in sensitivity. Based on the literature, it would be reasonable, however, to view these changes in this way, *i.e.*, accelerated aging due to UVR. Using our normal age-related changes in SWS cones as a baseline (Figure 4), the results indicate that five years of additional exposure to ambient UVR (unfiltered by a natural or prostheic lens) produces a loss in sensitivity that is equivalent to over 30 years of normal aging of the SWS cones.

The results from these IOL patients revealed large individual differences, as has been observed in virtually all studies of normal aging. These variations might be expected from variations in lifestyle and concomitant variations in UVR exposure. Six of eight patients had a statistically significant loss in sensitivity of SWS cones with the difference ranging from a factor of 1.3 to 8.3. Interviews with patients suggest that the sensitivity loss is greater in the younger individuals who spend more time outdoors, but the effect depends most on use of UVR-filtering eyewear. The patient for whom there was no difference between the two eyes indicated that he golfed several times a week, but he "religiously" wore UVR-absorbing sunglasses recommended by his ophthalmologist. In contrast, the patient with the greatest loss in sensitivity in the eye without a UVR-absorbing IOL was a farmer who frequently worked outdoors without protective sunglasses. The overall trend of these individual differences is clear and the quantitative data statistically significant -- higher UVR exposure leads to loss of sensitivity in SWS cones.

In addition to the implications of these data for understanding senescent changes in human vision, the data are also of interest in view of recent climatic changes that are resulting in higher UVR levels from reductions in the thickness of the stratospheric ozone layer. Because more UVR reaches the surface of the earth now than in the recent past, the hazards to the eye are likely to have increased. With increased UVR exposure, the eye, like the skin, might well experience accelerated aging.

ACKNOWLEDGEMENTS

The author is indebted to many colleagues whose contributions are evident from their joint authorship on articles described in this review. Gratitude is also extended to Janice L. Nerger, David H. Peterzell, Brooke E. Schefrin, Marcus Plach and Vicki J. Volbrecht for critically reading an earlier draft of this chapter. This research was supported by the National Institute on Aging (grant AG04058).

REFERENCES

Abramov, A., Hainline, L., Turkel, J., Lemerise, E., Smith, H., Gordon, J. & Petry, S., 1984, Rocket ship psychophysics. Assessing visual function in young children. *Invest. Ophthalmol. Vis. Sci.*, **25**: 1307.

Bachem, A., 1956, Ophthalmic ultraviolet action spectra. *Am. J. Ophthalmol.*, **41**: 969.

Balazsi, A.G., Rootman, J. Drance, S.M., Schulzer, M. & Douglas, G.R., 1984, The effect of age on the nerve fiber population of the human optic nerve. *Am. J. Ophthalmol.*, **97**: 760.

Boettner, E.A. & Wolter, J.R., 1962, Transmission of the ocular media. *Invest. Ophthalmol.* **1**: 776.

Bone, R.A., Landrum, J.T. & Tarsis, S.L., 1985, Preliminary identification of the human macular pigment. *Vision Res.*, **25**: 1531.

Bone, R.A., Landrum, J.T., Fernandez, L. & Tarsis, S.L., 1988, Analysis of macular pigment by HPLC: Retinal distribution and age study. *Invest. Ophthalmol. Vis. Sci.*, **29**: 843.

Brandhorst, H., Hickey, J., Curtis, H. & Ralph, E., 1975, Interim solar cell testing procedures for terrestial applications. *NASA Report TM X-71771*, Lewis Research Center.

Devaney, K.O. & Johnson, H.A., 1980, Neuron loss in aging visual cortex of man. *J. Gerontol.*, **35**: 836.

Eisner, A., Fleming, S.A., Klein, M.L. & Mauldin, W.M., 1987, Sensitivities in older eyes with good acuity: Cross-sectional norms. *Invest. Ophthalmol. Vis. Sci.*, **28**: 1824.

Elsner, A.E., Berk, L., Burns, S.A. & Rosenberg, P.R., 1988, Aging and human cone photopigments. *J. Opt. Soc. Am. A*, **5**: 2106.

Fite, K.V., Bengston, C.L. & Donaghey, B., 1991, Age, sex, and light damage correlates of lipofuscin accumulation in the outer retina of Japanese quail. (Abstract) *Invest. Ophthalmol. Vis. Sci. Suppl.*, **32**: 1095.

Gartner, S. & Henkind, P., 1981, Aging and degeneration of the human macula. 1. Outer nuclear layer and photoreceptors. *Br. J. Ophthalmol.*, **65**: 23.

Ham, W.T., Mueller, H.A., Ruffolo, J.J., Guerry, D. & Guerry, R.K., 1982, Action spectrum for retinal injury from near-ultraviolet radiation in the aphakic monkey. *Am. J. Ophthalmol.*, **93**: 299.

Harwerth, R.S. & Sperling, H.G., 1975, Effects of intense visible radiation on the increment-threshold spectral sensitivity of the rhesus monkey eye. *Vision Res.*, **15**: 1193.

Hansen, R.M. & Fulton, A.B., 1989, Psychophysical estimates of ocular media density of human infants. *Vision Res.*, **29**: 687.

Haegerstrom-Portnoy, G., 1988, Short-wavelength-sensitive-cone sensitivity loss with aging: A protective role for macular pigment? *J. Opt. Soc. Am. A*, **5**: 2140.

Jameson, D. & Hurvich, L.M., 1968, Opponent-response functions related to measured cone pigments. *J. Opt. Soc. Am.*, **58**: 429.

Johnson, C.A, Adams, A.J., Twelker, J.D. & Quigg, J.M., 1988, Age-related changes of the central visual field for short-wavelength sensitive pathways. *J. Opt. Soc. Am. A*, **5**: 2131.

Keunen, J.E.E., van Norren, D. & van Meel, G.J., 1987, Density of foveal cone pigments at older age. *Invest. Ophthalmol. Vis. Sci.*, **28**: 985.

Kilbride, P.E., Hutman, L.P., Fishman, M. & Read, J.S., 1986, Foveal cone pigment density difference in the aging human eye. *Vision Res., 26*: 321.

Kirschfeld, K., 1982, Carotenoid pigments: their possible role in protecting against photooxidation in eyes and photoreceptor cells. *Proc. Roy. Soc.B, 216*: 71.

Kremers, J.J.M. & van Norren, D., 1989, Retinal damage in macaque after white light exposures lasting ten minutes to twelve hours. *Invest. Ophthalmol. Vis. Sci., 30*: 1032.

Krinsky, N.I., 1979, Carotenoid protection against oxidation. *Pure Appl. Chem., 51*: 649.

Lerman, S., 1984, Biophysical aspects of corneal and lenticular transparency. *Curr. Eye Res., 3*: 3.

Marshall, J., 1978, Ageing changes in human cones. *In:* K. Shimizu, and J.A. Oosterhuis, eds. *XXIII Concilium Ophthalmologicum.* Amsterdam: Elsevier North-Holland.

Norren, D.V. & Meel, G.J.V., 1985, Density of human cone photopigments as a function of age. *Invest. Ophthalmol. Vis. Sci., 26*: 1014.

Norren, D.V. & Vos, J.J., 1974, Spectral transmission of the human ocular media. *Vision Res., 14*: 1237.

Parver, L.M., Auker, C.R. & Carpenter, D.O., 1980, Choroidal blood flow as a heat dissipating mechanism in the macula. *Am. J. Ophthalmol., 89*: 641.

Pugh, E.N. & Mollon, J.D., 1979, A theory of the Π_1 and Π_3 color mechanisms of Stiles. *Vision Res., 19*: 293.

Schefrin, B.E., Plach, M., Utlaut, N. & Werner, J.S., 1991, Sites responsible for age-related sensitivity losses of an S-cone pathway. (Abstract) *Invest. Ophthalmol. Vis. Sci. Suppl., 32*: 1274.

Schefrin, B.E. & Werner, J.S., 1990, Loci of spectral unique hues throughout the life span. *J. Opt. Soc. Am. A, 7*: 305.

Sample, P.A., Esterson, F.D., Weinreb, R.N. & Boynton, R.M., 1988, The aging lens: In vivo assessment of light absorption in 84 eyes. *Invest. Ophthalmol. Vis. Sci., 29*: 1306.

Stiles, W.S., 1953, Further studies of visual mechanisms by the two-colour increment threshold method. *Coloq. Probl. Opt. Vis. Union Int. Phys. Pure Appl., 1*: 65.

Volbrecht, V.J. & Werner, J.S., 1987, Isolation of short-wavelength-sensitive cone photoreceptors in 4-6-week-old human infants. *Vision Res., 27*: 469.

Wald, G., 1949, The photochemistry of vision. *Doc. Ophthalmol., 3*: 94.

Wald, G., 1964, The receptors of human color vision. *Science, 145*: 1007.

Weale, R.A., 1963, *The Aging Eye.* London: HK Lewis.

Weale, R.A., 1982, Senile ocular changes, cell death, and vision. *In* R. Sekuler, D. Kline, and K. Dismukes, eds. *Aging and Human Visual Function.* New York, Liss.

Weale, R.A., 1983, Senile cataract. The case against light. *Ophthalmology, 90*: 420.

Weale, R.A., 1988, Age and the transmittance of the human crystalline lens. *J. Physiol., 395*: 577.

Werner, J.S., 1982, Development of scotopic sensitivity and the absorption spectrum of the human ocular media. *J. Opt. Soc. Am., 72*: 247.

Werner, J.S., Donnelly, S.K. & Kliegl, R., 1987, Aging and the human macular pigment density; Appended with translations from the work of Max Schultze and Ewald Hering. *Vision Res., 27*: 257.

Werner, J.S., Peterzell, D.H. & Scheetz, A.J., 1990, Light, vision and aging. *Optom. Vision Sci., 67*: 214.

Werner, J.S. & Spillmann, L., 1989, UV-absorbing intraocular lenses: safety, efficacy, and consequences for the cataract patient. *Graefe's Arch. Clin. Exp. Ophthalmol., 227*: 248.

Werner, J.S. & Steele, V.G., 1988, Sensitivity of human foveal color mechanisms throughout the life span. *J. Opt. Soc. Am. A, 5*: 2122.

Werner, J.S., Steele, V.G. & Pfoff, D.S., 1989, Loss of human photoreceptor sensitivity associated with chronic exposure to ultraviolet radiation. *Ophthalmology, 96*: 1552.

Young, R.W., 1976, Visual cells and the concept of renewal. *Invest. Ophthalmol. Vis. Sci., 15*: 700.

Young, R.W., 1982, The Bowman lecture, 1982: Biological renewal. Applications to the eye. *Trans. Ophthalmol. Soc. U.K., 102*: 42.

Young, R. W., 1988, Solar radiation and age-related macular degeneration. *Surv. Ophthalmol., 32*: 252.

Young, R.W., 1991, *Age-Related Cataract.* New York: Oxford University Press.

CELLULAR AND MOLECULAR ASPECTS OF NEURONAL DIFFERENTIATION

G. Augusti-Tocco, S. Biagioni, M. Plateroti, G. Scarsella, and A.L. Vignoli

Dipartimento di Biologia Cellulare e dello Sviluppo
Università "La Sapienza"
Rome, Italy

The function of nervous system is dependent on the formation during development of a complex structure, arising from the emergence of diverse cell populations and from their specific connections. Specific cell interactions taking place during development give origin to a tissue architecture, which shows peculiar aspects in the different regions of the nervous system. The expression of the genetic program encoding specific cell types and their organization in the various structures of the nervous system is dependent on early developmental events.

Recent studies on the expression of homeoboxes sequences (Kussel and Gruss, 1990) and proto-oncogene int-1 (Wilkinson et al., 1987) has shown a very precise sequence of expression along the neural tube axis; this has been suggested as a possible molecular mechanism for the early divergence of specific developmental programs in different regions of the nervous system, with the emergence of specific neuronal populations and specific tissue architecture. At the same time increasing evidence is being obtained on the importance of epigenetic events (such as synthesis of specific molecules regulating neuronal survival and differentiation or acting as substrate and guidance factors for fiber outgrowth), which are also believed to play a major role in the plasticity of the nervous system (Thomson, 1990).

In the nervous system a high level of complexity is also found at the cellular level. In fact a distinctive feature of adult neurons is their polarity, based on the formation of cellular compartments, such as cell body, dendrites, axons and nerve terminals, which are endowed with specific functional roles. In nervous system development thus we can distinguish three basic processes:

1) outgrowth of neurites,
2) expression of specific components related to neurotransmission mechanism,
3) formation of specific connections between appropriate cells.

Outgrowth of neurites is a fundamental step in neuronal differentiation, since it not only allows neuron connection to target cells, but also is the anatomical basis for establishing neuron polarity, after neurite differentiation as axons or dendrites. The functional specialization of neuronal compartments is hovewer dependent on selective distribution of organelles and molecular components, synthesized in the perikaryon. Therefore in neuronal differentiation a major role is played not only by regulative processes, which activate the expression of specific gene products (e.g. neurotransmitter biosynthetic enzymes), but also by mechanisms specifying their cellular localization.

On the other hand increasing evidence is available on dual role played by neuronal

The Changing Visual System, Edited by P. Bagnoli and
W. Hodos, Plenum Press, New York, 1991

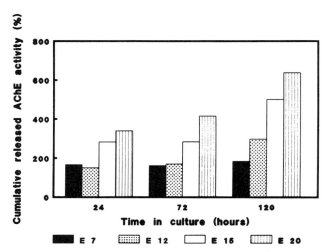

Fig. 1. Cumulative AChE activity released in culture medium by chick DRG neurons dissociated from lumbar and sacral ganglia at different developmental stages. At all stages examined, approximately 50,000 neurons were plated on collagen-coated dishes and cultured in Ham's F12 medium supplemented with 50 ng/ml NGF and 2% Ultroser G (IBF), as a substitute for serum. The released AChE activity, assayed by Ellman's method (1961), is expressed as percent of cellular activity.

specific molecules at different developmental stages (e.g. neurotrophic action played by neurotransmitters; Lipton and Kater, 1989), suggesting that destination of cellular components may vary according to an established developmental program.

An interesting example in this context is represented by acetylcholinesterase

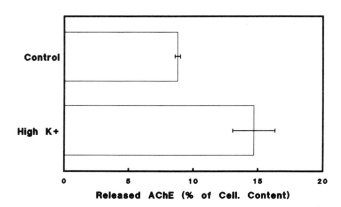

Fig. 2. AChE release induced by high potassium in DRG neurons obtained from E18 chick embryos. The cells were cultured for 48 hours and after replacement of fresh complete medium (see Fig. 1), were treated with 100 mM K+ for 1 hour. In control cultures potassium was replaced with choline chloride. Lactate dehydrogenase was also assayed in culture medium as a marker of aspecific leakage of cellular components; its level was practically undetectable in all experiments on AChE release reported here. Values are the means of four experiments ± S.E.M. and are expressed as percent of cellular AChE activity.

(AChE). The interest in AChE in fact arises from several observations, such as its early expression in non cholinergic structures of the nervous system, which have led to postulate novel roles for this enzyme in morphogenesis (Drews et al., 1986; Small, 1989; Layer, 1990).

Moreover this enzyme has a polymorphic structure; it can be found in the cells as monomer or in various multimeric association and as amphiphilic or hydrophilic form. The various molecular forms are differently represented in different cell types; and are associated to different cellular compartments. Their diversity arises from posttranscriptional regulation and their differential localization requires also mechanisms for directing their destination to cellular compartments (Massouliè and Toutant, 1988).

We have focused our attention on the secretion of the enzyme by various neuronal populations. AChE secretion does not occurr uniformly for all molecular forms present in the cells; G4 is selectively involved in this process in all cell types studied (Toutant and Massouliè, 1988). This suggests that AChE secretion requires signals for selective guidance of molecular species to functionally different cellular compartments. This is further supported by our findings on neuroblastoma lines (Melone et al., 1987). A comparative study on N18TG2 and the derived neuroblastoma x glioma hybrid 108CC15 has shown high secretion of AChE and very scarce association to plasma membrane in the parental line; in the hybrid cells the situation is reversed, and plasma membrane association of the enzyme is markedly enhanced (as shown by ultrastructural studies), while secretion is reduced. The functional properties of the two cell lines (that is the ability to form synaptic contacts by the 108CC15 hybrid cells, which is lacking in the parental N18TG2) has suggested a possible relation of AChE cellular distribution with developmental stages or alternative differentiative programs (Melone et al., 1987).

We have extended our studies on AChE secretion to nervous system structures characterized by a different neurotrasmission apparatus: dorsal root ganglia (DRG), as neurons expressing AChE and other cholinergic markers (Biagioni et al., 1989; Castrignanò et al., 1989), but not involved in the formation of cholinergic circuits, and spinal cord neurons, where AChE is most likely involved in the well known process of neurotransmitter inactivation.

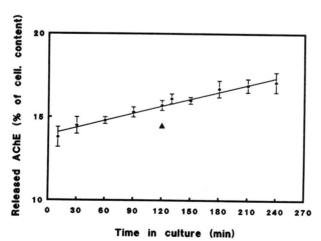

Fig. 3. Effect of veratridine on AChE release by DRG neurons obtained from E18 chick embryo. After 48 hours of culture the medium was replaced and released AChE activity was evaluated on aliquots of the medium. Veratridine (10^{-3}M), a drug which specifically open sodium channels localized on nerve fibers, was added 120 min after starting release determinations (as indicated by arrowhead). Values are means of four experiments ± S.E.M. and are expressed as percent of cellular AChE activity.

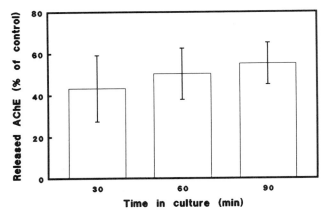

Fig. 4. Effect of nocodazole on AChE release by DRG neurons from E18 chick embryo. After 48 hours in culture, neurons were preincubated for 90 min with 5×10^{-6}M nocodazole, a drug interfering with microtubule polymerization. The medium was then replaced and aliquots withdrawn at indicated times for determination of AChE release in the absence of the drug. Values are means of four experiments ± S.E.M. and are expressed as percent of release in control cultures not exposed to the nocodazole.

We have previously shown that in DRG AChE level continously increases during development (Biagioni et al., 1989). From these studies it has also become evident that utilization of the enzyme undergoes changes during development. In fact the percentage of secreted AChE does not remain constant, but strikingly increases at late developmental stages (Fig. 1), suggesting that in adult DRG neurons AChE function is mainly accomplished through a secretive pathway.

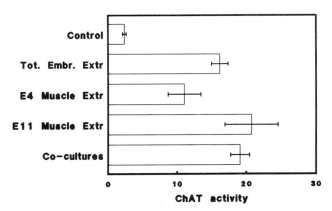

Fig. 5. Effect of chick embryo extracts and co-cultures with myotubes on spinal cord neurons ChAT activity. Spinal cord neurons (10^6cells), from E8 chick embryos, were plated on poly-L-lysine coated dishes and cultured for five days in Ham's F12 medium supplemented with factors, as indicated by Bottenstein and Sato (1979). Tissue extracts were generally prepared from E11 chick embryos homogenized in a 1:1 w/v of Puck solution and centrifuged at 10,000xg. In co-culture experiments the neurons were plated on a myotube layer obtained from fusion of E11 chick embryo myoblasts. ChAT activity was evaluated by Hamprecht and Takehiko method (1974) and is expressed as pmol of AcCh synthesized/hour/ 10^6cells (means ± S.E.M. of four experiments).

Further characterization of this process in cultured DRG neurons, from final stages of development (E18), has shown the existence of a constitutive component and a regulated one. As shown in Fig. 2, in fact, AChE secretion is nearly doubled when cells are exposed to a depolarizing stimulus as high potassium (100 mM) in the culture medium. Regulated secretion, however, does not seem to occur in the nerve terminals, since veratridine, a depolarizing agent specifically active on nerve fibers, does not modify the kinetic of AChE secretion (Fig. 3).

On the other hand exposure of DRG neurons to nocodazole for 90 min is followed by a 60% reduction of AChE secretion over a 30 min period (Fig. 4). This inhibition is lower after long time intervals, most likely due to gradual recovery of the nocodazole damage. Integrity of microtubule structures thus appear to be necessary for directing AChE transposition to a secretory vesicle compartment. N18TG2 neuroblastoma cells behave very similarly as far as high potassium stimulation and nocodazole inhibition is concerned. Hovewer these cells provide further evidence that AChE secretion is not related to formation of nerve fibers, as indicated by veratridine experiments on DRG, since it remains constant under culture conditions which stimulate or not fiber outgrowth (manuscript in preparation). From these data one can tentatively conclude that during development AChE secretion is modulated by signals other than those regulating its synthesis and seems to be inversely related to cell commitment as cholinergic neurons.

Another interesting question in this context is whether in cholinergic neurons AChE secretion may be modulated by signals released from other cells. The action of tissue extracts on the expression of specific molecules by cholinergic neurons is well known (Berg, 1978; Smith et al., 1986). It thus appeared obvious to investigate whether also AChE secretion may be in some way modulated by embryonic tissue extracts.

Cultures of dissociated spinal cord neurons from 8 day chick embryos have been used to test the effect of whole embryo and tssue extracts. Both extracts enhance in cultured spinal cord neurons the expression of the biosynthetic enzyme, choline acetyltransferase (ChAT); in this respect they mimic the effect of co-culturing spinal cord neurons with muscle cells (Fig. 5). As far as AChE is concerned, neurons kept five days in culture in the presence of either whole embryo or muscle and brain extracts show about a

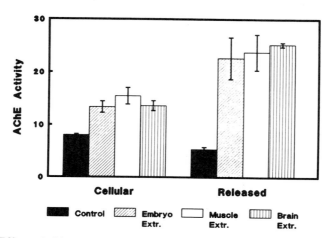

Fig. 6. Effect of chick embryo extracts on cellular and released AChE of spinal cord neurons. Spinal cord neurons, from E8 chick embryos, were cultured for five days in medium supplemented with 2% Ultroser and 2% tissue extracts (see Fig. 5). Medium was then replaced, omitting tissue extracts, and AChE release was determined over the following 24 hours. AChE activity is expressed as mU, nmoles/min of substrate hydrolyzed, and the reported values are means ± S.E.M. of at least eight experiments.

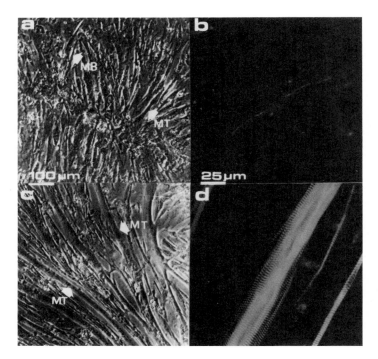

Fig. 7. Effects of whole chick embryo extract on expression and cellular organization of alpha-actinin. Myoblasts dissociated from E11 chick pectoral
muscles were cultured on collagen-coated dishes for seven days in
DMEM supplemented with 10% horse serum in the presence (c,d) or
absence (a,b) of 2% chick embryo extract. The cells were stained by
indirect immunofluorescence using an anti-alpha-actinin monoclonal
antibody (b,d). Phase contrast micrographs (a,c) show that fusion is
markedly enhanced by embryo extract, as indicated by the presence of
myoblasts and smaller myotubes in pannel a; pannel c shows a much
more advanced fusion, as indicated by the large size of myotubes
present.
Immunofluorescence shows that only myotubes are stained (pannel b);
the intensity of staining is greatly enhanced in myotubes in the presence
of embryo extract, when well defined bands of staining are evident
(pannel d).
(a,c: phase contrast micrographs; b,d: fluorescence micrographs; MB:
myoblast; MT: myotube).

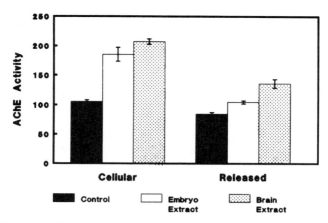

Fig. 8. Effect of chick embryo extracts on cellular and released AChE in muscle cells. Myotubes obtained from E11 chick embryo pectoral muscles, were cultured for seven days in the presence of 2% Ultroser G and 2% tissue extracts (see Fig. 6 and 7). AChE release was determined as described in Fig. 6.

doubling in their cellular enzyme content (Fig. 6). Furthermore, when considering enzyme secretion the data shown indicate a 4-5 fold enhancement.

Muscle cells also synthesize and release AChE (Rotundo and Fambrough, 1980; Senni et al., 1987); tissue extracts induce also in these cells the expression and specific cellular organization of markers, such as myosin (Cossu and Molinaro, 1987) and alpha-actinin. As shown in Fig. 7 (a,c), in fact, the fusion of myoblasts is greatly enhanced by whole embryo extract and the characteristic cellular organization of alpha-actinin can be observed only in myotubes obtained in the presence of extract (Fig. 7 b,d). On the other hand stimulation of AChE secretion, by tissue extracts, appears to be a specific response of neurons; in fact their effect on AChE secretion by cultured myotubes is significantly different as compared to that on neurons. In cultured muscle cells AChE cellular content is nearly doubled, as in neurons; while the increase in the secreted fraction is considerable lower (Fig. 8). Therefore the distribution of enzyme in the cellular and secreted fraction is different in the control and extract treated cultures. Addition of extract to the culture medium thus results in a significant decrease (P< 0.01) of AChE secretion.

The presented data clearly indicate that tissue extracts contain signal molecules capable of eliciting differential response in different cell types. This specific response with respect to AChE secretion, is an interesting observation since this phenomenon, although its functional roles is still unknown, appears a common property of AChE synthesizing cells. The site of AChE secretion in spinal cord neurons is presently unknown; the data reported on DRG and neuroblastoma cultures indicate that nerve terminals are not involved in this process. Furthermore dopaminergic central neurons have been shown to release AChE from their dendrites (Taylor et al., 1990). On this basis it is conceivable to propose that AChE secretion may represent a novel form of neuronal communication which may play an important role during development. On the other hand the reduced release of AChE secretion by myotubes in the presence of tissue extracts may be related to the more advanced process of fusion, which requires assembly of more complex forms, to be associated to the basal lamina.

In conclusion the data described above support the hypothesis that association of AChE to a secretory vesicle compartment may represent an event which is specifically regulated in relation to differentiation program and developmental stage. Its modulation in different neuronal population respond in a specific manner to external signal, and may represent an additional cellular communication system.

ACKNOWLEDGMENTS

This work was supported by grants from MURST and CNR.

REFERENCES

Berg, D. K., 1978, Acetylcholine syntesis by chick spinal cord neurons in dissociated cell culture, Dev. Biol., 66:500.

Biagioni, S., Odorisio, T., Poiana, G., Scarsella, G., and Augusti Tocco, G., 1989, Acetylcholinesterase in the development of chick dorsal root ganglia, Int. J. Devl. Neurosci., 7:267.

Bottenstein, J. E., and Sato, G. H., 1979, Growth of a rat neuroblastoma cell line in serum-free supplemented medium, Proc. Natl. Acad. Sci. U.S.A., 75:2546.

Castrignano', F., De Stefano, M. E., Leone, F., Mulatero, B., Tata, A. M., Fasolo, A., and Augusti Tocco, G., 1990, Ontogeny of acetylcholinesterase, substance P and calcitonin gene-related peptide-like immunoreactivity in chick dorsal root ganglia, Neuroscience, 34:499.

Cossu, G., and Molinaro, M., 1987, Cell heterogeneity in myogenic lineage, Current Topics in Devl. Biol., 23:185.

Drews, U., Schimdt, H., Oettling, G., and Vanittanakom, P., 1986, Embryonic cholinesterase in the chick limb bud, Acta Histochem.(Jena), 32S:133.

Ellman, G. L., Courtney, K. D., Andres, V., and Featherstone, R. M., 1961, A new and rapid colorimetric determination of acetylcholinesterase activity, Biochem. Pharmac., 7:88.

Hamprecht, B., and Takehiko, A., 1974, Differential assay for choline acetyltransferase, Analyt. Biochem., 57:162.

Kessel, M., and Gruss, P., 1990, Murine development control gene, Science, 249:374.

Layer, P. G., 1990, Cholinesterases preceding major tracts in vertebrate neurogenesis, BioEssays, 12:415.

Lipton, S. A., and Kater, S. B., 1989, Neurotransmitter regulation of neuronal outgrowth, plasticity and survival, TINS, 12:265.

Massoulie', J., and Toutant, J. P., 1988, Vertebrate cholinesterases : structure and types of interaction, Handbook of experimental pharmacology, 86:167.

Melone, M. A. R., Longo, A., Taddei, C., and Augusti-Tocco G., Acetylcholinesterase in neuroblastoma and neuroblastoma x glioma hybrid cells: cellular localization and molecular forms, Int. J. Devl. Neurosci., 5:417.

Rotundo, R. L., and Fambrough, D. M., 1980, Synthesis, transport and fate of AChE in cultured chick embryo muscle cells, Cell, 22:583.

Senni, M. I., Castrignano', F., Poiana, G., Cossu, G., Scarsella, G., and Biagioni, S., 1987, Expression of adult fast pattern of acetylcholinesterase molecular forms by mouse satellite cells in culture, Differentiation, 36:194.

Small, D. H., 1989, Acetylcholinesterases: zymogens of neuropeptide processing enzymes?, Neuroscience, 29:241.

Smith, R. G., Vaca, K., and Appel, S. H., 1986, Selective effects of skeletal muscle extracts fraction on motoneuron development in vitro, J. Neurosci., 6:439.

Taylor, S. J., Jones, A. A., Haggblad, J., and Greenfield, S. A., 1990, "On-line" measurement of acetylcholinesterase release from the substantia nigra of the freely-moving guinea-pig, Neuroscience, 37:71.

Thomson, A. M., 1990, Epigenesis and plasticity in the nervous system, TINS, 13:389.

Toutant, J. P., and Massoulie', J., 1988, Cholinesterases: tissue and cellular distribution of molecular forms and their physiological regulation, Handbook of experimental pharmacology, 86:225.

Wilkinson, D. G., Bailes, J. A., and McMahon, A. P., 1987, Expression of the proto-oncogene int-1 is restricted to specific neural cells in the developing mouse embryo, Cell, 50:79.

VGF: A TISSUE SPECIFIC PROTEIN AND A MARKER OF NGF-INDUCED NEURONAL DIFFERENTIATION

Andrea Levi, Nadia Canu, Eugenia Trani,
Marta Benedetti and Roberta Possenti

Institute of Neurobiology C.N.R.
Viale C. Marx 15, 00156 Rome, Italy

Introduction

Biochemical studies on the process of neuronal differentiation have largely profited from the establishment of cell lines which acquire a neuronal phenotype in response to various agents. In the last decade PC12 cells, derived from a rat pheochromocytoma, have become the first choice for studies of neuronal differentiation in tissue culture (Greene and Tishler 1982, Guroff 1985, Levi and Alemà 1991), especially since these cells differentiate in response to a well defined growth factor: nerve growth factor, NGF (Levi-Montalcini 1987). As a result, the molecular characterization of the structure of the two kinds of NGF receptor, and recent theories on the possible mechanism of action of NGF have relied heavily on the use of these cells and mutant subclones derived from them (Hempstead et al. 1989, Hempstead et al. 1991, Kaplan et al. 1991). These studies have been the basis for understanding, in general, how the specificity of action of the various member of the neurotrophin family is achieved (Bothwell M. 1991, Hallbook et al. 1991). NGF, like its close relatives, is supposed to act not only on subpopulations of cells derived from the neural crest (Levi Montacini 1987, Whittemore et al.1987, Thoenen et al. 1987, Vantini et al. 1989), but also on several cell types which display high affinity binding for this growth factor (Cattaneo 1986, Otten et al. 1989, Aloe and Levi Montalcini 1979, Levi-Montalcini et al. 1990). Its effects are multiform, in that trophic, tropic, differentiative and mitogenic actions of NGF have been reported. PC12 cells which do not require NGF in order to survive in culture, and which can be considered as being the common precursor to adrenal medullary cells and sympathetic neurons, are best suited for investigating the very early responses that eventually lead to the acquisition of a neuronal phenotype. Both transcription-independent and trascription-dependent phenomena contribute to this phenomenon (Greene et al. 1982), and in the past few years great efforts have been made in identifying those genes whose expression is modulated in PC12 cells exposed to NGF.

It is possible to divide the genes regulated by the binding of NGF to its receptor into two main categories: those whose induction plays a direct role in the process of the neuronal differentiation and those whose expression is directly linked to the expression of the differentiated phenotype so that their product probably contributes to neurone-specific functions. To the first group belong genes whose products are transcription factors and which by some yet unresolved process specifically induce the transcription from neuronal specific promoters (immediate early Herschman 1989, Sheng and Greenberg 1990, Bradbury et al.1991). The second kind of gene may be considered markers of the acquired neuronal phenotype and will probably be involved in those specialized functions that distinguish NGF-treated PC12 cells from untreated cells. A further generalization (which probably suffers from a number of exceptions) is that the first group of genes, often defined as immediate early, do not require ongoing protein synthesis in order to be activated, and that their increased transcription relies on modulation of the transcription machinery already present in untreated PC12 cells. On the contrary, neuronal-specific genes depend for their transcription on the accumulation of the products of the immediate early genes. This loosely followed rule allows an operational distinction to be made between these two groups of genes by interfering with the protein synthesis machinery of PC12 cells. Several genes have been identified which comply to the above mentioned criteria for the late, neuronal-specific genes (Levi et al. 1985, Anderson and Axel 1985, Leonard et al. 1986, Machida et al.1989). In this paper we will review the properties of a gene termed VGF (Levi et al 1985) which can be considered a good example of a gene activated with delayed kinetics (as opposed to the immediate early genes), in a translation dependent way and coding for a polypeptide which participates, in a still obscure way, in the specialized function of inducible, regulated secretion.

VGF expression is modulated by NGF through transcriptional control of the promoter

VGF cDNA was first isolated by screening (via differential hybridization) a cDNA library from PC12 cells treated for 24 hr with NGF (Levi et al. 1985). According to the conditions utilized for the screening i.e. a small sized library and the use of total cDNAs as labelled probes, VGF is both an abundant mRNA in NGF treated cells and a strongly induced one. Fig 1 shows that VGF mRNA is

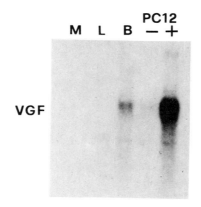

PC12

M L B — +

VGF

Fig 1. Northern blot analysis of oligo-dT selected (lanes M,L,B) or total RNA (PC12 -/+), probed with VGF cDNA.
In lanes M, L and B 10 ug of of polyA+ RNA from smooth muscle, liver and brain of adult rats were examined by Northern procedure with nick translated VGF cDNA; PC12 - and + represent 10 μg of total RNA extracted from untreated PC12 cell (-) or cells exposed 8 hours to 100 ng/ml of NGF (+).

induced approximately 50 fold upon NGF treatment of PC12 cells, and that it is present, albeit in low amounts, in brain, but not in liver and smooth muscle.

A detailed Northern analysis of the induction of VGF in PC12 exposed to NGF (Levi et al. 1985, Levi et al. 1988, Salton et al. 1991) can be summarized as follows: 1) increased levels of VGF mRNA as compared to controls can be detected after a few hours of NGF treatment, with the maximal induction peaking at about 8-9 hours. Substantial levels, well above those of untreated cells, are present in fully differentiated PC12 cells. 2) The maximal induction of VGF occurs at concentration of NGF that saturates the low affinity NGF receptors. 3) Treatment of PC12 cells with protein synthesis inhibitors strongly reduces the induction of VGF mRNA (see below).

Two criteria were used to define VGF as a marker of the differentiated phenotype: the expression of VGF mRNA and VGF protein should be restricted to cells of neuronal origin and the induction of the mRNA should correlate with the differentiation of PC12 cells. Table 1 summarizes a survey of different cell lines and tissues in which VGF expression has been detected.

The correlation with coexpression of the p75 NGF receptor is only partial and does not necessarily imply a cause-effect relationship.

It has been noted that a number of growth factors and agents are able to stimulate early biochemical responses from PC12 cells (ranging from induced phosphorylation of protein substrata to the induction of immediate early genes), in a way that closely resemble

Table 1.   VGF and 75kD NGF-Receptor in various neuro and endocrine tissues.

	VGF	NGF-RECEPTOR[3]
Amygdala[1]	+	+
Hippocampus[1]	+	+
Hypothalamus[1]		
SCN	+	(+)
SON	+	+
PVN	+	+
Thalamus[1]	+	+
Tuberomammilary N[1]	+	ND
Cortex cells[1]	+	ND
Dorsal Root Ganglia [2]	+	+
Myoentheric Plexus [2]	+	ND
Sympathetic Ganglia[2]	+	+
Adenohypophisys[2]	+	+
Adrenal Medulla [2]	+	+
Entheric endocr. cells[2]	+	ND

ND: Not Determined
(1) van den Pol et al. 1989
(2) Ferri et al. 1991
(3) Pioro and Cuello 1990

those elicited by NGF but subtle differences must account for the failure of these factors in inducing neuronal differentiation of PC12 cells (for a review see Levi and Alemà 1991). Table 2 demonstrates that despite the similarity of the early response under different conditions, only exposure of the cells to NGF strongly induces VGF mRNA, other agents exerting only a modest effect. This is true even

Table 2.   Correlation of VGF induction and differentiation in PC12 cells.

Factors	Relative VGF mRNA Induction	Morphological Different.
Control	1	-
NGF	50	+++
bFGF	5	++
IL-6	7	++
cAMP	7	±
TPA	7	-
EGF	6	-

for Interleukin 6 and bFGF which have been reported to partially promote PC12 cells differentiation (Satoh et al 1988, Togari et al. 1985).

It should be noted that in the promoter region of the VGF gene a CRE sequence (cAMP responsive element) is present (Salton et al. 1991), but increasing intracellular cAMP levels has only modest effect on transcription from the VGF promoter.

The VGF-RNA induction as detected by northern analysis could depend on increased transcription from the promoter and/or increased stability of the mRNA. In order to discriminate between these two possibilities we performed run on experiments to measure ongoing transcription in nuclei isolated from PC12 cells that were exposed for different times to NGF. Figure 2 demonstrate that, at least in part, increased levels of VGF mRNA can be accounted for by increased transcription; moreover inhibition of protein synthesis via cycloeximide strongly reduces, even if does not completely abrogate, the transcription of the VGF gene.

It is presently unclear whether translation-independent phenomena also contribute to NGF-induced upregulation of VGF gene expression or whether the experimental conditions employed failed to completely prevent residual protein synthesis. Having demonstrated transcriptional control of VGF gene expression by NGF, different sequences of the putative VGF promoter region were linked to a reporter gene (Chloramphenicol Acethyl Transferase CAT). Figure 3 shows the CAT activity in extracts of PC12 cells transfected with the VGF promoter CAT construct and treated with different agents.

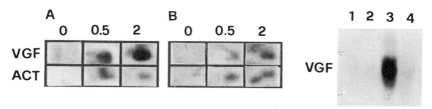

Fig 2. Transcription of VGF and β-actin in PC12 cells at different times of exposure to NGF in the presence or absence of protein synthesis inhibitors.
Left panel: Run on analysis was performed on nuclei isolated from PC12 cells treated for different time with 100 ng/ml of NGF in the absence (A) or in the presence of 100 µg/ml of cycloeximide (B). 0, 0.5 and 2 represent hours of treatment. The in vitro labelled nascent RNA was hybridized to cDNA for VGF and β-actin transferred to nitrocellulose after electrophoresis on agarose gel. Right panel: 10 µg of cytoplasmic RNA was utilized for Northern analysis. Lane 1: untreated cell; lane 2: cycloeximide; lane 3: NGF for 2 hours; lane 4: NGF in presence of cycloexamide.

The overall picture that emerges is the following: 1) within 800 bp 5' to the start of transcription, DNA elements are present which are responsible for the induction of VGF by NGF and by cAMP. Since saturating concentration of each of these agents act additively to induce the expression of the transfected constructs, NGF and cAMP must act, at least in part, through non overlapping mechanisms. 2) DNA sequences important for regulation of the VGF gene must also lie outside of the 800 bp 5' region examined until now, since the transfected promoters fail to be induced by the phorbol ester TPA (see figure 3 and table 2) and are induced by NGF about 10 fold less than the endogenous gene. That the regulatory region of regulated genes is composed by a mosaic of small elements is a recurrent finding that well accounts for fine tuning of a promoter (Dynan 1989).

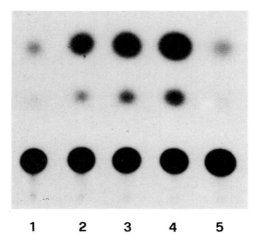

Fig. 3   Transcription from VGF promoter in transfected PC12 cells.
Transcription from the VGF promoter was assessed by CAT assay upon transfection of a plasmid containing about 800 bp of the VGF genomic sequence 5' to the start of transcription. Extract from PC12 cells were prepared 72 hours after transfection and 48 hours following treatment with various agents. Lane 1: no treatment; lane 2: 100 ng/ml NGF;   lane 3: 1 mM dbcAMP;   lane 4: NGF plus dbcAMP;   lane 5: 100 nM phorbol ester TPA.

Further experimental data (not shown) demonstrated that nuclear extracts from PC12 cells contain specific factors which bind to different regions of the promoter that cooperate for the expression of VGF in PC12 cells.
        The ability of the 800 region of the VGF promoter to drive the tissue specific expression of a reporter gene (Piccioli et al. 1991) is presently been pursued in transgenic mice (Cattaneo et al. work in progress).

These results, notwithstanding their preliminary nature, are a good point from which further studies on the induction of the neuronal phenotype in PC12 cells, and in neural cells in general (Rossi et al. in preparation), may be commenced.

VGF protein belongs to the regulated secretion compartment

We could not find sequences homologous to VGF in several databases screened, so we had no indirect clues of its possible function. Nevertheless, conceptual translation of the VGF cDNA sequence into protein sequence revealed a number of interesting features. Firstly, the presence of a stretch of eight hydrophobic residues starting from position 9   followed by a potential cleavage site for a signal sequence strongly suggests that the primary protein product may be translocated to the endoplasmic reticulum. Secondly, the numerous pairs of dibasic residues embedded in the sequence, which could be potential sites for digestion by trypsin-like proteases, as well as a high content of proline residues are reminiscent of a class of secreted proteins specifically expressed in neuro-endocrine tissue and known as Secretogranin/Chromogranin (Rosa et al. 1985, Ahn et al 1987). This similarity is strengthened by the presence in VGF, as in secretogranin I, of a potential site for tyrosine sulfation (a tyrosine preceded by a Glu-rich sequence see Benedum et al. 1987).

Antibodies against VGF protein were produced as a tool for studying its function. Bacterially expressed recombinant VGF was used as an immunogen for production of rabbit antisera. Three distinct regions of the polypepdide encompassing amminoacids 4-240, 80-340 and 443-588 gave rise to high titer antisera which recognized a doublet of apparent m.w. 90 and 76 kDa in Western blots, strongly induced by NGF in PC12 cells (Possenti et al. 1989). Similar bands are detected in various cell lines of neuronal origin derived from rat, mouse or human. In general, antibodies directed against the COOH domain of the protein recognize the antigen with a larger spectrum of interspecies crossreactivity while the antisera directed against the NH_2 region are more specific for the rat protein (fig 4 left panel).

Sequence analysis of the human cDNA for VGF, presently in progress, will confirm whether this different recognition by the antisera reflects differences in the homology between the primary structure of the VGF protein in human vs rat.

Pulse and chase experiments (Possenti et al. 1989) have demonstrated that the lower band of the doublet is produced by limited proteolysis of the upper band, this process occurring in a late compartment of the secretory pathway.   Similarly sulfation of

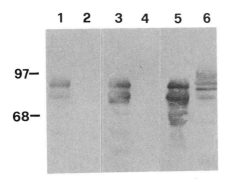
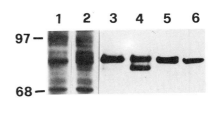

Fig. 4. Recognition of rat and human VGF by antisera to different domains of the protein VGF (left panel). Postranslational processing of VGF polypeptide (right panel).
Left panel: low speed supernatants from hypotonically lysed, NGF-treated PC12 cells (lanes 1, 3, 5) and from TT cells (a human carciroma of the thyroid) (lanes 2, 4, 6) were examined by Western procedure. Lanes 1 and 2 probed with antisera to the amminoacids 4-240 of VGF; lanes 3 and 4 as above probed with antisera to amminoacids 80-340, lanes 5 and 6 with antisera to region 443-588 of VGF protein.
Right panel: Total extracts from PC12 cells pulse-labelled (for 15 minutes) with ^{3}H proline in the absence (line 1) or after 16 hours treatment with 100 ng/ml of NGF (line 2), were examined by autoradiography after SDS Page. Lane 3 and 4 VGF immunoprecipitated after the pulse or after a further two hours chase respectively. Lanes 5 and 6 as above from cells labelled in the presence of the Golgi destructive drug monensin (Kaariainen et al. 1980).

the VGF protein is a postranslational modification which takes place at a late stage of VGF maturation (Possenti unpublished). As expected, treatments that interfere with the correct intracellular trafficking prevent the processing of VGF (fig 4 right panel).

   Preliminary data (Trani unpublished) suggest that the proteolytic cleavage site is in the amino terminal region. We have been unable to detect glycosylation of VGF by different approaches, this negative result together with absence of consensus sequence for glycosylation strongly suggests that such a postranslational modification cannot account for the higher than predicted molecular weight of the protein in SDS PAGE. Since in vitro

Fig. 5   Intracellular localization of the VGF protein in rat, mouse and human cell lines.
Indirect immunofluorescence staining of fixed and pearmibilized cells with anti-VGF antisera and goat anti-rabbit fluorescein labelled secondary antibody was utilized to detect VGF protein in different cell background. For the staining antisera directed against the COOH terminal region of VGF was utilized. Similar staining was obtained with the other antisera in the case of rat and mouse-derived cell lines. A: NGF-treated PC12 cells (pheochromocytoma, rat), B: GH3 cells (hypophysis derived, rat), C: HTC cells (hepathoma derived, rat), D: SKSNBE (neuroblastoma, human), E: CHP212 (neuroblastoma, human), F: TT (thyroid medullary carciroma, human) G: N18 (neuroblastoma, mouse), H: NIE115 (neuroblastoma, mouse)

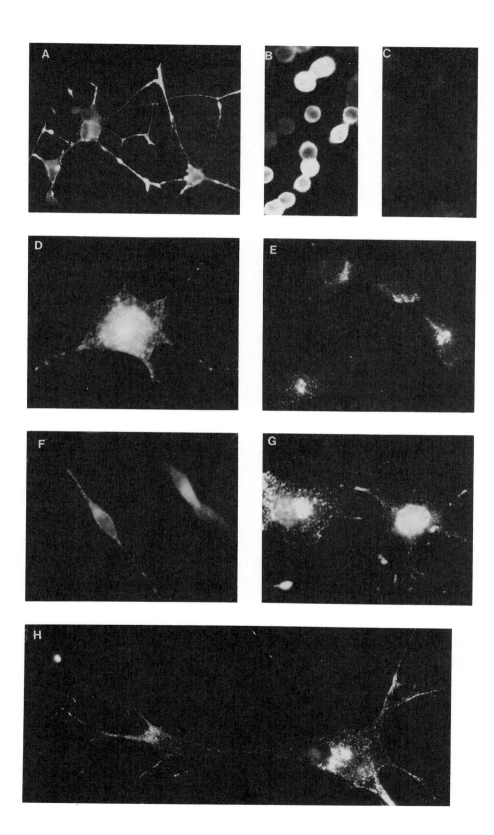

translated VGF mRNA gives rise to a polypeptide of similar M.W., we conclude that the unusual composition in amino acids of VGF (very rich in proline and cysteine residues) is responsible for its aberrant mobility in denaturing SDS Page.

A first hint on the possible biological function of VGF came by determining its intracellular localization via indirect immunofluorescence. Fig 5 shows the punctuate staining of different cell types with anti-VGF antibodies. No immunoreactivity was detected in non pearmibilized cells (not shown) and the immunofluorescence is compatible with VGF being present in the Golgi and in various vesicles often seen in long processes of differentiated PC12 cells and in neurons. A more precise localization of VGF protein was achieved by subcellular fractionation on sucrose gradients. VGF co-bands with proteins (like chromogranins) which are present in secretory vesicles (Possenti et al. 1989). Moreover the inaccessibility to proteolytic enzymes suggests that VGF is completely sequestered within closed structures that further studies have identified as dense-core vesicles (Cutler et al. in preparation). Finally it has been demonstrated that VGF is secreted upon stimulation of PC12 cells by different secretagogue agents, which induce depolarization of the plasma membrane. In conclusion, this polypeptide belongs to the class of proteins released via the regulated pathway.

Concluding remarks

VGF is a gene transcriptionally regulated by NGF. A number of clues suggest that VGF can be considered as a marker of NGF differentiated PC12 cells and, in general, of a subpopulation of mature neurons and endocrine cells, most of which express the low affinity NGF receptor. This point will be strengthened by unambiguous determination of its physiological function. Two main hypothesis which take into account its secretion via the regulated pathway, and its similarity to the secretogranins/chromogranins, have been made concerning the function of VGF. As already proposed for these proteins VGF could play a structural role in the assembly or function of secretory granules. In this case the high number of potential sites for proteolytic cleavage may reflect the necessity to dispense with this protein after secretion. Alternatively the whole protein or peptides derived from it may act as neuromodulators.

Irrespectively of the biological function of the VGF protein, the tissue specific expression of the gene as well as the induction of its transcription by NGF, have been exploited to gain insight into the molecular mechanism which govern regulation of gene expression in neuronal differentiation. The most challenging problem, in this respect, is probably to understand how the specificity of the response to differentiative stimuli is achieved. It is likely, even if not proved, that a postranslational modification of transcription factors already present inside the cells leads to the synthesis of new transcription factors, a specific combination of which is eventually responsible for the expression of differentiation-specific genes. Identification of DNA sequences necessary and sufficient for the tissue-restricted, growth factor-modulated gene expression will help to characterize transcription factors which bind to them and eventually to understand the relationship between the very early responses of the cell to the appearance of the differentiated phenotype.

Acknowledgements

We thanks M.T. Ciotti and C. Maialetti for the skillful technical assistence. Supported by grants from C.N.R. P.F. Invecchiamento e P.F. Biotecnologie e Biostrumentazioni.

References

Anderson, D.J., Axel, R. 1985 Molecular probes for the development and plasticity of neural crest derivatives. *Cell* 42: 649-662 .

Anh, T.G., Cohn, D.W., Gorr, S.U. Ornstein, D.L., Kashdan, M.A., Levine, M.A. 1987. Primary structure of bovine pituitary secretory protein I (chromogranin A) deduced from cDNA sequence. *Proc. Natl. Acad. Sci. USA* 84: 5043-5047.

Aloe, L., Levi-Montalcini, R. 1979. Nerve growth factor-induced transformation of immature chromaffin cells in vivo into sympathetic neurons: effects of antiserum to nerve growth factor. *Proc. Natl. Acad. Sci. USA* 76: 1246-1250.

Benedum, U.M., Lamouroux, A., Konecki, D.S., Rosa, P., Hille, A., Baeuerle, P.A., Frank, R., Lottspeich, F., Mallet, J., Huttner, W.B. 1987. The primary structure of human secretogranin I (chromogranin B): comparison with chromogranin A reveals homologous terminal domains and a large intervening variable region. *EMBO J.* 5: 1203-1211.

Bothwell, M., 1991. Keeping track of the Neurotrophin Receptors. *Cell* 65: 915-918.

Bradbury, A., Possenti, R., Shooter, E.M., Tirone, F. 1991. Molecular cloning of PC3, a putative secreted protein whose mRNA is induced by nerve growth factor and depolarization. *Proc. Natl. Acad. Sci. USA* 88: 3353-3357.

Burstein, D.E., Greene, L.A. 1978. Evidence for RNA synthesis-dependent and -independent pathways in stimulation of neurite outgrowth by nerve growth factor. *Proc. Natl. Acad. Sci. USA* 75: 6059-6063.

Cattaneo, A. 1986. Thymocytes as potential target cells for nerve growth factor. In: *Molecular Aspects of Neurobiology*, Levi-Montalcini, R. et al. eds., Springer-Verlag, Berlin, pp. 31-36.

Dynan, W. S. 1989. Modularity in promoters and enhancers. *Cell* 58: 1-4.

Ferri, G.L., Levi, A., Possenti, R. 1991. A novel neuroendocrine gene product: selective VGF expression in endocrin and neuronal population. *Brain Reserch* Submitted.

Gizang-Ginsberg, E., Ziff, E.B. 1990. Nerve growth factor regulates tyrosine hydroxylase gene transcription through a nucleoprotein complex that contains c-*fos. Genes Dev.* 4: 477-491.

Greenberg, M.E., Greene, L.A., Ziff, E.B. 1985. Nerve growth factor and epidermal growth factor induce rapid transient changes in proto-oncogene transcription in PC12 cells. *J. Biol. Chem.* 260: 14101-14110.

Greene, L.A., Tischler, A.S. 1982. PC12 pheochromocytoma cultures in neurobiological research. *Adv. Cell. Neurobiol.* 3: 373-414.

Greene, L.A., Burstein D.E., Black, M.M. 1982. The role of trnsciption-depended priming in nerve growth factor promoted neurite outgrowth. *Dev. Biol.* 91: 305-316.

Guroff, G.1985. PC12 cells as a model of neuronal differentiation. In: *Cell Culture in Neuroscience.* eds. J.E. Bottenstein, J. Sato. Plenum Press, N.Y. pp. 245-266.

Hallbook, F., Ibanez, C. F., Persson, H., 1991. Evolutionary studies of the nerve growth factor family reveal a novel member abundantly expressed in Xenopus ovart. *Neuron* 6: 845-858.

Hempstead, B.L., Kaplan D., Martin-Zanca, D., Parada, L.F., Chao, M.V. 1991. High affinity NGF binding requires co-expression of the *trk* proto-oncogene product and the low affinity NGF receptor. *Nature* 350: 678-683.

Hempstead, B.L., Scheifer, L.S., Chao, M.V. 1989. Expression of functional nerve growth factor receptors after gene transfer. *Science* 243: 373-375.

Herschman, H.R. 1989. extracellular signals, transcriptional responses and cellular specificity. *Trends Biol. Sci.* 14: 455-458.

Kaplan, D.R., Martin-Zanca, D., Parada, L.F. 1991. Tyrosine phosphorylation and tyrosine kinase activity of the *trk* proto-oncogene product induced by NGF. *Nature* 350: 158-160.

Koizumi, S., Contreras, M.L., Matsuda, Y., Hama, T., Lazarovici, P., Guroff, G. 1988. K252a: a specific inhibitor of the action of nerve growth factor on PC12 cells. *J. Neurosci.* 8: 715-721.

Lazarovici, P., Levi, B.-Z., Lelkes, P.I., Koizumi, S., Fujita, K., Matsuda, Y., Ozato, K., Guroff, G. 1989. K252a inhibits the increase in c-*fos* transcription and the increase in intracellular calcium produced by nerve growth factor in PC12 cells. *J. Neurosci. Res.* 23: 1-8.

Leonard, D.G.B., Ziff, E.B., Greene, L.A. 1987. Identification and characterization of mRNA regulated by nerve growth factor in PC12 cells. *Mol. Cell. Biol.* 7: 3156-3167.

Levi, A., Alemà, S. 1991. The mechanism of action of nerve growth factor. *Annu. Rev. Pharmacol. Toxicol* 31: 205-228.

Levi, A., Eldridge, J.D., Paterson, B.M. 1985. Molecular cloning of a gene sequence regulated by nerve growth factor. *Science* 229: 393-395.

Levi, A., Possenti, R., Eldridge, J., Paterson, B.M., 1988. Studies on a gene sequence sequence whose expression is regulated by NGF in PC12 cells. *In Neuronal Plasticity and Trophic Factors*. Biggio, G.et al. eds. Liviana Press 45-52.

Levi-Montalcini, R. 1987. The nerve growth factor 35 years later. *Science* 237: 1154-1162.

Levi-Montalcini, R., Aloe, L., Alleva, E. 1990. A role for nerve growth factor in nervous, endocrine and immune systems. *Progress in NeuroEndocriImmunology*. 3: 1-10.

Lillien, L.E., Claude, P. 1985. Nerve growth factor is a mitogen for cultured chromaffin cells. *Nature* 317: 632-634.

Machida, M. C., Rodland, K.D., Matrisian, L., Magun, B.E., Ciment, G. 1989. NGF induction of the gene encoding the protease Transin accompanies neuronal differentiation in PC12 cells. *Neuron* 2: 1587-1596.

Masiakowski, P., Shooter, E.M. 1988. Nerve growth factor induces the genes for two proteins related to a family of calcium-binding proteins in PC12 cells. *Proc. Natl. Acad. Sci. USA* 85: 1277-1281.

Milbrandt, J. 1987. A nerve growth factor-induced gene encodes a possible transcriptional regulator. *Science* 238: 797-799.

Milbrandt, J. 1988. Nerve growth factor induces a gene homologous to the glucocorticoid receptor gene. *Neuron* 1: 183-188.

Mori, N., Stein, R., Sigmund, O., Anderson, D.J. 1990. A cell type-preferred silencer element that controls the neural-specific expression of the SCG10 gene. *Neuron* 4: 583-594.

Otten, U., Ehrhard, P., Peck, R. 1989. Nerve growth factor induces growth and differentiation of human B lymphocytes. *Proc. Natl. Acad. Sci. USA* 86: 10059-10063.

Piccioli,P., Ruberti, F., Biocca, S., Di Luzio, A., Werge, T.M., Bradbury,A., Cattaneo, A. 1991. Neuroantiboby: Molecular cloning of a monoclonal antibody against substance P for the expression in the central nervous system. *Proc. Natl. Acad. Sci.* 88: 5611-5615.

Pioro, E.P., Cuello, A.C. 1990 Distibution of nerve growth factor receptor-like immunoractivity in the adult rat central nervous system. Effect of colchicine and correlation with the cholinergic system-I Forebrain *Neuroscience* 34: 57-87.

Pioro, E.P., Cuello, A.C. 1990 Distibution of nerve growth factor receptor-like immunoractivity in the adult rat central nervous system. Effect of colchicine and correlation with the cholinergic system-II Brainstem, cerebellum and spinal cord. *Neuroscience* 34:89-110.

Possenti, R., Eldridge, J.D., Paterson, B.M., Grasso, A., Levi, A. 1989. A protein induced by NGF in PC12 cells is stored in secretory vesicles and released through the regulated pathway. *EMBO J.* 8: 2217-2223.

Prentice, H.M., Moore, S.E., Dickson, J.G., Doherty, P., Walsh, F.S. 1987. Nerve growth factor induced changes in nerve cell adhesion molecule NCAM in PC12 cells. *EMBO J.* 6: 1859-1863.

Rosa, P., Fumagalli, G., Zanini, A., Huttner, W.B. 1985. The major tyrosine-sulfated protein of the bovine anterior pituitary is a secretory protein present in gonadotrophs, thyrotrophs, mammotrophs and corticotrophs. *J. Cell Biol.* 100: 928-937.

Salton, S.R.J., Fischberg, D.J., Dong, K.W.1991. Structure of the gene encoding VGF, a nervous sistem specific mRNA that is rapidly and selectively induced by nerve growth factor in PC12 cells. *Mol. Cell. Biol.* 11:2335-2349.

Satoh, T., Nakamura, S., Taga, T., Matsuda, T., Hirano, T., Kishimoto, T., Kaziro, Y.1988 Induction of neuronal differntiation in PC12 cells by B-cell stimulatory factor 2/ intrleukin 6., *Mol. Cell. Biol.* 8:3546-3549.

Seeley, P.J., Rukenstein, A., Connolly, J.L., Greene, L.A. 1984. Differential inhibition of nerve growth factor and epidermal growth factor effects on the PC12 pheocromocytoma line. *J. Cell Biol.* 98: 417-426.

Sheng, M., Greenberg, M.E. 1990. The regulation and function of c-*fos* and other immediate genes in the nervous system. *Neuron* 4: 477-485.

Thoenen, H., Bandtlow, C., Heumann, R. 1987. The physiological function of nerve growth factor in the central nervous system: comparison with the periphery. *Rev. Physiol. Biochem. Pharmacol.* 109: 145-178.

Tirone, F., Shooter, E. 1989. Early gene regulation by NGF in PC12 cells: induction of an interferon-related gene. *Proc. Natl. Acad. Sci. USA* 86: 2088-2092.

Togary, A., Dickens, G., Kuzuya, H., Guroff, G. 1985. The effect of fibroblast growth factor on PC12 cells. *J. Neurosci.* 5: 307-316.

Unsicker, K., Krisch, B., Otten, J., Thoenen, H. 1978. Nerve growth factor-induced fiber outgrowth from isolated rat adrenal chromaffin cells: impairment by glucocorticoids. *Proc. Natl. Acad. Sci. USA* 75: 3498-3502.

Vantini, G., Schiavo, N., Di Martino, A., Polato, P., Triban, C., Callegaro, L., Toffano, G., Leon, A. 1989. Evidence for a physiological role of nerve growth factor in the central nervous system of neonatal rats. *Neuron* 3: 267-273.

Whittemore, S.R., Seiger, A. 1987. The expression, localization and functional significance of β-nerve growth factor in the central nervous system. *Brain Res. Reviews.* 12: 439-464.

NERVE GROWTH FACTOR (NGF) PREVENTS THE EFFECTS OF MONOCULAR DEPRIVATION IN THE RAT

Luciano Domenici[1], Nicoletta Berardi[1], Giorgio Carmignoto[2], Tommaso Pizzorusso[3], Vincenzo Parisi[1], and Lamberto Maffei[1,3]

[1]Istituto di Neurofisiologia CNR, 56100 Pisa, Italy
[2]Fidia Research Laboratories, Abano Terme, Italy
[3]Scuola Normale Superiore, Pisa, Italy

Hubel and Wiesel [1,2] demonstrated that the mammalian visual cortex is susceptible to manipulation of the visual experience during the first part of the postnatal development (critical period). When visual signals are available but not identical in the two eyes, as in the case of monocular deprivation, cortical neurons do not retain their binocular input and stop responding to the deprived eye [3,4,5]. In addition, the visual acuity and the contrast sensitivity of the deprived eye decrease dramatically (amblyopia)[6,7]. These functional changes correspond anatomically to an alteration of the columnar organization. The cortical territories occupied by the afferents from the non deprived laminae of the LGN increase in size at the expense of the afferents coming from the deprived laminae[8]. In addition, cell bodies in the deprived laminae of LGN shrink[9].

It is generally assumed that the phenomena occurring after a monocular deprivation (MD), are the outcome of competitive activity-dependent interactions between the geniculate afferents. Cortical synapses receiving a strong input, as it is the case for the non deprived eye, are strengthened and stabilized while those receiving a weaker input are depressed and may be removed.

Activation of the postsynaptic site is an essential prerequisite for the long-term modifications of synapses caused by MD. And indeed a number of factors acting at the postsynaptic site have been found to prevent, at least partially, the effects of MD and to have a role in synapse stabilization during visual development[10-14].

However, the crucial question, what the axons from LGN are competing for still remains to be answered.

We have formulated the hypothesis that the competition might be for a neurotrophic factor, released or produced in an electrical activity dependent manner. Activity in the deprived fibers would be inappropriate for the necessary production and/or uptake of neurotrophic factor and their synaptic efficacy would decrease. Cortical cells would then stop responding to the deprived eye and the visual acuity for the deprived eye would dramatically decrease. Neurons in the deprived laminae of LGN would suffer for the absence of neurotrophic factor and would shrink.

We have tested this working hypothesis by investigating the effects of intraventricular NGF injection on the visual cortex of monocularly deprived rats. NGF is a well known neurotrophic factor both in the PNS[15] and in the CNS[16,17,18].

The data are clear in indicating that when NGF is exogenously provided the effects of monocular deprivation do not take place.

These results have been previously presented in a general review on the role of neurotrophic factors in the mammalian visual cortex plasticity[19].

METHODS

Subjects and surgery

Fifty three Long Evans hooded rats were used. Seventeen rats were normal (group I). Thirty six rats were monocularly deprived for one month by means of eyelids suture starting immediately before eye opening (postnatal day 14, P14). In the rat this corresponds to a deprivation spanning the whole length of the critical period [20, 21]. In fifteen rats only monocular deprivation was performed (group II). In fifteen rats deprivation was combined with the intraventricular injection of a solution containing ß-NGF (1-1.6 μg/μl in buffered saline; group III). In six rats cytochrome C (1 μg/μl in buffered saline) was injected with the same protocol as NGF (group IV). The volume injected was 2 μl. Injections were performed every other day for one month by means of a microsyringe connected to a cannula (gauge 26) inserted through a hole 1 mm lateral and in correspondence with bregma, to reach the lateral ventricle. When a dye (Pontamine Sky Blue) was injected by this procedure it was invariably found in the ventricles. Eyelid suture and intraventricular injections were performed under ether anaestesia. The diffusion of NGF was estimated by placing a piece of fibrine (Spongestan) soaked with iodinated NGF (specific activity 64.1 μCi/μg) onto the cortical surface in correspondence with bregma (N=3 rats). The diffusion of iodinated NGF was approximately 3 mm from bregma 24 hours later.

Recording sessions

At the end of the deprivation period, single neuron responses or visual evoked potentials (VEP) were recorded in urethane anaesthetized rats (6 cc/Kg, 20% solution, Sigma) by means of a micropipette filled with NaCl (3 M), inserted in the binocular portion of the primary visual cortex (binocular area 17 or area OC1B) contralateral to the deprived eye. Both eyes were fixed by means of metal rings surrounding the external portion of the eye bulbes. Visual stimuli consisted

of light bars projected on a reflecting screen or in
gratings of different orientation and spatial frequency
computer generated on a display (HP 1300 A, mean luminance 12
cd/m^2) positioned 20 cm from the rat eyes and centered on
the cell receptive fields, previously determined. The
gratings were alternated in phase with a fixed temporal
frequency, chosen in the range 1-2 Hz for extracellular unit
recordings and 2-4 Hz for VEPs. The signals were filtered and
amplified in a conventional manner, computer averaged and
analyzed.

Extracellular unit recording

Five rats of group I (normal rats), five rats of group II
(deprived rats), five rats of group III (deprived NGF treated
rats) and three rats of group IV (deprived cytochrome C
treated rats) were used, all aged P 45 or older. On isolating
a cell, the location of the receptive field in the visual
space and the optimal stimulus orientation and direction of
movement were determined. Neurons were classified as
orientational if the cell response was maximal for a given
orientation (preferred orientation) and indistinguishable
from spontaneous activity for the orthogonal stimulus
orientation. The ocular dominance was then assessed with bars
or gratings of optimal orientation. Neurons in ocular
dominance class 1 were driven only by the stimulation of the
contralateral eye; neurons in ocular dominance classes 2-3
were binocular and preferentially driven by the contralateral
eye; neurons in class 4 were equally driven by the two eyes;
neurons in class 5-6 were binocular and preferentailly driven
by the ipsilateral eye and neurons in class 7 were driven
only by the ipsilateral eye. A chi-square test, 4 degrees of
freedom was used to evaluate the differences between ocular
dominance distributions.

Two of the NGF treated rats were recorded during the
treatment (postnatal day 42) in order to evaluate possible
transient effects of NGF on neuronal excitability and on the
quality of the cell visual response.

Visual evoked potentials

VEPs were recorded in five rats of group I, ten rats of group
II, ten rats of group III and three control rats (deprived
cytochrome C treated rats). For each condition (visual
cortex, viewing eye, spatial frequency, contrast) at least
400 responses were averaged. For each record the amplitude,
phase and relative power of the first twelve harmonics were
measured. For the temporal frequencies employed, signals
consisted mainly of the second harmonic (relative power
higher than 70%). For this reason, the amplitude of the
second harmonic in each record (1/2 the peak to trough
amplitude) was taken as the amplitude of VEP for that
condition. To assess the spatial resolution value (visual
acuity) gratings of maximum (available) contrast were used
(70 %); the spatial frequency was progressively increased
until the signal was indistinguishable from the noise. If
necessary, lenses of appropriate dioptric power were placed
in front of the eyes of the rat. The visual acuity was taken
as the highest spatial frequency still evoking a reliable

response. The contrast threshold at a given spatial frequency was evaluated by extrapolating to zero voltage (noise level) the linear regression through a contrast response curve (VEP amplitude vs log stimulus contrast)[22]. The contrast sensitivity is the reciprocal of the contrast threshold. The noise level for a given condition (temporal frequency of alternation, viewing eye, visual cortex) was taken as the amplitude of the second harmonic in records where the stimulus was covered with a translucent screen.

RESULTS

The functional properties of cat and monkey visual cortex are still immature at the beginning of the critical period[20,21]. To control whether this holds also in the rat we assessed the ocular dominance distribution of cortical cells and the visual acuity in four rats at postnatal day 20. We found that, as in other mammals[23] the great majority of cortical neurons are equally dominated by both eyes (ocular dominance class 4), most of the cells are not orientational and the receptive fields are large. In addition, the visual acuity measured by VEPs recording is nearly half its normal value in adults.

Effects of monocular deprivation: extracellular unit recordings

At the end of the critical period a total of 350 cells were recorded in normal rats (group I, 100 cells), monocularly deprived rats, either untreated (group II, 100 cells) or treated with cytochrome C (group IV, 50 cells) and monocularly deprived rats treated with NGF (group III, 100 cells).

In Figure 1 we report the pooled data obtained from rats of group I, II, III.

In normal rats (hatched columns) the majority of the cells are driven predominantly or exclusively by the contralateral eye (75%) and the proportion of binocular cells is 80%.

In MD rats (Fig. 1, black columns) the proportion of cells driven by the contralateral eye falls to 20% while the ipsilateral eye dominates 65% of cells. Binocularity is nearly halved (43%) with respect to normal rats.

The ocular dominance distribution in NGF treated rats (Fig. 1, white columns) is not significantly different (chi square, p> 0.05) from the ocular dominance distribution in normal adult rats: 66% of the cells are dominated by the contralateral deprived eye and 87% are binocular.

The treatment with cytochrome C was completely ineffective in preventing the effects of monocular deprivation: the ocular dominance distribution in cytochrome C (not reported in Figure) treated rats is indistinguishable from that of untreated monocularly deprived rats.

Thus exogenous supply of NGF prevents the shift in ocular dominance distribution induced by monocular deprivation.

A crucial point was to assess whether the treatment with NGF had altered other functional properties of visual cortical cells such as the selectivity for the stimulus orientation.

The selectivity for the stimulus orientation is reported in Fig. 2 (A) for the same cells out of which the ocular dominance histograms had been compiled. It is evident from the figure that the distribution of cells according to orientation selectivity is not altered by NGF treatment. It has to be noted that no substantial difference was found between the orientational selectivity of cells recorded in NGF treated rats before or after the end of the treatment.

It is known that pharmacological treatments altering the cells spontaneous discharge eliminate the effects of monocular deprivation on the ocular dominance distribution[11,12]. To assess whether NGF treatment affected the cells resting discharge we measured the spontaneous activity of visual cortical neurons in normal rats and in rats under NGF treatment (Fig. 2B). We found that the mean spontaneous discharge (computed from several records one-two minutes long) did not vary significantly (two tailed t test, p>0.05) from the cell sample in normal rats (N=15, mean=10 ± 5 spikes/sec) to the sample in NGF treated rats, either within treatment (N= 15, mean value=7 ± 4 spikes/sec) or after the end of the treatment (N=25, mean value=10 ± 8 spikes/sec).

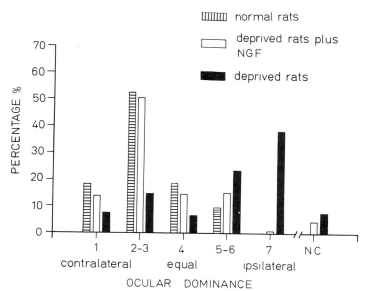

Figure 1. Ocular dominance distributions representing data from all normal rats (hatched columns), all MD rats (black columns), all MD rats treated with NGF (white columns).

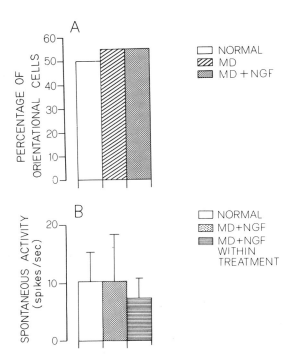

Figure 2. Histograms compiled from the neurons recorded in the primary visual cortex and classified according to their orientational selectivity (A) and their spontaneous discharge (B).

A. Histogram represents neurons recorded in the primary visual cortex of normal (open column), monocularly deprived (MD, hatched column) and monocularly deprived NGF treated (MD+NGF, dotted column) rats.

B. Histogram compiled from neurons recorded in the primary visual cortex of normal (open column), monocularly deprived NGF treated (dotted column, MD+NGF) and monocularly deprived NGF treated rats within treatment (hatched column, MD+NGF within treatment). Neurons are classified according to their spontaneous discharge, evaluated over periods lasting one minute (for each cell, data from three periods were averaged off-line).

Effects of monocular deprivation: visual evoked potentials

In adult pigmented rats, the curve relating VEP amplitude to stimulus spatial frequency (VEP spatial frequency curve) is approximately low pass shaped for spatial frequencies higher than .1 c/deg, with the estimated visual acuity being around 1.2 c/deg[24], in accordance with the behavioral visual acuity[25].

The visual acuity we found for normal rats and for the non deprived eye of MD rats (table 1) is in accordance with the data in the literature.

In figure 3 pooled data from normal rats, MD untreated rats and MD rats treated with NGF are shown separately for the ipsi and contralateral cortex. The shaded area represents the range of VEP amplitudes (mean values, inner solid line plus or minus one SD) recorded from the non deprived eyes at various spatial frequencies. The mean visual acuity was 1.1 c/deg (N= 7, SD = 0.1) for the contralateral cortex and 1 c/deg (N= 7, SD = 0.1) for the ipsilateral cortex (ipsi and contralateral to the stimulated eye).

One month of monocular deprivation strongly reduced the visual acuity of the deprived eye in all rats monocularly deprived and with no treatment. The mean visual acuity for the deprived eye was 0.4 c/deg (N= 8, SD = 0.1) in the contralateral cortex, and 0.3 c/deg (N= 8, SD = 0.1) in the ipsilateral cortex. In addition, the signal amplitude was significantly reduced (t-test $p < 0.01$) at all spatial frequencies tested in both cortices (Fig. 3 A and B; open circles).

To test whether the reduced signal amplitude was due to a loss in contrast sensitivity, we measured in two normal rats and two MD rats the contrast threshold for various spatial frequencies in the deprived and in the normal eye. Contrast thresholds for the deprived eye were increased at spatial frequencies ranging from 0.1 to 1 c/deg.

In rats with intraventricular NGF injections, one month of monocular deprivation produced a much weaker effect. Indeed, both the mean visual acuity and the mean VEP amplitude (Fig. 3 A and B; filled triangles) were not significantly (t-test $p > 0.1$) different from the corresponding values in the normal eye. In addition, the contrast sensitivity for the deprived eye recorded in two rats of the same group was within the normal range for spatial frequencies lower than 0.8 c/deg.

The injection of cytochrome C was not effective in preserving the visual acuity and the contrast sensitivity of the deprived eye. The mean visual acuity for the deprived eye in this group was 0.4 c/deg (N= 3, SD = 0.15).

Thus, intraventricular injection of NGF prevents, at least partially, loss of both visual acuity and contrast sensitivity in the deprived eye.

TABLE 1. Visual acuity for the normal rats and for the non
deprived eye of MD rats.
Visual acuity assessed for both eyes in five normal rats
(NOR) and for the non deprived eye (D) of ten monocularly
deprived rats. VEPs were recorded in the binocular portion of
both visual cortices. Ipsi and contra refer to the visual
cortex where the recordings have been made (i.e. ipsilateral
and contralateral to the stimulated eye). Mean values ± SD
have been reported for each group.

| Rat | Visual acuity (c/deg) | |
	ipsi	contra
NOR 1	0.9	1.2
NOR 2	1.2	1.0
NOR 3	0.9	1.1
NOR 4	1.0	1.0
NOR 5	1.0	1.1
Mean	1.0	1.08
SD	0.12	0.08
D 1	1.1	1.2
D 2	1.0	
D 3		1.0
D 4	1.0	1.0
D 5	1.0	1.1
D 6	1.1	
D 7	0.9	1.1
D 8	0.9	
D 9		1.0
D10		1.1
Mean	1.0	1.07
SD	0.08	0.08

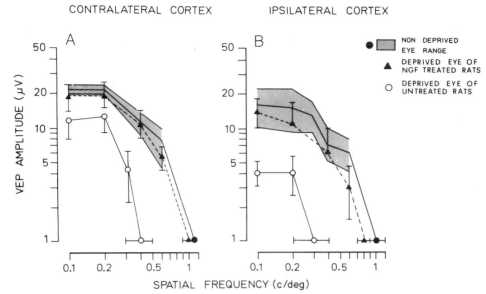

Figure 3. Effects of monocular deprivation on visual evoked potentials (VEP) recorded in untreated rats and NGF treated rats. The mean VEP amplitude is reported as a function of the stimulus spatial frequency. The contrast of the visual stimuli was 30-40% with the exception of the deprived eye of untreated rats, in which case it was 40-50%. A. VEP recorded in the cortex contralateral to the stimulated eye. B. VEP recorded in the cortex ipsilateral to the stimulated eye. The shaded area is the range found for the VEP amplitude in response to stimulation of the non deprived eye (N= 7) mean values (inner solid line) ± one standard deviation. Filled triangles: mean VEP amplitude for the deprived eyes of NGF treated rats (N=8). Open circles: mean VEP amplitude for the deprived eye of untreated rats (N=8). Vertical bars represent the standard deviation. The symbols on the abscissa correspond to the mean visual acuity, i.e. the highest spatial frequency still able to evoke a reliable signal with maximum contrast (filled circles, non deprived eye; filled triangles, deprived eye of NGF treated rats; open circles, deprived eye of untreated rats); the horizontal bars are the standard deviation. The mean noise level was 2 µv, SD= 1 µv.

DISCUSSION

Monocular deprivation in rats during the critical period[19,20] results in a loss of binocular neurons and a shift in the ocular dominance distribution toward the open eye. As in other mammals[6,7], the contrast sensitivity for the deprived eye decreases substantially, and the visual acuity is reduced by more than a factor of two.

We have found that the neurotrophic factor NGF, when exogenously supplied to monocularly deprived rats, prevents both the shift in ocular dominance distribution and the loss of visual acuity and contrast sensitivity in the deprived eye. This suggests that NGF preserves the functional input from the deprived eye to the visual cortex.

The data from control animals (cytochrome C treated) indicate that the effects of NGF are not aspecific, resulting, e.g. from animal handling or anaesthesia. A specific role for NGF in the development of the mammalian visual cortex is in accordance with the presence of both NGF[26,27] and NGF receptors[28,29,30] in the neocortex of newborn, as well as adult rats and primates. Interestingly, the content of NGF in the rat neocortex[25] and primate occipital cortex[26] is higher during the first part of the critical period, later decreasing to adult level.

The mechanisms underlying these actions of NGF in the visual system are unknown, although several possible explanations can be proposed.

For example NGF could increase the electrical activity of cortical neurons, as may occur with PC12 cells[31]. An increased electrical activity of visual cortical cells would be expected to antagonize the effects of monocular deprivation, as described by Shaw and Cynader[12] for glutamate infusion. Such an explanation seems unlikely, since single cell recordings during NGF treatment failed to detect either an increase in spontaneous discharge or an alteration in cell responses to visual stimuli. These findings also suggest that NGF does not impair the transmission of either excitatory[12] or inhibitory[11] visual information.

Another possibility is that NGF interferes with the normal development of the visual cortex . Were this to be the case, the functional properties of the visual cortex in adult NGF-treated rats should be abnormal and even resemble those found for young pups at the beginning of NGF treatment. This is not the case, since both ocular dominance distribution and visual acuity are normal in NGF treated rats.

A third hypothesis takes into account a possible effect of NGF on the cholinergic input to the visual cortex. It is well known that NGF has a neurotrophic action on the cholinergic neurons of the CNS[16,17,18], although a neurotrophic action of NGF on other CNS neurons has been reported[32]. Preliminary results (Dr. G. Vantini, Fidia Research Laboratories, Abano Terme, Italy) in the visual cortex of monocularly deprived rats show that ChAT activity is not substantially changed after treatment with NGF.

The most probable explanation for the findings presented here is that NGF preserves the functional input from the deprived eye to the visual cortex through a specific, direct action on visual neurons. Additional experiments, particularly of molecular biology, will be needed to clarify the mechanisms of this action.

Of particular interest is the result that an exogeneous supply of NGF prevents the amblyopic effects of monocular deprivation. It is well known that a number of ophthalmological pathologies, such as monocular anisometropia or strabismus during the critical period may cause amblyopia in human subjects. NGF puts itself on the stage as a factor to be tested in view of a possible therapeutic approach to treat amblyopia in man.

ACKNOWLEDGMENTS

We thank M. Antoni, G. Cappagli, V. Alpigiani, and A. Tacchi for technical assistance. Dr. G. Tinivella made the computer program for VEP acquisition and analysis. N. Berardi is associate Professor at the Dept General and Environmental Physiology, University of Napoli, Napoli, Italy. Fidia Research Laboratories (Abano Terme, Italy) kindly provided NGF.

REFERENCES

1. T.N.Wiesel, D.H. Hubel, Single cell responses in striate cortex of kittens deprived of vision in one eye, J Neurophysiol 26: 1003 (1963).
2. D.H. Hubel, T.N. Wiesel, S. Le Vay, Plasticity of ocular dominance columns in monkey straite cortex, Phil Trans R Soc London (Biol) 278: 377 (1977).
3. U.C. Drager, Observation of monocular deprivation in mice, J. Neurophysiol 41: 28 (1978).
4. F.H. Baker, P. Crigg, G.K. Von Nordon, Effects of visual deprivation and strabismus on the response of neurons in the visual cortex of the monkey, including studies on the striate and prestriate cortex in normal animals, Brain Res 66: 185 (1974).
5. S.M. Sherman, P.T. Spear, Organization of visual pathways in normal and visually deprived cats, Phys Rev 62: 738 (1982).
6. A. Snyder, R. Shapley, Deficit in the visual evoked potentials of cats as a result of visual deprivation, Exp Brain Res 37: 73 (1979).
7. D.C. Smith, Developmental alterations in binocular competitive interactions and visual acuity in visually deprived cats, J Comp Neurol 198: 667 (1981).
8. C.J. Shatz, M.P. Stryker, Ocular dominance in layer IV of the cat's visual cortex and the effects of monocular deprivation, J Physiol 281: 267 (1978).
9. R.W. Guillery, D.J. Stelzner, The differential effects of unilateral lid closure upon the monocular and binocular segments of the dorsal geniculate nucleus in the cat, J Comp Neurol 139: 413 (1970).
10. T. Kasamatsu, J.D. Pettigrew, Depletion of brain catecholamines: failure of ocular dominance shift after

monocular occlusions in kittens, Science 194: 206 (1976).

11. A.S. Ramoa, M.A. Paradiso, R.D. Freeman, Blockade of intracortical inhibition in kitten striate cortex: Effects on receptive field properties and associated loss of ocular dominance plasticity, Exp Brain Res 73: 285 (1989).

12. C. Shaw, M. Cynader, Disruption of cortical activity prevents ocular dominance changes in monocularly deprived kittens, Nature 308: 731 (1984).

13. M.F. Bear, W. Singer, Modulation of visual cortical plasticity by acetylcholine and noradrenaline, Nature 320: 172 (1986).

14. A. Kleinschmidt, M.F. Bear, W. Singer, Blockade of "NMDA" receptors disrupts experience-dependent plasticity of kitten striate cortex, Science 238: 355 (1987).

15. R. Levi-Montalcini, Nerve-Growth Factor 35 years later, Science 237: 1154 (1987).

16. M. Seiler, M.E. Schwab, Specific retrograde transport of nerve growth factor (NGF) from neocortex to nucleus basalis in the rat, Brain Res 300: 33 (1984).

17. L.F. Kromer, Nerve growth factor treatment after brain injury prevents death, Science 235: 214 (1987).

18. J. Hartikka, F. Hefti, Development of septal cholinergic neurons in culture: plating density and glial cells modulate effects of NGF on survival, fiber growth, and expression of transmitterspecific enzymes, J Neurosci 8: 2967 (1988).

19. L. Maffei, N. Berardi, G. Carmignoto, A. Cellerino, L. Domenici, A. Fiorentini, T. Pizzorusso, Role of neurotrophic factors in the plasticity of the visual system, in:"Regeneration and plasticity in the visual system: proceedings of the Retina Research Symposia, 4", D. Man-Kit Lam and G. Bray, eds., MIT Press, in press.

20. L.A. Rothblat, M.L. Schwartz, The effect of monocular deprivation on dendritic spines in visual cortex of young and adult albino rats: evidence for a sensitive period, Brain Res 161: 156 (1979).

21. L.A. Rothblat, M.L. Schwartz, P.M. Kasdan, Monocular deprivation in the rat: evidence for an age-related defect in visual behavior, Brain Res 158: 456 (1978).

22. F.W. Campbell, L. Maffei, M. Piccolino, The contrast sensitivity of the cat, J Physiol 229: 719 (1973).

23. K. Albus, W. Wolf, Early post-natal development of neuronal function in the kitten's visual cortex: A laminar analysis, J Physiol 348: 153 (1984).

24 L.C.L. Silveira, C.A. Heywood, A. Cowey, Contrast sensitivity and visual acuity of the pigmented rat determined electrophysiologically, Vision Res 27: 1719 (1987).

25. D. Birch, G.H. Jacobs, Spatial contrast sensitivity in albino and pigmented rats, Vision Res 19: 933 (1978).

26. T.H. Large, S.C. Bodary, D.O. Clegg, G. Weskamp, U. Otten, L.F. Reichardt, Nerve growth factor gene expression in the developing rat brain, Science 234: 352 (1986).

27. M. Hayashi, A. Yamashita, K. Shimizu, Nerve growth factor in the primate central nervous system: regional distribution and ontogeny, Neuroscience 36: 683 (199).

28. Q. Yan, E.M. Johnson, An immunohistochemical study of the nerve growth factor receptor in developing rats, J Neurosci 8: 3481 (1988).

29. S. Koh, R. Loy, Localization and development of NGF sensitive rat basal forebrain neurons and their afferent projections to hippocampus and neocortex, J Neurosci 9: 2999 (1989).

30. E.P. Pioro, A.C. Cuello, Distribution of nerve growth factor receptor-like immunoreactivity in the adult rat central nervous system. Effect of colchicine and correlation with the cholinergic system-I. Forebrain, Neuroscience 34: 57 (1990).

31. G. Mandel, S. Cooperman, R.A. Maue, Selective induction of brain type II Na channels by nerve growth factor, Proc Natl Acad Sci 85: 924 (1988).

32. G. Carmignoto, P. Candeo, R. Cannella, C. Comelli, L. Maffei, Effect of NGF on the survival of rat retinal ganglion cells following optic nerve section, J Neurosci 9: 1263 (1989).

EVIDENCE FOR A ROLE OF NGF IN THE VISUAL SYSTEM

Maria Cristina Comelli, Paola Candeo, Roberto Canella,
Adalberto Merighi[#], Lamberto Maffei[*], Giorgio Carmignoto

Fidia Research Laboratories, Via Ponte della Fabbrica 3/A,
35031 Abano Terme, Italy; [*]Istituto di Neurofisiologia del
CNR, Via S. Zeno 51, 56100 Pisa, Italy, and [#]Dipartimento
di Morfofisiologia Veterinaria, Università di Torino, Via
Nizza 52, 10126 Torino, Italy

INTRODUCTION

It is generally accepted that the development, maintenance and
survival of specific neuronal populations, both in the peripheral (PNS)
and central nervous system (CNS), is dependent upon the supply of
diffusable trophic molecules, produced in limiting amounts by neurons
and/or glia in their target fields (for review, see Thoenen et al.,
1987). The prototype of neuronotrophic factors, Nerve Growth Factor
(NGF) is essential for neural crest-derived sensory and peripheral
symphathetic neurons (Levi-Montalcini and Angeletti, 1968) and for
cholinergic neurons of forebrain nuclei in the CNS (Hefti, 1986;
Vantini et al., 1989). In all these NGF-responsive peripheral and central neurons, NGF binds to specific cell surface receptors (NGFRs)
expressed both on cell bodies and axonal terminals in the innervated
target area (Greene and Shooter, 1980). The immunocytochemical mapping
of the NGFR with the 192-IgG monoclonal antibody (Chandler et al.,
1984) has demonstrated that the receptor is expressed by many different
neuronal population in the CNS (Yan and Johnson, 1989; Pioro and
Cuello, 1990), suggesting that NGF, or an NGF-like molecule have a
trophic role for many other cell types beyond the cholinergic ones.
The first evidence that NGF may also be active in the visual system was
obtained in the early eighties when it was demonstrated that NGF, when
intraocularly supplied to axotomized retinal ganglion cells (RGCs) in
the goldfish, enhanced the process of axonal regneration in the transected optic nerve (ON). More recent studies (Yan et al., 1989; Pioro
and Cuello, 1990) have demonstrated that the NGFR is expressed in many
nuclei of the visual system receiving a retinal input both in developing and adult rats.

In addition the messenger RNA encoding for NGFR has been reported
to be present in the retina of avian (Large et al., 1989) and of many
different mammalian species, including primates (Schatteman et al.,
1988). It has been demonstrated that NGF, when intraocularly supplied
to axotomized RGCs in the goldfish, enhances processes of axonal regeneration in the transected optic nerve (ON) (Turner et al., 1980; Yip
and Johnson, 1982). These were the first evidence suggesting that NGF
may also be active in the visual system.

Here we will review our results obtained over the last few years
on the expression and distribution of NGFR in the rat visual system. We

The Changing Visual System, Edited by P. Bagnoli and
W. Hodos, Plenum Press, New York, 1991

will also briefly describe the effects produced by exogenously supplying NGF to axotomized rat RGCs and to monocularly deprived kittens. All together, these results allow us to hypothesize that NGF itself, or an NGF-like molecule, plays an important role in the mammalian visual system.

MATERIALS AND METHODS

Optic nerve (ON) section. Adult Long Evans rats had their right ON intracranially transected. Animals received intraocular injections of either NGF or cytochrome c (cyt c) (3 ug in 3 ul per injection on either day). Seven weeks after ON section, the ONs were serially cut and prepared for electron microscopy (for details, see Carmignoto et al., 1989).

Monocular deprivation (MD). Under halothane anesthesia, kittens were monocularly deprived by lid suture of the right eye at the 30th day of age. At the same time a cannula connected to a 2002 Alzet mini-pump filled with 0.5 ug/ul of either NGF or cyt c was inserted into the anterior ventricle. Kittens were divided in control untreated (n=2), cyt c (n=3) and NGF (n=3) treated groups.

After two weeks of MD, extracellular action potentials were recorded from single units of area 17 with tungsten microelectrodes (Digitimer), conventionally filtered, amplified and audiomonitored. Each cell recorded was assigned to one group of the seven point scale of Hubel and Wiesel (1977). The degree of shift in ocular dominance after monocular deprivation was expressed by the Binocularity (B), which is defined as the number of cells in groups 2, 3, 4, 5, and 6 divided by the number of all visually responsive cells, and the open eye dominance (OED) (Paradiso et al., 1983) in the hemisphere contralateral to the open eye, as follows:

$$OED = \frac{(n° \text{ cells gr 1}) + 2/3 \text{ (n° cells gr 2)} + 1/3 \text{ (n° cells gr 3)}}{total \text{ n° cells}}$$

Symmetrical penetrations were made in both hemispheres.

RESULTS

NGFR in the visual system. We have recently demonstrated that in the rat retina the messenger RNA encoding for NGFR is expressed troughout development and in adulthood (Carmignoto et al., 1991).In addition we have localized immunocytochemically localized NGFR by using the 192-IgG monoclonal antibody. As shown in Fig. 1A, NGFR immunoreactivity in the adult rat retina is associated with Muller cell bodies located in the inner nuclear layer (INL) and with their end feet processes in the ganglion cell layer (GCL). Immunopositive cell bodies located in the ganglion cell layer are also present. On the basis of soma diameter and dentritic arborization at least some of these cells can be classified as RGCs. Fig. 1B shows an example of a cell with a soma diameter of approximately 14 um. Fig. 1C shows an example of a cell with a soma diameter of approximately 21 um and the typical arborization of a type 1 RGC.

At least some RGCs were also capable of anterogradely and retrogradely transporting the NGFR along optic nerve fibers (Carmignoto et al., 1991). Our results are consistent with other studies in both developing and adult rats where the NGFR-like immunoreactivity was demonstrated to be mainly associated to fibers and terminals in all the visually related nuclei (Yan and Johnson, 1989; Pioro and Cuello, 1990), i.e., the Superior Colliculus, dorsal and ventral part of the Lateral Geniculate Nucleus, Suprachiasmatic nucleus, and nuclei of the

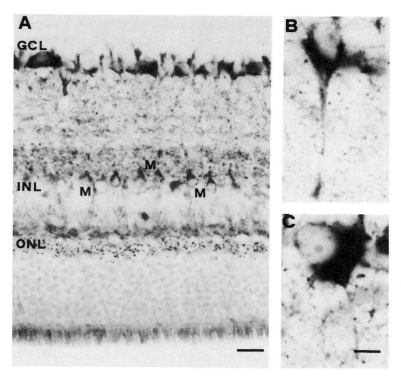

Fig. 1 A. Coronal section of an adult rat retina processed with the anti-NGFR antibody. The immunoreactivity is associated with Muller cell bodies (M) in the inner nuclear layer (INL) and with their end feet (asterisks) in the ganglion cell layer (GCL). Also some cells in the GCL are strongly immunopositive. Scale bar: 30 um. B. RGC with a soma diameter of 14 um. C. Type 1 RGC with a soma diameter of 21 um. Scale bar: 8 um.

pretectal area (Yan and Johnson, 1989; Pioro and Cuello, 1990). However, all these nuclei are known to receive projections that are not exclusively related to RGCs. Therefore the possibility arises that, at least in part, the immunoreactivity in these nuclei does not belong to the retinal input.

To exclude such a possibility we have carried out a series of experiments in which, after transection of the ON, we have been able to demonstrate that the NGFR immunopositive fibers and terminals in the dorsal part of the LGN belong exclusively to RGCs. Conversely in the ventral part of the LGN, as in the other visually related nuclei, NGFR resulted to be in part associated to other projections beside the retinal ones (Carmignoto et al., 1990).

In addition we have studied the regulation of the messenger RNA encoding for NGFR in the retina, at different surviving times following ON section. Our observations showed that the NGFRmRNA is increased 3-fold in the axotomized rat retina at 5 weeks following ON section (Comelli et el., 1990) with respect to the normal, contralateral one. This result supports the hypothesis that RGCs are dependent on NGF, or an NGF-like molecule for their survival. The increased expression of the NGFR seems to be related both to surviving RGCs and to Muller cells, as suggested by the pattern of immunostaining obtained with the anti-NGFR antibody.

<u>Effect of exogenous administration of NGF in the visual system</u>. The presence of the NGFR on RGCs, and the increased expression of the NGFR following ON section, suggests that RGCs are sensitive to the action of NGF. Following either intracranial section of the ON in the rat (Carmignoto et al., 1989) or an ischemic insult in the cat (Siliprandi et al., 1990), a consistent number of RGCs was found to survive the insult when intraocularly supplied with NGF. This rescuing effect was evident also on ON fibers, as demonstrated by the higher number of myelinated fibers found in NGF treated animals, when compared to controls (Carmignoto et al., 1989). The exogenous supply of NGF to axotomized RGCs also promoted axonal regeneration in the ON. Fig. 2 is a representative example of corresponding regions in a control (A) and NGF-treated animal (B), 7 weeks after axotomy. In the NGF-treated animal unmyelinated axons, a marker of RGC axonal regeneration (Richardson et al., 1986; Hall et al., 1989), were much more numerous and distributed throughout the nerve than in controls. At least some of these axons belong to RGCs, being able to anterogradely transport HRP injected into the eye (Comelli et al., 1991, manuscript in preparation). In NGF-treated rats, a higher number of newly myelinated fibers was also found, with respect to controls (Fig. 3).

Recently we have also studied the effect of intraventricular injections of NGF on visual cortical plasticity, hypothesizing that the ocular dominance shift of cortical neurons towards the open eye which follows monocular deprivation in kittens is due to competition between geniculo-cortical afferents for NGF, or an NGF-like molecule, produced by cortical neurons and/or glia. According to this hypothesis modifications of the activity related to the deprived eye, in terms of either level of synaptic activity or lack of correlation between pre- and post-synaptic activation, could lead to a reduced support of the trophic factor deriving from the cortical cell. The end result would be a diminished synaptic efficiency, eventually followed by withdrawal of terminals and consequent loss of function. The availability of exogenously administered NGF could, therefore, counteract the effect of monocular deprivation.

Our results suggest that two weeks of monocular deprivation in 30-day old kittens causes the great majority of cortical neurons to became monocularly responsive to the normal open eye, with only few neurons remaining binocularly responsive (B=0.06±0.021; OED=0.910±0.055;

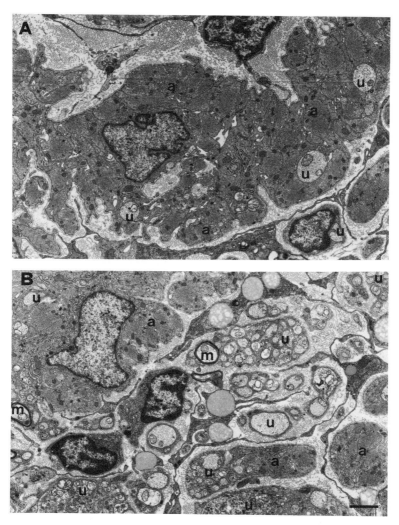

Fig. 2 Corresponding regions of a transected and regenerating ON from
a control (A) and a NGF treated animal (B), seven weeks after
ON section. u: unmyelinated axons; m: myelinated axons; a:
astrocytic processes. Scale bar: 1 um.

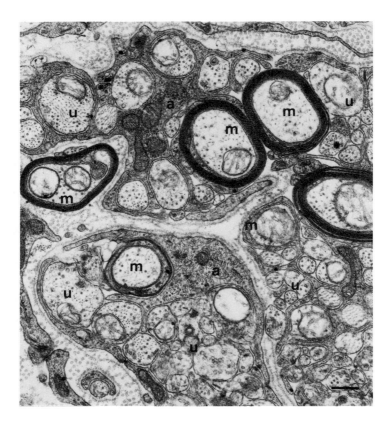

Fig. 3   Examples of newly myelinated fibers in the ON of an NGF treated
          animal, seven weeks following ON section.
          u: unmyelinated fibers; m: newly myelinated fibers; a:
          astyrocytic processes. Scale bar: 0.2 um.

90 cells; n=2). In monocularly deprived kittens treated with NGF, the ocular dominance shift was much less prounounced (B=0.443±0.01; OED=0.576± 0.01; 171 cells; n=3), while treatment with cyt c was completely ineffective (B=0.089±0.006; OED=0.900±0.016; 165 cells; n=3). Other studies have shown that treatment with NGF was also effective in preventing the effects of monocular deprivation in the rat visual cortex (Berardi et al, 1990; Berardi et al., 1991; see also Domenici et al., this volume).

DISCUSSION

   NGF in the visual system. Extensive studies have now established that NGF is a target-derived factor for cholinergic forebrain neurons (for review: Thoenen et al., 1987). Recently, NGFR and NGF mRNA have been identified in many different CNS areas (Maisonpierre et al., 1991; Yan et al., 1989). In the visual system NGF seems to play an important role, at least at two different levels. In the retina, NGF promotes the survival of RGCs, following either ON section in the rat (Carmignoto et al., 1989) or an ischemic insult in the cat (Siliprandi et al., 1990). The results reported here indicate that regeneration of rat RGC axons is also enhanced by NGF intraocular administration. The ability of NGF to exert biological effects is associated with an initial interaction with specific NGFRs. Using immunocytochemistry, the NGFR was found on Muller cells and RGCs, as well as on RGC terminals of the adult rat in nuclei related both to the primary and accessory visual pathway. These RGC axon terminals are also able to take up, internalize and retrogradely transport ^{125}I-NGF following injection into either the superior colliculus or lateral geniculate nucleus (Carmignoto et al., 1991). Taken together these data support the hypothesis that NGF, or an NGF-like molecule, is produced by the target regions of RGCs, taken up, internalized and retrogradely transported to the cell bodiesthereby acting as a classical neurotrophic factor for RGCs.
   Exogenous NGF is also effective at the level of the visual cortex. The wide expression of the NGFR in visually-related nuclei, including the visual cortex, and the prevention by NGF treatment of the ocular dominance shift of area 17 neurons following MD suggest that NGF could be more generally involved in the phenomenon of neuronal cortical plasticity. The ocular dominance shift of cortical neurons consequent to MD could be due to competition among terminals of either eye for limited quantities of NGF produced by cortical neurons and/or glia. This implies that NGF receptors are expressed by geniculo-cortical axonal terminals. It cannot, however, be excluded that in this model NGF may not necessarily act in a classical way for geniculo-cortical afferents. NGF may regulate visual cortical plasticity by interacting with a different neuronal system, such as intrinsic cortical cells or cholinergic projections from the basal forebrain, both being also known to express the NGFR. Therefore, identification of the target cells for NGF effect as well as the cellular mechanisms underlying such an effect represent important goals for future studies.
   In conclusion, our results concerning the effect of exogenous NGF on the ocular dominance shift of area 17 neurons following MD give support to the hypothesis that synthesis and/or release of trophic molecules may be regulated by neural activity (for review see Purves, 1988) and raise the attractive possibility that NGF and, in general terms, neurotrophic factors are specifically involved in experience--dependent neuronal plasticity.

   NGF and NGFRs. The mechanism by which NGF elicits its neuronotrophic effects have not been fully resolved, but seems to be dependent on a receptor coupling event. A low molecular weight (75-kD) receptor is expressed by NGF responsive cells and has been classified as a low-affinity NGFR (dissociation constant Kd=10^{-9} M) (Chao et al., 1986; Radeke et al., 1987). Although with different efficiency, the low-affinity NGFR also binds BDNF (Rodriguez-Tebar et al., 1990) and NT-3 (Ernfors et al., 1990), the other two members of the so-called "NGF-family" of neurotrophins. Furthermore, the biological responsiveness to NGF depends upon its interaction with a high-affinity binding site (Kd = 10^{-11}M). The functional significance of the low-affinity receptor on a variety of peripheral and central neuronal populations is, therefore, still unclear. However, injections of the 192-IgG monoclonal antibody that recognizes the low-affinity NGFR (Meakin et al., 1991) induce immunosympathectomy in developing rats by in vivo sequestration of the p75 low-affinity NGFR (Johnson et al., 1986), suggesting that this molecule plays a crucial role in mediating responses to the neurotrophins. Support for this hypothesis derives from recent results showing that NGF binding specificity is conveyed by the trk oncogene product p140, the high molecular weight NGFR (Parada et al., 1991; Barbacid et al., 1991). Interestingly, the trk protein per se displays the binding properties of the a low-affinity receptor. Thus, high affinity NGF binding requires co-expression of the p75 low-affinity receptor and the trk proto-oncogene (Hempstead et al., 1991), with NGF responsive cells expressing both molecules.

Data on the NGFR distribution in the rat visual system were obtained using the 192-IgG monoclonal antibody recognizing the low-affinity NGFR (Meakin et al. 1991). Thus, no conclusions can be drawn concerning the expression of the p140 receptor in this system.

The NGFR expressed in the adult rat retina and visually related nuclei might also recognize other neurotrophins. The messenger RNAs encoding all components of the "NGF-family" of neuronotrophic factors, i.e. NGF, BDNF, and NT-3, have been detected in the retina of the adult rat (Maisonpierre et al., 1990), raising the possibility that these factors can be differentially involved in the establishment and maintenance of RGC connections.

However, the effects produced by exogenous NGF on both the survival of lesioned RGCs and the enhancement of axonal regeneration indicate that in the adult rat at least a subset of RGCs is NGF-sensitive, and would be expected to express the high-affinity NGFR.

REFERENCES

Berardi, N., Carmignoto, G., Domenici, L., and Maffei, L., 1990, The intraventricular NGF injections prevents the effects of monocular deprivation in the rat, J. Physiol., 422:9P.

Berardi, N., Carmignoto, G., Cremisi, F., Domenici, L., Maffei, L., Parisi, V., and Pizzorusso, T., 1991, NGF prevents the change in ocular dominance distribution induced by monocular deprivation in the rat visual cortex, J. Physiol., 434:14P.

Carmignoto, G., Maffei, L., Candeo, P., Canella, R., and Comelli, C., 1989, Effect of NGF on the survival of rat retinal ganglion cells following optic nerve section, J. Neurosci., 9:1263.

Carmignoto, G., Candeo, P., Comelli, M.C., Calderini, G., and Maffei, L., 1990, Expression of Nerve Growth Factor Receptor (NGFR) on adult rat retinal ganglion cell (RGC) terminals. 20th Annual Meeting of The Society for Neuroscience, Abstract 343.19.

Carmignoto, G., Comelli, M.C., Candeo, P., Cavicchioli, L., Yan, Q., Merighi, A., and Maffei, L., 1991, Expression of NGF Receptor and NGF Receptor mRNA in the developing and adult rat retina, Exp Neurol., 111:302.

Carmignoto, G., Canella R., Candeo P., and Comelli M.C., 1991, Expression of NGF receptor by retinal ganglion cells in the adult rat,

Proceeding 5th World Congress of Biological Psychiatry, Florence, 9-14 June, 1991, Excerpta Medica International Congress Series, in press.

Chandler, C.E, Parsons, L.M., Hosang, H., and Shooter E.M., 1984, A monoclonal antibody modulates the interactions of Nerve Growth Factor to PC12, J. Biol. Chem., 259:6882.

Chao, M.V., Bothwell, M.A., Ross, A.H., Koprowski, H., Lanahan, A.A., Buck, C.R., and Sehgal, A., 1986, Gene transfer and molecular cloning of the human NGF receptor, Science, 232:518.

Comelli, M.C., Bonfanti, L., Merighi, A., Carmignoto, G., and Maffei, L. 1990, The expression of Nerve Growth Factor Receptor (NGFR) mRNA is developmentally regulated and increased after optic nerve section, 20th Annual Meeting of the Society for Neuroscience, Abstract 343.18.

Ernfors, P., Ibànez, C.F., Ebendal, T., Olson, L., and Persson, H., 1990, Molecular cloning and neurotrophic activities of a protein with structural similarities to nerve growth factor: developmental and topographical expression in the brain, Proc. Natl. Acad. Sci. USA, 87:5454.

Greene, L.A., and Shooter, E.M., 1980, The nerve growth factor: biochemistry, synthesis and mechanism of action, Annu. Rev. Neurosci., 3:353.

Hall, S. and Berry, M., 1989, Electron microscopy study of the interaction of axons and glia at the site of anastomosisi between the optic nerve and cellular or acellular sciatic nerve grafts, J. Neurocytol., 18:171-184.

Hefti, F., 1986, Nerve growth factor promotes the survival of septal cholinergic neurons after fimbrial transections, J. Neurosci., 6:2155.

Hempstead, B.L., Martin-Zanca, D., Kaplan, D.R., Parada, L.F., and Chao, M.V., 1991, High affinity NGF binding requires coexpression of the trk proto-oncogene and the low affinity NGF receptor, Nature, 350:678.

Hubel, D.H., Wiesel, T.N., LeVay, S., 1977, Plasticity of ocular dominance columns in monkey striate cortex, Phil. Trans. R. Soc. B., 278:377.

Johnson, E.M., Osborne, P.A., Taniuchi, M., 1989, Destruction of sympathetic and sensory neurons in the developing rat by a monoclonal antibody against the nerve growth factor (NGF) receptor, Brain Res., 478:166-170.

Kaplan, D.R., Hempstead, B., Martin-Zanca, D., Chao, M.V., and Parada, L.F., 1991, The trk proto-oncogene product: a signal transducing receptor for Nerve Growth Factor, Science, 252:554.

Klein, R., Parada, L.F., Coulier, F., and Barbacid, M., 1989, trkB, a novel tyrosine protein kinase receptor expressed during mouse neural development, The EMBO J., 8(12):3701.

Large, T.H., Weskamp, G., Helder, J.C., Radeke, M.J., Misko, T.P., Shooter, E.M., and Reichardt, L.F., 1989, Structure and developmental expression of the nerve growth factor receptor in the chicken central nervous system, Neuron, 2:1123.

Levi-Montalcini, R., and Angeletti, P.U., 1968, Nerve growth Factor, Physiol Rev., 48:534.

Maisonpierre, P.C., Belluscio, L., Friedman, B., Alderson, R.F., Wiegand, S.J., Furth, M.E., Lindsay, R., and Yancopoulos, G.D., 1990, NT-3, BDNF, and NGF in the developing rat nervous system: parallel as well as reciprocal patterns of expression, Neuron, 5:501.

Meakin, S.O., and Shooter, E.M., 1991, Molecular investigations on the high-affinity nerve growth factor receptor, Neuron, 6:153.

Paradiso, M.A., Bear, M.F., Daniels, J.D., 1983, Effects of intracortical infusion of 6-Hydroxy-dopamine on the response of kittens visual cortex to monocular deprivation, Exp. Brain Res., 51:413.

Pioro, P., and Cuello, A.C., 1990, Distribution of nerve growth factor receptor-like immunoreactivity in the adult rat central nervous system. Effect of colchicine and correlation with the cholinergic system-I. Forebrain, Neuroscience, 1:57.

Purves, D., 1988, Body and Brain. A trophic theory of neural connections. Cambridge, MA: Harvard University Press.

Radeke, M.J., Misko, T.P., Hsu, C., Herzenberg, L.A., and Shooter, E.M., 1987, Gene transfer and molecular cloning of the rat nerve growth factor, Nature, 325:593.

Richardson, P.M., Issa, V.M. and Shemie, S., 1982, Regeneration and retrograde degeneration of axons in the rat optic nerve, J. Neurocytol., 11:949-966.

Rodriguez-Tebar, A., Dechant, G., and Barde, Y.A., 1990, Binding of brain-derived neurotrophic factor to the nerve growth factor receptor, Neuron, 4:487.

Siliprandi, R., Canella, R., Comelli, M.C., Zanoni, R., and Carmignoto, G., 1990, Nerve Growth Factor (NGF) effects on the function of cat retinal ganglion cells following ischemia, Invest. Opthalmol. Vis. Sci., 31(Suppl):139.

Schatteman, G.C., Gibbs, L., Lanahan, A.A., Claude, P., and Bothwell, M., 1988, Expression of NGF receptor in the developing and adult primate central nervous system, J. Neurosci., 8:860.

Thoenen, H., Bandtlow, C., and Heumann, R., 1987, The physiological function of nerve growth factor in central nervous system: comparison with the periphery, Rev. Physiol. Pharmacol., 109:145.

Turner, J.E., Delaney, R.K., and Johnson, J.E., 1980, Retinal ganglion cell response to nerve growth factor in the regenerating, and intact visual system of the goldfish ("carassius auratus"), Brain Res., 197:319.

Yan, Q., and Johnson, E.M.Jr, 1989, Immunohistochemical localization and biochemical characterization of nerve growth factor receptor in adult rat brain, J. Comp. Neurol., 290:585.

Yip, H.K., and Grafstein, B., 1982, Effect of nerve growth factor on regeneration of goldfish optic axons, Brain Res., 238:329.

IPSILATERAL PROJECTIONS DURING DEVELOPMENT AND REGENERATION OF

THE OPTIC NERVE OF THE CICHLID FISH HAPLOCHROMIS BURTONI

Claudia Wilm

Fac. of Biology, Dept. of Neurophysiology
Univ. of Bielefeld, P.O.Box 8640
4800 Bielefeld 1, Germany

INTRODUCTION

Projections from the retina into the ipsilateral tectum are not only restricted to mammals, but are widely distributed among vertebrates (for review see Wilm and Fritzsch, 1990). The mechanisms for the development of ipsilateral projections are less clear.

In mammals and birds a substantial ipsilateral projection into the colliculus superior (tectum opticum) develops initially (for review see Cowan et al., 1984). Later in development this projection is reduced or completely eliminated. Several authors suggested that part of the ipsilateral projection in mammals and the entire ipsilateral projection in the chick represent pathfinding errors of growing axons at the chiasma. Mammals are less suited for the confirmation of this hypothesis, because sorting mechanisms for the development of an ipsilateral projection have been likely evolved. Therefore, a clear distinction between fibers which grow by chance and fibers which are determined to grow ipsilaterally is difficult.

A suitable model, however, to answer the question, whether ipsilateral projections could be developed without the determination of a certain ganglion cell population to grow ipsilaterally, are bony fish like the cichlid Haplochromis burtoni.

Adult fish possess a completely crossed projection, except few fibers into the preoptic area at the midline of both brain halves (Wilm and Fritzsch, 1990). The following questions should be stressed in detail:

1. Can, comparably to amniotes, in this species of bony fish an enhanced ipsilateral projection be developed generally? (This issue was never thoroughly studied in any bony fish using a very sensitive tracer like DiI).

2. Under which experimental conditions can an enhanced ipsilateral projection be developed?

3. Under which conditions can this experimentally induced ipsilateral projection persist?

RESULTS AND DISCUSSION

The retinal projection was labeled with DiI in aldehyde fixed animals. The development of the retinal projection was studied between 6 and 10 days after fertilization and in 33 days old juveniles. Between 6 and 10 days the contralateral projection grew in a wide front without pioneers from the rostral pole across the centre of the tectum. At maximum 15 fibers projected via the optic tract into the ipsilateral tectum in any animal. In contrast, in amniotes several hundreds or thousands of retinal fibers project ipsilaterally. Even if it is taken into account that less ganglion cells project into the tectum during early development in fish than in birds or mammals, less than 15 ipsilateral fibers clearly do not represent an "enhanced" ipsilateral projection.

In bony fish, however, retina and tectum grow continuously, probably during their entire life. Although there were only few ipsilateral fibers during early development it could be probable that a few retinal fibers grow with each wave of newly formed ganglion cells ipsilaterally. But these ipsilateral fibers are subsequently eliminated. If in amniotes the contralateral projection is eliminated during the stage when an enhanced ipsilateral projection is developed, this enhanced projection persists, supposedly because of reduced competition (Cowan et al., 1984). This experiment could show, wether in bony fish ipsilateral fibers are continuously generated. I removed one eye in larvae and reared the animals up to 9 months. The eye increased in diameter from about 1 mm to 8 mm. Comparably to mammals the removal of one eye could lead to an enhanced ipsilateral projection in adult animals. Only 1 out of 19 animals showed this enhanced projection, which is not a considerable evidence for the hypothesis that substantial numbers of retinal fibers grew ipsilaterally during later development.

There are 2 main differences between the visual system of amniotes and that of bony fish. Probably these differences relate to the different ontogeny. The first difference is the mode of growth of retinal fibers. In amniotes hundred- thousands to millions of retinal fibers grow during few days through the chiasma. The visual system of bony fish on the other hand grows slowly, over years.

The second difference is the order of fibers in the optic nerve. Fibers in the optic nerve of mammals show less topological order. Axons of neighboring ganglion cells can be widely scattered in the optic nerve. In contrast, the optic nerve of cichlids is the best ordered nerve of vertebrates (Maggs and Scholes, 1986). And in addition growing fibers are restricted to a well defined region of the optic nerve. Slow growth and high order could be essential for the low incidence of errors in this bony fish. Therefore I studied next, whether the disturbance of the normal growth pattern of retinal fibers is sufficient for the development of an enhanced ipsilateral projection. For that purpose I crushed the optic nerve behind the eye in juvenile animals. The lesion disturbed the normal order of retinal fibers and retinal fibers regenerated throughout, rather than in a well defined region of the optic nerve. After 15 days a substantial ipsilateral projection had developed which covered the entire tectum. As well ganglion cells with small as ganglion cells with large dendritic fields projected ipsilaterally and they resided from the entire retina. While during ontogeny only few fibers had projected ipsilaterally, a substantial ipsilateral projection developed during regeneration. No certain ganglion cell population was determined to project ipsilaterally. Changing the ordered growth pattern in the optic nerve was apparently sufficient for the development of the ipsilateral projection.

This picture changed dramatically after 3 to 4 weeks. The ipsilateral projection disappeared from the caudal and central tectum. Many fibers ended blindly in the caudal tectum. After 2 months the ipsilateral projection could no longer be traced with HRP or fluorescent dextran-amines. Apparently the intact contralateral projection of this tectum inhibited the ipsilateral projection to establish permanent connections.

To study the ipsilateral projection after removal of the native contralateral projection I simultaneously lesioned one optic nerve and removed the other eye. Now the ipsilateral projection persisted in the entire tectum even after 1 1/2 years. Complex terminal fields had been developed.

An ipsilateral projection also persisted when both optic nerves were crushed. From each eye retinal fibers regenerated into both tecta. In 80% of these animals the ipsilateral projection persisted, but was less pronounced than for a complete removal of the native contralateral projection. Four months the ipsi- and contralateral projections were separated into patches.

After nerve crush, retinal fibers regenerated into both tecta, contra- and ipsilaterally. Ipsilateral fibers could not establish stable terminations as long as the contralateral projection remained undisturbed. A stable ipsilateral projection developed either after removal of the native contralateral projection of this tectum or after its disturbance, that is after bilateral nerve crush. After bilateral nerve crush, both projections in one tectum initially overlapped but then segregated.

SUMMARY

1. During development of the visual projection no enhanced ipsilateral projection occurred in Haplochromis burtoni in contrast to amniotes. This corresponds to the high degree of order of fibres in the optic nerve of cichlids. The slow and continuous proliferation of ganglion cells resulted into a nearly error free crossing of fibers from the first outgrowth of ganglion cell axons.

2. Disorganization of the fibre order by crushing the optic nerve and thereby induced disturbed growth pattern lead to considerable numbers of ipsilaterally regenerating fibers.

3. For the stabilization of the ipsilateral projection in this experimental situation it is essential that the native contralateral projection is either disturbed or completely eliminated. Ipsilateral and contralateral projection subsequently separated from one another. Therefore, the development of a permanent ipsilateral projection, is a two-step process: at first fibers grow ipsilaterally at the diencephalon and at second the ipsilateral projection has to establish stable connections.

4. Finally this model implies that ipsilateral projections may develop as a stochastic process in vertebrates in which large numbers of relatively disordered fibers arrive together at the chiasma. How far this actually occurs during the development of the visual projection of many vertebrates because of missing or sloppy correction mechanisms for aberrant projections remains to be elucidated.

References

Cowan, W.M., Fawcett, J.W., O'Leary, D.D.M., and Stanfield, B.B., Regressive events in neurogenesis. Science, 225:1258-1256 (1984).

Maggs, A., and Scholes, J., Glia domains and nerve fibre patterns in the fish retinotectal pathway. J. Neurosci., 6:424-438 (1986).

Wilm, C., and Fritzsch, B., Ipsilateral retinofugal projections in a percomorph bony fish: their experimental induction, specificity and maintenance. Brain Behav. Evol., 36:271-299 (1990).

ABNORMAL ORGANIZATION OF THE HUMAN RETINA IN A GENETIC DISORDER (BLOCH-

SULZBERGER SYNDROME)

A. Silva-Araújo*, J.M. Lopes**, J. Salgado-Borges*,
M.A. Tavares***

*Department of Ophthalmology, Medical School of Porto
**Department of Pathology, Medical School of Porto
***Department of Anatomy, Medical School of Porto

INTRODUCTION

Bloch-Sulzberger syndrome (incontinentia pigmenti) is an autosomal dominant X-linked disorder, characterized by pleiotropic clinical manifestations[1] which, being related with an ecto-mesodermic dysplasia, frequently displays visual changes[1]. The most typical end-stage of the ocular involvement leading to disruption of the retina cytoarchitetonics and allied functional impairment is due to the presence of a retrolental mass – either designated as persistence and hyperplasia of the primary vitreous, pseudoglioma or retrolental fibroplasia – with detachment of a dysplasic retina[2-7].

Different authors point that these morphological changes correspond to the end-stage of early post-natal triggered vascular abnormalities[4,6,8,9], whose cause still remains obscure. In fact, retinal vascular changes and disarrangement of pigmentar epithelium (RPE) are the most outstanding morphological changes[3,4,10]. However, the fully characterization of the origin of the pigmented cells, specific localization of gliotic areas and discrimination between neo-vessels vs persistence of embryonic vessels, were not previously fully established mainly due to the non-specificity of the anatomopathologic methods available for the study of this entity. To date, recently developed immunocytochemical methods can provide a new insight on the above mentioned issues.

By applying specific immunocytochemical stainings this study tries to go one step further in aiming to characterize the extent of the retinal disarrangement and allied optic nerve changes in two familiar cases of this entity.

MATERIAL AND METHODS

Morphological evaluations were performed in the left eyes of two patients (mother/daughter) which underwent enucleation at the age of 12 months due to suspected retinoblastoma. Both eyes were fixed in 10% buffered formaldehyde and paraffin sections were stained with hematoxylin-eosin; other paraffin embedded sections were dewaxed in xylene, rehydrated in graded ethanols to distilled water and immunostained for light microscopy using glial fibrillary acidic protein (GFAP), factor

The Changing Visual System, Edited by P. Bagnoli and
W. Hodos, Plenum Press, New York, 1991

VIII and low-molecular weight cytokeratin, by applying avidin-biotin methods.

RESULTS AND DISCUSSION

Many retinal abnormalities have been previously described in this syndrome [1]. To our knowledge these descriptions were based on studies performed with classical histological methods. In the present study the morphological organization/disorganization of the retinas of both eyes was strikingly similar. In accord with other cases reported in the literature [2-7] they were completely detached, funnel-shaped, thickened and folded, delineating cystic-like structures.

The retinas appeared incorporated in a whitish membrane-like formation extended into the retrolental space which protruded into a dense and collapsed vitreous. This membrane, located at the vitreo-retinal interface, was appended and continuous with the inner retinal layers; it consisted of cells with immunoreactivity to PGFA or factor VIII (Figs. 1,2), disclosing thus its vascular and glial origin, respectively. Probably due to the presence of such structure, the infolded retina showed a marked disruption of the inner layers where marked gliosis was evident (Fig. 1); yet, despite these profound morphological changes it was possible to identify areas where the nerve fiber layer, the ganglionar cell layer and the inner plexiform layer were rather preserved. However, the outer retinal layers formed a series of tubular-like structures or rosettes thrown secondarily into folds. Amid these areas the gliotic changes were also remarkable and contained "nests" of pigmented cells immunoreactive for low-molecular weight cytokeratin well in keeping with their putative RPE origin (Fig. 3). Furthermore the subretinal space with clusters of RPE cells also immunoreactive for cytokeratin, was completely filled with a proteinaceous gel. The RPE, with increased lipofuscin pigment, showed proliferative areas displaying papilar or placoid appearance. The optic nerves showed areas of intense neovascularization and sectorial gliosis diffusely reactive for PGFA (Fig. 4).

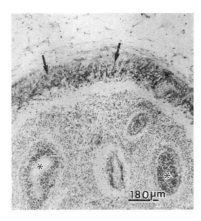

Fig. 1 - Retinal rosettes(*) and gliosis of vi-treo-retinal-inter-face (arrows) deco-rated by PGFA. Avidin-Biotin.

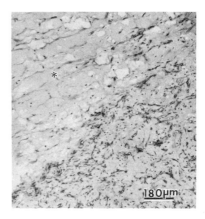

Fig. 2 - Endothelial cells, of the neo-vascu-lar epiretinal mem-brane, immunoreac-tive for factor VIII. Condensed cor-tical vitreous (*). Avidin-Biotin.

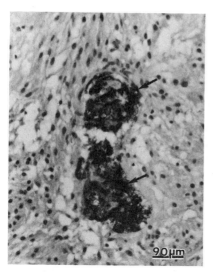 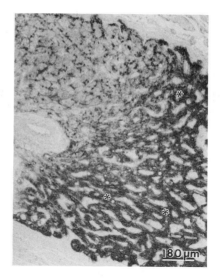

Fig. 3 - Intra-retinal RPE
cells (arrows),
strongly reactive
for low-molecular
weight cytokeratin,
enmeshed in gliotic
areas. Avidin-Biotin.

Fig. 4 - Sectorial gliosis
(*) of the optic
nerve diffusely
reactive for PGFA.
Avidin-Biotin.

There is still controversy in the establishment of the etiopathogenic factors underlying this disorder; major drawbacks are, as for the cases herein described, the wide umbrella of retinal abnormalities coexisting in the end-stage of the retinal dysplastic detachement. According to some authors the retinal dysplasia and allied detachement could result from abnormalities of the RPE [10], which modulates the retina development. Alternatively, others favour that the failure of the post-natal development of the temporal part of the retina might be the cause of capillary non-perfusion areas leading to pre-retinal fibrogliosis [4,8,9]. As for retinopathy of prematurity we think that the persistence of the vascular abnormalities and organization of the avascular retina into a contracting scar are main pathogenic events for the retinal desorganization and detachement. However, the associated intra-retinal RPE proliferation observed in both cases might support the aforementioned abnormalities of the retinal vessels.

Regardless the mechanisms underlying this situation the severe changes of the retinal organization leading to the end-stage of retinal detachement and disruption of the retinal circuitries, are important morphological bases for the functional impairment which is associated with this situation.

REFERENCES

1. R. G. Carney Jr., Incontinentia pigmenti: a world statistical
   analysis, Arch. Dermatol. 112: 535 (1976).

2. J. G. Cole, H. G. Cole, Incontinentia pigmenti associated with
   changes in the posterior chamber of the eye, Am. J. Ophthalmol. 47:
   321 (1959).

3. C. A. Brown, Incontinentia pigmenti: the development of pseudo-glioma, Br. J. Ophthalmol. 72: 452 (1988).

4. J. François, Incontinentia pigmenti (Bloch-Sulzberger syndrome) and retinal changes, Br. J. Ophthalmol. 68: 19 (1984).

5. S. T. Jones, Retrolental membrane associated with Bloch-Sulzberger syndrome (incontinentia pigmenti), Am. J. Ophthalmol. 62: 330 (1966).

6. A. Spallone, Incontinentia pigmenti (Bloch-Sulzberger syndrome): seven cases reports from one family, Br. J. Ophthalmol. 71: 629 (1987).

7. P. H. Zweifach, Incontinentia pigmenti. Its association with retinal dysplasia, Am. J. Ophthalmol. 62: 716 (1966).

8. R. C. Watzke, T. S. Stevens, R. G. Carney, Retinal vascular changes of incontinentia pigmenti, Arch. Ophthalmol. 94: 743 (1976).

9. R. B. Jain, G. S. Willets, Fundus changes in incontinentia pigmenti (Bloch-Sulzberger syndrome): a case report, Br. J. Ophthalmol. 62: 622 (1978).

10. O. Mensheha-Manhert, M. M. Rodrigues, J. A. Shields, G. M. Shannon, R. P. Mirabelli, Retinal pigment epithelium in incontinentia pigmenti. Am. J. Ophthalmol. 79: 571 (1975).

VISUAL SYSTEM IN SOME SYSTEMIC DISEASES

Fatma Ferkan Demircioğlu

Gazi University
School of Medicine
Beşevler, Ankara, Turkey

BEHÇET'S DISEASE

Behçet's disease was initially described by a Turkish dermatologist, Behçet, in 1937 as a triad of oral ulcers, genital ulcers and hypopyon uveitis and it has subsequently been confirmed in the medical literature.[1] Oral ulcers are the most common clinical feature. They are recurrent and painful, ranging from 2 mm to 12 mm in size, often coming in crops. The genital ulcerations have similar features, but are less often diagnosed.[1,2] The skin disease can be erythema nodosum, superficial thrombophlebitis, pyoderma, or a phenomenon called pathergy, which is defined as the presence of a pustule after breaking of the skin by a needle, such as in blood drawing. The arthritis is an asymmetric, nondeforming, large joint polyarthritis that is frequently steroid responsive. Cardiac involvement and central nervous system disease have been reported.[3] Vascular disease is common and can present as a migratory superficial thrombophlebitis, major vessel thrombosis, superior and inferior vena cava syndrome, arterial thrombosis, aortic aneurysm or even peripheral gangrene.[2–4] Familial occurrences and platelet disturbances have been cited as important predisposing factors in the pathogenesis of Behçet's disease.[5–8]

The most common ocular manifestations are iridocyclitis, with or without hypopyon, and retinal vasculitis.[1–9] Conjunctivitis, keratitis, and scleritis have occasionally been described but are less common.[1–9] The most common ocular manifestation is an uveitis. This presents either with or without a hypopyon. Early series commonly described hypopyon uveitis, but more recent series have decreased the frequency of hypopyon uveitis. Posterior segment lesions have also been described in Behçet's disease.[9] The characteristic posterior segment lesion is retinal vasculitis which may involve both veins and arteries with arterial occlusions and retinal necrosis. Occasionally, secondary neovascularization and retinal detachment will develop. The disease is most often bilateral. The pathology of the lesion is a perivascular infiltrate with lymphocytes and plasma cells associated with retinal necrosis. Early lesions show a sparse round cell infiltrate of the retina, choroid, and chamber angle, while later lesions show extensive loss of retinoarchitecture with neovascularization. The end stage of the disease is a blind, painful eye with secondary glaucoma, rubeosis, and retinal detachment. The natural history of Behçet's disease is poor. The majority of patients will lose all or part of their vision within five years.

HYPERTENSION

The present perception about the pathogenesis and maintenance of hypertension is 1that there are abnormalities in the control systems that fail to reduce hypertension to normal when tension elevates.[10] The hypertension produces damages in the arteries and vascular system. It causes premature morbidity and mortality, heart failure, renal failure, strokes, heart attack and fundus changes.[11,12] Traditionally, the arteriolar changes of hypertension have been considered to result from vasospasm, whereas the arteriosclerotic changes result from thickening of the arteriolar wall.[13] It is impossible to consider them separately. Diffuse arteriolar narrowing is a hallmark of hypertensive retinopathy. With long standing hypertension, elastic tissue of the intima of the arteriole forms multiple concentric layers. The muscular layer can be replaced by collagen fibers, and the intima can be replaced by hyaline thickening. These changes result in the "onion skin" appearance. As the arteriolar wall becomes thickened, the light reflex loses its brightness and becomes broader, duller and more diffuse such as "copper wire" in appearance. As the process continues, the arteriole assumes the appearance of a "silver wire." Increasing thickening of the vessel wall causes venous compression, the appearance of arteriovenous nicking (Gunn's sign) and deflection of the venule as it crosses the arteriole (Salus's sign).[13] Retinal micro-aneurysms and macro-aneurysms may also be associated with hypertension. Malignant hypertension characteized by fibrinoid necrosis of the arterioles which is not common in the retinal arterioles. Retinal hemorrhages such as "cotton-wool" spots, retinal capillary occlusion and papilledema are seen in this type of hypertension.

Numerous attempts have been made to organize the retinal changes of hypertension into a clinically useful classification. The Keith-Wagener-Barker classification was based on the level of severity of retinal findings of a group of patients with hypertension.[9,13,14] Their classification encompassed four categories. In patients with grade I, there is minimal narrowing of the retinal arterioles, increasing in central light reflex with some irregularity of the walls of the arterioles. This group of patients generally have mild hypertension. In patients with grade II, retinal abnormalities include the changes listed for group one, with more definite focal narrowing in "copper and silver wiring" appearance, arteriovenous nicking (Gunn's sign) and the deflection of the venule as it crosses the arteriole (Salus's sign). Patients in this group are generally asymptomatic. In patients with grade III, abnormalities include the previous ones along with hemorrhages and exudates. Hemorrhages may occur in the inner retinal layer in a characteristic flame pattern and focal ischemia in the nerve fiber layer may result in "cotton-wool" microinfarcts. Many of these patients have cardiac, cerebral, or renal dysfunctions. In patients with grade IV, the previously listed abnormalities are more severe. The cotton-wool spots around the macula are termed a "macula star." The optic nerve head becomes swollen and edematous and there is papilledema.[9,13,14] The cardiac, the cerebral and the renal disease are more severe. The patients who have retinopathy had five-year untreated survivals of 85, 50, 13 and 0 percent.[14] Until the etiology of essential hypertension is known, its treatment and the reduction of the development of its visual disturbances will necessarily be empiric, but through increasing insight into the mechanism of hypertension and into the pharmacology of the drugs used to treat it, we are emerging from a period of "blind empiricism" into an era of enlightened empiricism.[14] Although improvement in the diagnosis and treatment of hypertension has reduced the mortality and morbidity rates, the management of hypertension remains a challenge for all physicians.

DIABETES MELLITUS

Diabetes mellitus is a kind of systemic metabolic disorder which involves the small vessels and capillary bed of the various major organs of the body.[15] During the period of this systemic disease, many of the patients with diabetes mellitus have severe visual, renal, cardiac and peripheral artery disturbances. Among these disturbances, the most important one is visual complication which is termed "diabetic retinopathy."[15-17] In diabetic retinopathy, the fundus abnormalities are divided into two subtypes. The initial or first stage of the fundus abnormalities is called "background diabetic retinopathy" or "nonproliferative diabetic retinopathy."[9] The late or second stage of the fundus abnormalities is termed "proliferative diabetic retinopathy" (PDR).

Background Diabetic Retinopathy

In background or nonproliferative diabetic retinopathy, all of the fundus abnormalities result from pathologic changes in the retinal blood vessels. Two pathophysiologic processes, the first, retinal vessel closure, and the second, abnormal retinal vascular permeability, are seen in background diabetic retinopathy.[9] The earliest detectable vessel closure in diabetic retinopathy occurs at the level of the retinal capillary bed. As a response to focal capillary closure, microaneurysm formations tend to cluster around these small nonperfusion areas. Dilation of the adjacent capillary bed often accompanies capillary closure in diabetic retinopathy. In general, arteriolar closure increases the risk of proliferative changes. Generalized venous dilation and branch or central retinal venous occlusion may develop. The other most frequent finding in background diabetic retinopathy is of retinal hemorrhages. The hemorrhages may assume a dot, blot or flame configuration. The hemorrhages indicate the preproliferative stage of the disease and increased risk of neovascularization. Foveolar hemorrhages cause a decrease in the retinal visual acuity. Another characteristic ocular manifestation in background diabetic retinopathy is intraretinal microvascular abnormalities (IRMA). IRMA describes the irregular segmental dilation of the retinal capillary bed. These dilated vessels represent intraretinal neovascularization or shunt vessels. The dilated vascular segments also occur in a partially occluded capillary bed in the same manner as the microaneurysms which constitute one of the fundus signs of retinal ischemia. They may also leak and cause retinal edema. IRMA also is considered a component of preproliferative retinopathy. One of the other important signs of background retinopathy is macular edema. The edema is caused by a breakdown of vessel–retinal barriers, allowing leakage of fluid and plasma into the surrounding retina. Macular edema divides into two subtypes. These are focal and diffuse types of edema. Focal edema refers to localized areas of retinal thickening resulting from microaneurysm or IRMA. Diffuse edema is more widespread retinal thickening caused by a generalized leakage from dilated capillaries throughout the posterior pole.[9] The other maculopathy besides macular edema is macular ischemia. Macular ischemia happens when arterioles as well as capillaries become occluded. In the extreme cases, most of the posterior pole may lose its retinal circulation and profound loss of vision may occur.

Proliferative Diabetic Retinopathy

Proliferative diabetic retinopathy, a term which refers to the presence of newly-formed blood vessels and/or fibrous tissue arising from the retina or optic disc.[9] Endothelial proliferation and new vessel formation are ischemia of the inner retinal layers secondary to closure of the retinal capillary bed. The natural course of proliferative diabetic retinopathy follows four fundamental processes. These changes are outlined as follows. Firstly, the proliferation and the regression typical of new vessels are seen.

Secondly, the proliferation of fibrous tissue accompanying the new vessel develops. Thirdly, the formations of adhesions develop between the fibrovascular proliferation and the posterior vitreous surface. At last, the contraction of the posterior vitreous surface occurs, associated with proliferations. At the end stage of the disease, marked loss of vision has occurred. This loss is best explained by proliferative diabetic retinopathy due to retinal ischemia.

REFERENCES

1. H.H. Behçet, Über rezidivierende aphthöse durch virus-verursachte geschwüre am mund, am auge und an den genitalien, *Derm. Wochenschr.*, 105:1152 (1937).
2. F.F. Demircioğlu, E. Böke, M. Demircin, S. Dağslai, T. Küğükali, Abdominal aortic aneurysm with inferior vena obstruction, *Angiology*, 40:227 (1989).
3. F.F. Demircioğlu, B. Komsuoğlu, S. Dündar, Myocardial functions in Behçet's syndrome, *Cerrahpaşa Tip Fak. Derg.*, 14:7 (1983).
4. F.F. Demircioğlu, E. Böke, M. Demircin, S. Dağsali, Aortic aneurysm due to Behçet's syndrome, *Turk. Arrh. Derm. Syph.*, 20:175 (1986).
5. S.V. Dündar, F.F. Demircioğlu, K. Özerkan, Familial Behçet's symdrome, *GATA Mil. Med. Acad. Bul.*, 21:287 (1979).
6. F.F. Demircioğlu, T. Gürsel, M.A. Gürer, V. Sepici, M. Bozkurt, A. Gülekon, Platelet aggregation in Behçet's disease, First National Congress of Behçet's Disease, (1987). Istanbul, Türkiye.
7. F.F. Demircioğlu, T. Gürsel, M.A. Gürer, V. Sepici, M. Bozkurt, A. Gülekon, Platelet functions in Behçet's disease, Second Mediterranean Congress of Angiology, ANG-(369), (1990). Antalya, Türkiye.
8. F.F. Demircioğlu, T. Gürsel, M.A. Gürer, V. Sepici, M. Bozkurt, A. Gülekon, The physiological basis of vascular endothelium in patients with vasculitis, NATO ASI, Vascular Endothelium, (1990). Corfu, Greece.
9. D.A. Jabs, R.P. Murphy, E.Y. Chew, G.H. Bresnick, M.D. Davis, The rheumatic diseases, hypertension, background diabetic retinopathy, proliferative retinopathy, in "Retina, Volume 2: Medical Retina," S.J. Ryan, A.P. Schachat, R.P. Murphy, A. Patz, eds., C.V. Mosby Company, St. Louis (1989).
10. F.F. Demircioğlu, Hypertension, *Karayollari Vakfi Derg.*, 1:38 (1988).
11. F.F. Demircioğlu, N. Ülkü, A. Metin, Epidemiology of cardiovascular disease in elementary schools in Ankara, *T.C.D.D. Hosp. Bull.*, 1:103 (1989).
12. S. Kuştimur, H. Elhani, F.F. Demircioğlu, Immunoglobulin leves in hypertension, *Türkiye Klinikleri*, 5:225 (1987).
13. F.F. Demircioğlu, Fundus changes in hypertensive patients, NATO ASI, The Changing Visual System: Maturation and Aging in the Central Nervous System, (1991). S. Martino al Cimino (Viterbo), Italy.
14. W.B. Anderson, Examination of the retina, in "The Heart," J.W. Hurst, R.B. Logue, eds., Sixth Edition, McGraw Hill Book Company, New York (1986).
15. Ş. Zileli, F.F. Demircioğu, N. Adalar, The relationship between glucose tolerance test and free fatty acids in patients with diabetes mellitus, *Hac. Med./Surg. Bull.*, 4:280 (1971).
16. F.F. Demircioğlu, A. Karamehmetoğlu, G. Gürsel, N. Nazli, Glucose tolerance, test and electrocardiogram, *Hac. Med./Surg. Bull.*, 9:137 (1976).
17. S. Kuştimur, H. Elhani, F.F. Demircioğlu, Serum immunoglobin levels in patients with diabetes mellitus under different treatments, *J. Turk. Bioch.*, 3:39 (1986).

EFFECTS OF INTRAOCULAR ACTIVITY BLOCKADE ON THE MORPHOLOGY OF DEVELOPING LGN NEURONS IN THE CAT

Kathrin Herrmann, Rachel O.L. Wong and Carla J. Shatz

Department of Neurobiology, Stanford University School of Medicine
Stanford, CA 94305

INTRODUCTION

Spontaneous neuronal activity is known to play a major role in the construction and final functioning of neuronal circuits, especially those that are formed through interactions of competing inputs. The requirement for neuronal activity in the formation of highly specific connections found in the adult has been well documented in the development of the cat visual system. Shatz and Stryker (1988) and Sretavan et al. (1988) showed that prenatal intracranial infusion of the sodium channel blocker tetrodotoxin, TTX, blocks the segregation of retinogeniculate afferents into eye-specific layers in the lateral geniculate nucleus, LGN, that normally form before birth in the cat. In addition, Stryker and Harris (1986) demonstrated that the formation of the ocular dominance columns in layer 4 of the cat visual cortex can be prevented if retinal ganglion cell discharges are eliminated by intraocular injections of TTX within the critical period postnatally. These studies have clearly shown that action potential activity is required for the elimination of excessive <u>axonal</u> branches and the remodeling of the <u>axonal</u> arbor. Little, however, is known about the role of activity on dendritic development. In this paper we wished to determine whether action potential activity from the retina also influences the morphological development of the <u>dendritic</u> arbors of LGN neurons.

MATERIAL AND METHODS

To investigate whether intraocular activity blockade affects the dendritic morphology of LGN neurons in the A- and A1-laminae, kittens received repeated (every 2-3 days) monocular injections of increasing amounts (1.0 to 2.5 µl) of TTX (Calbiochem, #584411, 5mM) starting at P7 (postnatal

The Changing Visual System, Edited by P. Bagnoli and
W. Hodos, Plenum Press, New York, 1991

day 7) under halothane (1-2% in O_2). At P28 (n=4) or P35 (n=2), three or four weeks after continuous action potential blockade, the animals were anesthetized with nembutal, and perfused with 0.1M phosphate buffer followed by 4% paraformaldehyde. To reveal the dendritic morphology of LGN neurons, we cut 200 μm thick vibratome slices of the fixed tissue, impaled single neurons in the LGN with intracellular electrodes filled with 5% Lucifer Yellow and subsequently photooxidized the dye into a stable DAB product (Maranto, 1982). Well stained cells were drawn with the aid of a camera lucida, and their location within the LGN was determined after Nissl staining. The morphology of neurons in the silenced and non-silenced laminae was compared by measurements of soma size, dendritic length, spine density and branching frequency. To help morphologically classify different neuron types in the LGN, we also injected fluorescent latex microspheres into area 18 of 2 animals, 3-6 days prior to perfusion, in order to retrogradely label and subsequently dye-fill presumptive Y cells (the only LGN neurons known to project to area 18). In addition to these TTX-treated animals, we also studied the morphology of LGN neurons in 1 week old normal, untreated kittens to establish their dendritic structure at the time when we started our TTX treatment, and to test directly whether TTX arrests the morphological development of LGN neurons.

RESULTS

The cat LGN is composed of a heterogeneous population of neurons, both physiologically and anatomically (e.g. Guillery, 1966, Friedlander et al., 1981). At 4 weeks of age, all morphologically distinct cell types present in the adult, could already be distinguished (Friedlander, 1982). For example, class 1 cells (see fig. 1), characterized by a large soma of up to 35 μm in diameter that gives rise to up to 10 primary, radially oriented dendrites, as well as class 2 and 3 cells with their characteristic grape-like appendages (Guillery, 1966) could be observed after dye filling. For the quantitative comparison of neurons in the TTX and non-TTX laminae, we analysed the class 1 cells (as presumed Y cells) separately from the other cell types, because they could be most readily identified. All the other cell classes were pooled and analysed as a single group.

Soma size of LGN neurons was significantly reduced in the TTX laminae as compared with the non-TTX laminae, confirming earlier reports based on Nissl staining (Kuppermann and Kasamatsu, 1984). Measurements of the soma area of cells from corresponding classes revealed that the size of all LGN neurons in TTX laminae was relatively smaller in the TTX as compared with the non-TTX laminae. This result points to the idea that the effects of monocular deprivation and TTX blockade on LGN soma size are different, because after monocular deprivation only Y cells are thought to be affected. However, neither dendritic field radius nor bránching frequency was affected by TTX treatment. Spine density, on the other hand, was lower in neurons of the TTX laminae, although this result was statistically significant only for class 1 cells.

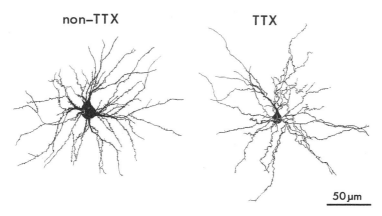

non–TTX   TTX

50 μm

Fig.1. Comparison of camara lucida drawings of class 1 neurons in the kitten TTX (right) and non-TTX (left) LGN laminae of a P28 kitten, subjected to continuous intraocular action potential activity blockade between P7 and P28.

The apparent failure of TTX treatment to interfere with dendritic growth may be because LGN neurons had already achieved a high degree of maturity by P7, the age when we started our TTX injections. However, by filling cells with Lucifer Yellow, we found that many cells at P7 still appeared immature and could not always be easily assigned to a specific cell class, although some clearly resembled those present at 4 or 5 weeks. Therefore, for the quantification of the dendritic parameters we pooled all these cell types together and compared the data with those from P28 and P35 neurons after TTX treatment. At P7, LGN neurons were significantly smaller in all measured parameters, such as soma size, dendritic field radius and spine density when compared to either the TTX or the non-TTX neurons, suggesting that these parameters can increase independently of action potential activity.

SUMMARY AND DISCUSSION

LGN neurons grow significantly within the first postnatal month, with respect to both soma size and dendritic parameters. After 3-4 weeks of continuous intraocular action potential blockade with TTX during the first postnatal month, LGN neurons in the silenced TTX laminae had a significantly smaller soma size, confirming earlier reports (Kuppermann and Kasamatsu,1984). The comparison between cell size measurements at P7, the age at which we started our TTX treatment, and P28 or 35 indicates, that LGN neurons in the silenced laminae do grow, but their increase in soma size is attenuated. However, neurons in the silenced (TTX) lamina, all developed numerous dendritic spines, elaborate branching patterns and dendritic field areas much larger than those at P7.

Therefore, even in the absence of afferent action potential activity, the dendrites of LGN neurons continue to grow to a similar complexity as that seen in the non-silenced or normal LGN laminae. Thus, under TTX blockade, LGN soma size is dramatically reduced, but, in contrast, dendritic parameters are not affected. Moreover, soma size is not likely to reflect the extent of the dendritic arborization, but is more likely to reflect the axonal arborization, since the effect of unilateral intraocular TTX injections is highly likely to cause LGN axonal branches to be smaller than normal, as it occurs with monocular visual deprivation (Le Vay et al., 1980). If so, then the mechanisms that control the refinement of axonal and dendritic arbors may be quite different. The same conclusion was obtained for retinal ganglion cells after comparing their dendritic growth in the presence or absence of action potential activity (Wong et al., 1991). These results indicate that action potentials from the retina are not required for the dendritic development of LGN neurons, but they do not imply that other forms of changes in membrane potential such as synaptic input from sources other than the retina , do not in fact play a role in this process. Finally, Archer et al. (1982) and Dubin et al., (1986) reported an incomplete segregation of ON and OFF responses in the LGN after postnatal monocular TTX blockade. Because, in general, the dendritic morphology of LGN neurons in the present study appears unaffected in TTX treated kittens, it is likely that the changes in the physiological behavior of LGN cells is due to aberrant ganglion cell input (Kalil et al., 1986) rather than abnormal remodeling in the dendritic structure itself.

Acknowledgements

Supported by a NATO fellowship (KH), a fellowship from Fight for Sight - Research Division of the National Society to prevent Blindness (KH), a C.J. Martin fellowship (NH&MRC) (ROLW), NSF grant BNS 8919508 (CJS), and a grant from the Alzheimer's Association (CJS).

REFERENCES

Archer, S.M., Dubin, M.W., and Stark, L.A., 1982, Abnormal development of kitten retinogeniculate connectivity in the absence of action potentials, Science, 217: 743.

Dubin, M.W., Stark, L.A., and Archer, S.A., 1986, A role for action-potential activity in the development of neuronal connections in the kitten retinogeniculate pathway, J. Neurosci.,6: 1021.

Friedlander, M.J., 1982, Structure of physiologically classified neurons in the kitten dorsal lateral geniculate nucleus, Nature, 300: 180.

Friedlander, M.J., Lin, C-S., Stanford, L.R., and Sherman, S.M., 1981, Morphology of functionally identified neurons in lateral geniculate nucleus of the cat, J. Neurophysiol., 46: 80.

Guillery, R.W., 1966, A study of Golgi preparations from the dorsal lateral geniculate nucleus of the adult cat, J. Comp. Neurol., 128: 21.

Kalil, R.E., Dubin, M.W., Scott, S., and Stark, L.A., 1986, Elimination of action potentials blocks the structural development of retinogeniculate synapses, Nature, 323: 156.

Kuppermann, B.D., and Kasamatsu, T., 1984, Changes in geniculate cell size following brief monocular blockade of retinal activity in kittens, Nature,306: 465.

Le Vay, S., Wiesel, T.N., and Hubel, D.H., 1980, The development of ocular dominance columns in normal and visually deprived monkeys, J. Comp. Neurol.,191: 1.

Maranto, A.R., 1982, Neuronal mapping: A photooxidation reaction makes lucifer yellow useful for electron microscopy, Science, 217: 953.

Shatz, C.J., and Stryker, M.P., 1988, Prenatal tetrodotoxin infusion blocks the segregation of retinogeniculate afferents, Science, 244: 87.

Sretavan, D.W., Shatz, C.J., and Stryker, M.P.,1988, Modification of retinal ganglion morphology by prenatral infusion of tetrodotoxin, Nature, 336: 468.

Stryker, M.P., and Harris, W.A., 1986, Binocular impulse blockade prevents the formation of ocular dominance columns in cat visual cortex, J. Neurosci., 6: 2117.

Wong, R.O.L., Herrmann, K., and Shatz, C.J., 1991, Remodeling of retinal ganglion cell dendrites in the absence of action potential activity, J. Neurobiol., in press.

DEVELOPMENT OF ORIENTATION-SPECIFIC NEURONAL RESPONSES

IN FERRET PRIMARY VISUAL CORTEX

Barbara Chapman and Michael P. Stryker

Neuroscience Graduate Program
Department of Physiology
University of California
San Francisco, CA 94143-0444
USA

Neurons in the primary visual cortex of higher mammals respond best to light-dark borders at particular orientations. These orientation-specific responses are present at birth in the monkey (Hubel et al., 1977), and can be recorded by the end of the first postnatal week in the cat (Hubel and Wiesel, 1963; for review see Fregnac and Imbert, 1984). Since it is difficult to perform electrophysiological recordings in very young animals, we have chosen to study the development of oriented visual cortical responses in the ferret. The ferret visual system is quite similar to that of the cat (Law et al., 1988), but the ferret is born approximately three weeks earlier in development.(Linden et al., 1981).

In order to study the normal development of orientation selectivity, we have looked at response properties of primary visual cortex neurons in ferrets of different ages. Radial microelectrode penetrations were made through cortical area 17 in anaesthetized, paralyzed animals, and extracellular responses of neurons to moving light bars were recorded. Orientation tuning histograms were compiled, showing the responses of each neuron to 36 different stimulus orientations. Since orientation tuning is a circular function with a period of 180°, we quantified the degree of orientation selectivity of each neuron by fourier transforming the data from the tuning histograms, and taking the percentage of the total harmonic power which was found at the second harmonic as a measure of orientation selectivity (Worgotter and Eysel, 1987). The measure correlates very well with the degree of orientation selectivity subjectively determined by examining the orientation tuning histograms, with neurons having greater than 30% of total power at the second harmonic showing clearly oriented responses.

The earliest age at which visual cortical responses could be recorded was postnatal day 23, a developmental stage comparable to day of birth in the cat (Linden et al., 1981). At this age no clearly orientation-specific responses were

The Changing Visual System, Edited by P. Bagnoli and
W. Hodos, Plenum Press, New York, 1991

found in primary visual cortex, although a small number of
cells may have shown slight orientation bias. This immature
state, with few if any oriented cortical cells, persisted
through the 5th postnatal week. During postnatal week 6 a
larger percentage of cells showed orientation specificity, and
by postnatal week 7 cortical responses had matured to an adult-
like state, with approximately 50% of cells showing clear
orientation preference.

To determine whether this development of oriented responses
occurs through an activity-dependent mechanism, we silenced
cortical neuronal activity during the time that orientation was
maturing. The sodium channel blocker tetrodotoxin (TTX) was
infused into area 17 through a 30 ga. cannula connected to an
osmotic minipump (Alzet 2002). Infusion of 2.5×10^{-12}
moles/hr TTX was found to silence all neuronal activity in an
area extending approximately 5 to 10 mm from the cannula tip.
TTX infusion was begun during the 4th postnatal week when
oriented responses are not seen in cortex, and continued
through post-natal week 7 by which time oriented responses
similar to those seen in adult animals would normally be
present. Four days after the infusion was terminated, neurons
within the TTX-treated area were found to respond vigorously to
visual stimulation, but these responses were not orientation
selective. Neurons in the opposite (untreated) cortex showed a
distribution of orientation selectivity identical to that in
normal adults (Mann-Whitney U: p=0.50, data not shown). These
results are shown in figure 1.

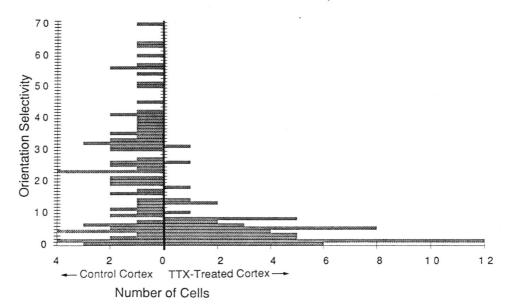

Fig. 1. Histograms showing the distributions of
orientation selectivity of neurons in primary visual
cortex of TTX-treated ferrets. Data from neurons in
the control (untreated) cortices are plotted to the
left of zero, data from the TTX-treated cortices are
plotted to the right. Higher values of orientation
selectivity (calculated as described in the text)
indicate more selective responses.

The distribution of orientation selectivities seen in the cortices of 7-8 week old animals treated with TTX starting during postnatal week 4 was statistically indistinguishable from the distribution seen in normal animals at 4 weeks of age (Mann-Whitney U: p=0.37, data not shown) suggesting that the activity blockade produced by the TTX treatment maintained the cortical neurons in an immature state. Thus the normal development of orientation specificity in ferret primary visual cortex neurons appears to depend on the presence of neuronal activity.

In normal adult ferrets, afferents projecting to a single orientation column have receptive fields covering an elongated region of space aligned with the preferred orientation of cortical cells in that column (Chapman et al., 1991). It is not clear whether this arrangement of afferents is a cause or a consequence of cortical cell orientation specificity, and the relative contributions of subcortical inputs versus intracortical connections to oriented cortical responses are not known. It will be of interest to study the development of this arrangement of afferent input to a cortical orientation column, and to determine whether the alignment of afferents seen in normal adults is also found in the animals which lack orientation selectivity because their normal cortical development has been disrupted by activity blockade.

REFERENCES

Chapman, B., Zahs, K. R. and Stryker, M. P., 1991, Relation of cortical cell orientation selectivity to alignment of receptive fields of the geniculocortical afferents that arborize within a single orientation column in ferret visual cortex, *J. Neurosci., 11(5)*: 1347-1358.
Fregnac, Y. and Imbert, M., 1984, Development of neuronal selectivity in primary visual cortex of cat, *Physiol. Rev., 64(1)*: 325-434.
Hubel, D. H. and Wiesel, T. N., 1963, Receptive fields of cells in striate cortex of very young, visually inexperienced kittens, *J. Neurophysiol., 26*: 994-1002.
Hubel, D. H., Wiesel, T. N. and LeVay, S., 1977, Plasticity of ocular dominance columns in monkey striate cortex, *Phil. Trans. R. Soc. Lond. B., 278*: 377-409.
Law, M. I., Zahs, K. R. and Stryker, M. P., 1988, Organization of primary visual cortex (area 17) in the ferret, *J. Comp. Neurol., 278*: 157-180.
Linden, D. C., Guillery, R. W. and Cucchiaro, J., 1981, The dorsal lateral geniculate nucleus of the normal ferret and its postnatal development, *J. Comp. Neurol., 203*: 189-211.
Worgotter, F. and Eysel, U. T., 1987, Quantitative determination of orientational and directional components in the response of visual cortical cells to moving stimuli, *Biol. Cybern. 57*: 349-355.

DEVELOPMENT OF THE TYROSINE HYDROXYLASE IMMUNOREACTIVE

CELL POPULATION IN THE RABBIT RETINA

Giovanni Casini and Nicholas C. Brecha

Depts. of Anatomy & Cell Biology and Medicine
UCLA and VAMC-West Los Angeles
Los Angeles, CA 90073

INTRODUCTION

Important steps in visual information processing in the retina occur in the inner plexiform layer (IPL). Amacrine cells, whose somata are located in the inner nuclear layer (INL) and ganglion cell layer (GCL), densely innervate the IPL and play multiple roles in the processing of visual signals through their synaptic contacts with bipolar, ganglion and other amacrine cells. Two main classes of amacrine cells have been recognized: narrow-field and wide-field. Narrow-field amacrine cells are likely to be involved in the direct transmission of visual information through the retina. Wide-field amacrine cells are particularly heterogeneous and can be subdivided into high and low cell density populations (Masland, 1988). The low density or sparsely distributed wide-field amacrine cells are thought to have more diffuse, regulatory or modulatory functions (for review see Masland, 1988, and the chapter in this volume entitled "Organization and development of sparsely distributed wide-field amacrine cells in the rabbit retina" by N. C. Brecha, G. Casini and D. Rickman).

To date, several different types of wide-field amacrine cells have been identified (see Casini and Brecha, 1991 for ref.), and tyrosine hydroxylase (TH, the rate-limiting enzyme of catecholamine biosynthesis) immunoreactive (IR) amacrine cells are a well-studied representative of the low cell density group (see Mitrofanis et al., 1988a for ref.). In adult rabbit retinas, these cells are located in the proximal INL, and TH-IR processes are distributed to laminae 1, 3, and 5 of the IPL (Brecha et al., 1984; Tauchi et al., 1990).

Previous investigations showed that newborn rabbit retinas contain very low levels of TH activity and endogenous dopamine (Lam et al., 1981). From postnatal day (PD) 6, both TH activity and dopamine levels increase slowly until PD 18. A dramatic increase then follows and adult levels are reached at PD 25 (Lam et al., 1981). In order to better understand the ontogeny of wide-field amacrine cells and to gain insights into the elaboration of their processes in the IPL, we used immunohistochemical methods to describe the changing morphology, density and distribution of TH-IR neurons during postnatal development in the rabbit retina.

METHODS

Antiserum. A mouse monoclonal antiserum directed to TH was used (clone 2/40/15; Boehringer-Mannheim, Indianapolis, IN). This antibody shows extensive species cross-reactivity, recognizing a single protein of the appropriate molecular weight

The Changing Visual System, Edited by P. Bagnoli and
W. Hodos, Plenum Press, New York, 1991

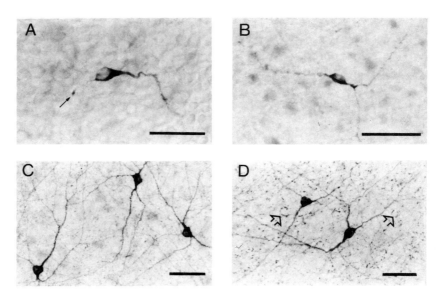

Fig. 1. Examples of TH-IR cells in whole-mounted rabbit retinas at PD 0 (A), PD 6 (B), PD 12 (C) and adult (D). A growth cone is seen in A (small arrow). Arrows in D indicate varicosities in lamina 1 of the IPL arranged in two "ring-like" structures. Scale bars: A, 25 μm; B, C and D, 50 μm.

(56,000-60,000) in immunoblots of total adrenal protein from quail, chick, rat and bovine adrenal (Rohrer et al., 1986).

Tissue preparation and immunohistochemical procedures. New Zealand albino rabbits obtained from commercial sources were used in this study. Care and handling of the animals were approved by the Animal Research Committee of the VAMC-West Los Angeles in accordance with all NIH animal guidelines.

Retinas were collected from rabbits at PD 0, 6, 12, 19, 26 and from adults (PD 90 or older). The retinas were dissected, fixed in a paraformaldehyde solution and prepared as whole-mounts using immunohistochemical protocols (Casini and Brecha, 1991). Dilution of the primary antiserum was 1:50 for PD 6 or younger retinas; 1:100 for the other retinas. Specificity of immune reactions was assessed by incubating the retinas with normal mouse serum in place of the primary antibody.

Quantitative analysis. TH-IR cell bodies were counted at 100 x in 1 mm^2 fields along two stripes oriented perpendicularly to the visual streak. Nearest neighbor analysis (Wässle and Riemann, 1978) was performed on samples of cells from approximately 2 mm^2 areas at different locations in the retina. Cell body areas were measured at 1000 x. Correction for shrinkage was not applied since the retinal whole mounts were attached to the slide before dehydration.

RESULTS

Morphology

In newborn retinas (PD 0), TH-IR cells are present in all retinal regions and display very weak immunoreactivity. Immunostaining is mainly confined to a thin rim of cytoplasm surrounding the nucleus. In most cases, one thick primary process, often with second-order ramifications, is present in the IPL adjacent to the INL corresponding best to lamina 1 of the IPL. Varicosities on these processes are not observed. Occasionally,

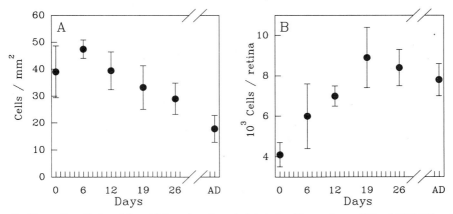

Fig. 2. Overall cell densities (A) and estimated total cell numbers (B) of TH-IR cells as a function of age. Both in A and in B, each point represents the mean ± s.d. of values from three retinas taken from different animals.

fine processes having growth cones are seen. (Fig. 1A). At PD 6, cell body and fiber immunoreactive staining is stronger. While some TH-IR cells display very immature characteristics as seen at PD 0, other cells have a more mature appearance with long immunoreactive processes and second- and third-order ramifications that bear a few varicosities (Fig. 1B). There is no apparent relationship between the degree of maturation of TH-IR neurons and their position in the retina.

At PD 12 (around the time of eye opening), the somal shape and ramification of processes of TH-IR cells have undergone important maturative changes, and TH-IR cells display general morphological characteristics similar to those of the adult. These cells usually have 2 to 5 primary processes, and there is a complicated network of TH-IR fibers in lamina 1 of the IPL (Fig. 1C). Some TH-IR processes carrying small varicosities also can be seen in lamina 3. In both laminae, many fibers ending in growth cones are present. At PD 19, the network of TH-IR fibers in lamina 1 of the IPL has attained an even higher degree of complexity. Processes are seen in lamina 5 and growth cones are not observed. At PD 26, TH-IR somata and the distribution and ramification patterns of TH-IR fibers have the typical morphological characteristics of those observed in adult animals. Some differences, however, still exist in comparison to the adult, since at PD 26 varicosities arranged in ring-like structures typical of the adult (Fig. 1D) are not seen, and the plexus of TH-IR fibers in lamina 5 of the IPL is less developed.

Quantitative analysis

Changes in cell body size, cell density (cells/mm^2) and distribution of nearest neighbor distances during postnatal development have been evaluated. The cell body size of TH-IR neurons gradually increases from PD 0 (somal area of about 55 μm^2) until adulthood (about 160 μm^2). Overall, TH-IR cell density markedly decreases from PD 0 - PD 6 (40 - 50 cells/mm^2) to adulthood (about 18 cells/mm^2) (Fig. 2A). Throughout development, highest cell densities are observed in the dorsal retina. Approaching adulthood, a small peak in cell density develops in the visual streak. Estimated TH-IR cell number increases from PD 0 (about 4000 cells/retina) to PD 19 (about 9000 cells/retina) and then remains relatively constant (Fig. 2B). Retinal area gradually increases from PD 0 (about 100 mm^2) to adulthood (about 500 mm^2). These observations suggest that the overall decrease in TH-IR cell density is mainly due to an increase of retinal surface area. There is a poor match between the distribution of nearest neighbor distances of TH-IR cells and a theoretical non-random distribution before PD 12. After PD 12, there is a shift towards a more regular distribution.

DISCUSSION

The development of TH-IR retinal neurons has been studied in several mammalian (cat: Wang et al., 1990; rat: Mitrofanis et al., 1988b; mouse: Wulle and Schnitzer, 1989; guinea pig: Parkinson et al., 1985; hamster and gerbil: Mitrofanis and Finlay, 1990) and non-mammalian (chick: Kagami et al., 1991) species. Overall, these studies indicate species differences in the time of appearance and developmental patterns of TH-IR cells.

In rabbits, TH immunoreactivity is present in retinal neurons at the time of birth, indicating that the transmitter phenotype of these neurons is established before birth. Generally, the commitment to specific transmitter phenotype is made before birth (Lam et al., 1981), but cellular maturation is completed at later ages. GABAergic and glycinergic neurons in the rabbit retina, for instance, display many of the adult biochemical characteristics at around the time of eye opening (Kong et al, 1980; Lam et al., 1980).

The weakness of immunoreactivity observed at PD 0 and the gradual increase in density of immunostaining during development fit with previous biochemical data showing low levels of both TH activity and endogenous dopamine in newborn rabbit retinas, with a gradual increase until PD 18 and a dramatic increase during the following week (PD 18 to PD 25) when adult levels are reached (Lam et al., 1981). These biochemical data and the morphological as well as quantitative findings of the present study indicate that maturation of TH-IR neurons in the rabbit retina is not complete until at least PD 25-26.

The present investigation demonstrates that TH-IR fibers arborize in the IPL over a span of many days. Processes grow in the correct IPL laminae and they are never seen in laminae that do not contain TH-IR processes in the adult. This observation suggests the presence, in different levels of the IPL, of specific factors that are able to guide the ingrowth of amacrine cell processes.

Most of the adult morphological characteristics of TH-IR cells are already present at the time of eye opening (around PD 12). The processes of TH-IR cells at this age appear to be in a very active state of growth, and quantitative data indicate that adult cell number and distribution are approached at this time. In relationship to general retinal development, synaptic specializations in the IPL are first seen at PD 8 - 9, there is a dramatic increase in synaptic density during the following two or three days and adult values are asymptotically reached at around PD 20 (McArdle et al., 1977). The rapid increase in synaptic density in the IPL corresponds to the time of eye opening. Functionally, light-evoked responses of some ganglion cells are first seen at PD 8, and by PD 10 the majority of ganglion cells can be activated by light. Complete maturation of ganglion cell receptive field properties is achieved by PD 20 (Masland, 1977). It seems likely that at eye opening TH-IR cells are involved in synapse formation in the IPL and, since most ganglion cells start forming their receptive field properties at this age, TH-IR neurons might also play a role in visual information processing. It appears, therefore, that the time of eye opening represents an important point during development for the differentiation of the IPL and functional maturation of the retina.

Although TH-IR neurons at PD 26 are similar in appearance to those of adult retinas, some fine details in the organization of the meshwork of immunoreactive processes are not seen until after the first month of age. These details include the consistent presence of TH-IR processes in lamina 5 of the IPL and organization of varicosities in ring-like structures in lamina 1. In cat and rat retinas, these "rings" have been shown to surround A II amacrine cells (Voigt and Wässle, 1978), and a regulatory or modulatory function of TH-IR amacrine cells on the rod pathway has been proposed (Jensen and Daw, 1984; Thier and Aïder, 1984; Voigt and Wässle, 1978; Masland, 1988).

TH-IR neurons in the rabbit retina constitute one type of catecholamine-accumulating cells (type 1) whose processes are distributed to lamina 1 of the IPL. A second type of catecholamine-accumulating cells (type 2) does not display TH immunoreactivity in the cell body, but possesses processes arborizing in laminae 1, 3 and 5 that are labeled by TH immunohistochemistry (Tauchi et al., 1990). Since TH-IR processes are initially found in laminae 3 and 5 of the IPL when processes in lamina 1 are already present and well established, the possibility exists that type 1 cells develop earlier than type 2 catecholamine-accumulating cells.

TH-IR cell densities and numbers calculated in adult retinas are consistent with those found by Brecha et al. (1984), and higher than those reported by Tauchi et al. (1990). The increase observed in retinal surface area during development is similar to that measured by Robinson et al. (1989) and suggests that the decrement in TH-IR overall cell density is due to retinal growth. Furthermore, the decrease of TH-IR cell density in the dorsal retina and the formation of a small density peak in the visual streak are probably due to nonuniform retinal growth (Robinson et al., 1989).

In summary, the present study describes morphological and quantitative changes of the TH-IR cell population during postnatal development in the rabbit retina. The results show that the neurochemical identity of these neurons is established by birth. Processes enter and ramify into the appropriate IPL laminae and by the time of eye opening they have already formed a relatively complex network in lamina 1 of the IPL. Eye opening represents an important time point for the development of TH-IR neurons. At PD 12, TH-IR cells are likely to be functional and might begin to play a role in visual information processing. Mature morphological and biochemical characteristics of these cells are reached at around PD 26, but some fine details of the organization of TH-IR meshwork are not established until well after the first month of age.

ACKNOWLEDGMENTS

We wish to thank D. Rickman and Dr. C. Sternini for their helpful comments on this manuscript. Supported by National Institutes of Health grant EY 04067 and VA Medical Research Funds.

REFERENCES

Brecha, N. C., Oyster, C. W., and Takahashi, E. S., 1984, Identification and characterization of tyrosine hydroxylase immunoreactive amacrine cells, Invest. Ophthalmol. Vis. Sci., 25:66.

Casini, G., and Brecha, N. C., 1991, Vasoactive intestinal polypeptide-containing cells in the rabbit retina: immunohistochemical localization and quantitative analysis, J. Comp. Neurol., 305:313.

Jensen, R. J., and Daw, N. W., 1984, Effects of dopamine antagonists on receptive fields of brisk cells and directionally selective cells in the rabbit retina, J. Neurosci., 4:2972.

Kagami, H., Sakai, H., Uryu, K., Kaneda, T., and Sakanaka M., 1991, Development of tyrosine hydroxylase-like immunoreactive structures in the chick retina: Three-dimensional analysis, J. Comp. Neurol., 308:356.

Kong, Y. C., Fung, S. C., and Lam, D. M. K., 1980, The postnatal development of glycinergic neurons in rabbit retina, J. Comp. Neurol., 193:1127.

Lam, D. M. K., Fung, S. C., and Kong, Y. C., 1980, The postnatal development of GABAergic neurons in the rabbit retina, J. Comp. Neurol., 193:89.

Lam, D. M. K., Fung, S. C., and Kong, Y. C., 1981, Postnatal development of dopaminergic neurons in the rabbit retina, J. Neurosci., 1:1117.

Masland, R. H., 1977, Maturation of functions in the developing rabbit retina, J. Comp. Neurol., 175:286.

Masland, R. H., 1988, Amacrine cells, Trends Neurosci., 11:405.

McArdle, C. B., Dowling, J. E., and Masland, R. H., 1977, Development of outer segments and synapses in the rabbit retina, J. Comp. Neurol., 175:253.

Mitrofanis, J., and Finlay, B. L., 1990, Developmental changes in the distribution of retinal catecholaminergic neurons in hamsters and gerbils, J. Comp. Neurol., 292:480.

Mitrofanis, J., Vigny, A., and Stone, J., 1988a, Distribution of catecholaminergic cells in the retina of the rat, guinea pig, cat, and rabbit: Independence from ganglion cell distribution, J. Comp. Neurol., 267:1.

Mitrofanis, J., Maslim, J., and Stone, J., 1988b, Catecholaminergic and cholinergic neurons in the developing retina of the rat, J. Comp. Neurol., 276:343.

Parkinson, D., Spira, A., Wyse, J.P., and Patten, M., 1985, The ontogenesis of the dopaminergic cell in the pre- and postnatal guinea pig retina, Int. J. Dev. Neurosci., 3:157.

Robinson, S. R., Dreher, B., and McCall, M. J., 1989, Nonuniform retinal expansion during the formation of the rabbit's visual streak: Implications for the ontogeny of mammalian retinal topography, Vis. Neurosci., 2:201.

Rohrer, H., Acheson, A. L., Thibault, J., and Thoenen, H., 1986, Developmental potential of quail dorsal root ganglion cells analyzed in vitro and in vivo, J. Neurosci., 6:2616.

Tauchi, M., Madigan, N. K., and Masland, R. H., 1990, Shapes and distributions of the catecholamine-accumulating neurons in the rabbit retina, J. Comp. Neurol., 293:178.

Thier, P., and Alder, V., 1984, Action of iontophoretically applied dopamine on cat retinal ganglion cells, Brain Res., 292:109.

Voigt, T., and Wässle, H., 1987, Dopaminergic innervation of AII amacrine cells in mammalian retina, J. Neurosci. 7:4115.

Wang, H. -H., Cuenca, N., and Kolb, H., 1990, Development of morphological types and distribution patterns of amacrine cells immunoreactive to tyrosine hydroxylase in the cat retina, Vis. Neurosci., 4:159.

Wulle, I., and Schnitzer, J., 1989, Distribution and morphology of tyrosine-hydroxylase immunoreactive neurons in the developing mouse retina, Dev. Brain Res. 48:52.

Wässle, H., and Riemann, H.J., 1978, The mosaic of nerve cells in the mammalian retina, Proc. R. Soc. Lond. (Biol.), 200:441.

EMERGENCE OF VISUAL CORTICAL AREAS: PATTERNS OF DEVELOPMENT OF NEUROPEPTIDE-Y IMMUNOREACTIVITY AND SOMATOSTATIN-IMMUNOREACTIVITY IN THE CAT

Dale Hogan and Nancy E.J. Berman

Department of Anatomy and Cell Biology, Univ. of Kansas Medical Center
Kansas City KS 66103, USA

A prominent feature in the evolution of neocortex in higher mammals is the appearance of multiple areas of cortex which function in the hierarchal and parallel processing of sensory input and motor output. One way each of these areas can be identified is by their characteristic and specific patterns of connectivity with cortical and subcortical areas. How axonal growth cones from neurons in the thalamus and other cortical areas recognize which presumptive cortical area is an appropriate target and enter it to form connections is not known. In the cat, the earliest born neurons of the neocortex form a transient structure termed the "subplate" (Luskin and Shatz, '85) which has been reported be necessary to allow thalamocortical afferents to enter the cortical plate of area 17 (Ghosh et al. '90). Thus, the subplate could play an important role in the formation of cortical connectivity

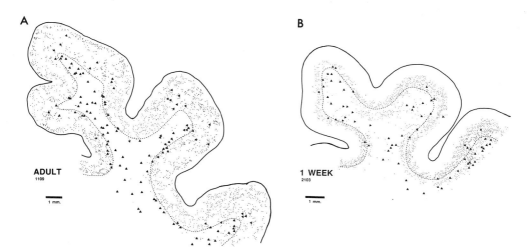

Fig. 1. Camera Lucida drawings of visual cortical areas in A) adult and B) 1 week old kitten. Each dot represents one SOM-ir neuron and each triangle represents one NPY-ir neuron. Drawings are composites of separate camera lucida drawings of non-adjacent sections from the same animal stained for NPY and SOM. SOM-ir is expressed in neurons only in mature cortical laminae and is overexpressed in lateral areas at one week of age as compared to the adult. The pattern of NPY expression, by contrast, does not vary significantly by age or visual area.

The Changing Visual System, Edited by P. Bagnoli and
W. Hodos, Plenum Press, New York, 1991

that leads to the emergence of multiple visual areas (Rakic, '88; Ghosh et al, '90). Several neuropeptides, including Neuropeptide-Y (NPY) and Somatostatin (SOM) have been reported to be markers of the subplate (Chun et al., '87; Chun and Shatz, '89) and also conjectured to be involved in its target recognition role (Lipton and Kater,'89). We speculated that if neuropeptide expression in the subplate is an important factor in target recognition by afferent projections, then this expression should vary across cortical areas. The cat visual cortex provides a unique opportunity to observe the emergence of cortical areas since areas 17, 18, 19 and the medial and lateral suprasylvian areas (MLS and LLS) can be examined on one coronal section. These areas have different patterns of projections and mature at different times during kitten development. We examined developing cat visual cortex using immunohistochemical techniques to determine whether the spatial and/or temporal pattern of expression NPY and SOM across the various areas implies that these neuropeptides are important in the emergence of these areas.

In the adult, there is no difference in the pattern of SOM-ir neurons in areas 17, 19, MLS or LLS (Fig. 1A). SOM-ir neurons are found in all layers of the cortex except layer I, and some interstitial cells are SOM-ir also. In area 18, there is a patchiness to the label in the middle cortical layers. This patchiness takes the form of "holes" in which there are no SOM-ir neurons.

During development, SOM-ir neurons appear only in the mature laminae of the cortex. At one week of age, SOM-ir neurons are found only in layers V and VI; by 2 weeks they are also found in layer IV; by 3 weeks, when the mature cortical lamination pattern is established, SOM-ir neurons are found in all cortical layers except layer I, as in the adult. In addition, there is a clear difference across cortical areas which is most striking at one week of age (Fig. 1B). There is no evidence of excess expression of SOM in areas 17, 18 and 19 at this age, but the number of immunoreactive cells increases from medial to lateral. The grey matter of MLS contains 50% more SOM-ir neurons than

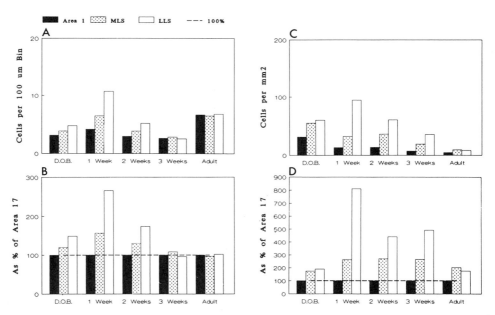

Fig. 2. Counts of SOM-ir neurons from kittens and adult cats. A) Neurons in grey matter counted in 100 μm bins drawn perpendicular to pia. B) SOM-ir neurons in lateral areas expressed as a percentage of area 17. C) Density of SOM-ir neurons in 500 μm of white matter underlying visual cortical areas. D) Density of SOM-ir neurons in white mater of lateral areas expressed as a percentage of area 17. Overexpression of SOM-ir by neurons in lateral areas peaks at 1 week of age and falls to adult levels by 3 weeks.

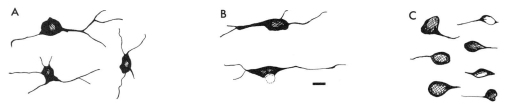

Fig. 3. Camera lucida drawings of individual SOM-ir neurons, randomly oriented. A). Multipolar type A neurons. B) Bipolar type B neurons, and C) Simple type C neurons. Scale bar = 10μm.

area 17 and LLS has almost 3 times as many SOM-ir neurons per section as areas 17 (Fig. 2A). This exuberance is even more marked in the white matter where MLS contains 3 times as many labelled cells and LLS has 8 times as many SOM-ir neurons as area 17 (Fig. 2B). This exuberant expression in the lateral visual areas occurs at the time when corticocortical connections are being established in these areas (Price and Zumbroich, '87). At 2 weeks of age, lateral exuberance is still present, but is much reduced (Fig. 2A & B). By three weeks of age, the differences between the medial and lateral areas have decreased, and the distribution of Som-ir neurons has reached the adult pattern.

We used the classification scheme of Mizukawa et al. ('87) to score the morphology of the SOM-ir neurons (Fig. 3). The most numerous labelled neuron was the "C-type". These neurons have a lightly stained perikaryon with a large unstained nucleus and usually only one short stained process. Less than 10% of the SOM-ir neurons were A-type, darkly stained multipolar neurons with complex stained processes or B-type, darkly stained fusiform bipolar neurons. Similar morphological types were seen in both kittens and adults. In kitten cortex, some SOM-ir neurons were seen which had the morphology typical of migrating neurons, i.e., fusiform cell bodies with a leading and trailing process parallel to cortical columns.

NPY has been known for some years to be widely colocalized with SOM in adult cat visual cortex (Demeulemeester et al., '88) and adult rat visual cortex (Papadopoulos et al., '87). In the adult cat visual cortex, NPY-ir neurons are far less numerous than SOM-ir neurons and appear to colocalize predominately with the SOM type A and B neurons. When we examined NPY distribution in kitten visual cortex, we observed that the total number of NPY-ir neurons per section increases postnatally in all areas (Fig. 4A). The number of NPY-ir neurons in the white matter rises through the fourth postnatal week, reaching adult levels at that time. However, there has not been a significant increase in the number of NPY-ir neurons in cortical grey matter between P0 and P21. Adult cortex has three

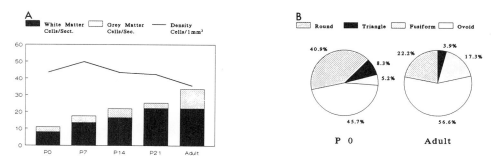

Fig. 4. A) Number of NPY-ir neurons per section at various postnatal ages and adult. Total height of each bar reflects corrected number of NPY-ir neurons per section (Abercrombie, '46). Area of sections determined using Summagraphics bit pad (Fairfield, CT) and Sigma Scan software (Jandel, Carta Madera, CA). NPY-ir neuron numbers per section rise with age, but their density remains relatively constant. B) Percentage of total neurons per section with cell bodies of specified shape at P0 and adult. NPY-ir neurons have flatter perikarya in the adult than at birth.

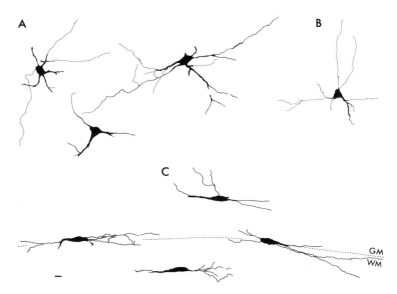

Fig 5. Camera lucida drawings of NPY-ir neurons in adult. A) Multipolar neurons from grey matter. B) Multipolar neuron in white matter. C) Bipolar neurons in layer VIb and white matter; dotted line represents grey matter-white matter border. Scale bar =10μm.

times as many NPY-ir neurons as that of neonates. We are currently studying the time course of this increase in older kittens. The density of cells remains relatively constant throughout development. The increase in number is directly correlated to the increasing brain size (Fig. 4A).

NPY-ir neuron morphologies fall into similar categories to that of SOM-ir neurons, most being either multipolar or fusiform bipolar (Fig. 5). Simple stained neurons similar to SOM-ir C type comprise less than 10% of labeled neurons in either neonates or adults. We observed an overall flattening of the shape of the neuronal perikarya between P0 and adult (Fig. 4B). This change in morphology is consistent with compression of neuronal perikarya by the increased density of the cortex, by formation of sulci, and by the increase in numbers of fibers and glia (Marin-Padilla, '72; Marin-Padilla, '78; Kostovic and Rakic, '80; Valverde and Facal-Valverde, '88). However, the death of neurons of certain morphological classes and subsequent replacement by NPY-ir neurons of other morphological classes (Meyer and Wahle, '87) cannot be ruled out except by [3H] thymidine studies.

The increase in NPY-ir cell numbers is accompanied by an increase in the density of NPY-ir axons. Developmentally, medial areas are invaded by immunoreactive processes first, with the lateral areas lagging about a week behind. As the axons grow into the cortex, they follow a radial pattern, growing straight up through the cortical plate and branching first in layer I. In the adult, dense fibers crisscross the whole extent of the cortex in secondary visual areas. In areas 17 and 18, stained processes avoid layer IV.

These results suggest that somatostatin expression by neurons of the subplate could be a factor in the emergence of secondary visual areas since SOM is expressed by neurons in the area of the subplate of the lateral suprasylvian visual areas at the time of establishment of major corticocortical afferent systems. NPY, by contrast, does not appear to be localized preferentially to the subplate but is found more widely spread in cortex and white matter. This evidence supports a more generalized role for NPY during development, perhaps similar to its adult functions. In the adult, NPY has been hypothesized to act on general cerebral function either via its role as a vasoconstrictor (Lundberg et al., '82) or its hypothesized cooperation in the dopaminergic pathways of general cerebral alertness and attention (Härfstrand et al., '86)

Acknowledgments: We wish to thank Erin R. Terwilleger and Wen-Li Liu for technical assistance. Research supported by MH38399, BNS881997, and RCD8954894.

REFERENCES

Abercrombie, M., 1946. Estimation of nuclear population from microtome sections. Anat. Rec. 94:239-247.

Chun, J.J.M., Nakamura, M.J., and Shatz, C.J., 1987. Transient cells of the developing telencephalon are immunoreactive neurons. Nature 325: 617-620.

Chun, J.J.M., and Shatz, C.J., 1989. Interstitial cells of the adult neocortex are the remnant of the early generated subplate neuron population. J.Comp. Neurol.282:555-569.

Demeulemeester, H., Vandesande, F., Orban, G.A., Brandon, C., and Vanderhaeghen, J.J., 1988. Heterogeneity of GABAergic cells in the cat visual cortex. J. Neurosci. 8:988-1000.

Ghosh, A., Antonini, A., McConnell, S.K., Shatz, C.J., 1990. Requirement for subplate neurons in the formation of thalamocortical connections. Nature 347:179-181.

Härfstrand, A., Fuxe, K., Agnati, L.F., Eneroth, P., Zini, I., Andersson, K., von Euler, G., Terenius, L., Mutt, V., and Goldstein, M., 1986, Studies on neuropeptide y-catecholamine interactions in the hypothalamus and in the forebrain of the male rat. Relationship to neuroendocrine function. Neurochem. Int. 8:355-376.

Kostovic, I. and Rakic, P., 1980. Cytology and time of origin of interstitial neurons in the white matter of infant and adult human and monkey telencephalon. J. Neurocytol. 9:219-242.

Lipton, S.A. and Kater, S.B., 1989. Neurotransmitter regulation of neuronal outgrowth, plasticity and survival. Trends Neurosci. 12:265-270.

Lundberg, J.M., Terenius,L., Hokfelt, T., Marthing, C.R., Tatemoto, K., Mutt, V., Polak, J., Bloom, S.R., and Goldstein, M., 1982. Neuropeptide-y (NPY) like immunoreactivity in peripheral noradrenergic neurones and effects of NPY on sympathetic function. Acta. Physiol. Scand. 116:477-480.

Luskin, M.B., and Shatz, C.J., 1985. Studies of the earliest generated cells of the cat's visual cortex: cogeneration of subplate and marginal zones. J. Neurosci. 5:1062-1075.

Marin-Padilla, M.,1972. Prenatal ontogenetic history of the principle neurons of the neocortex of the cat (Felis domestica). A Golgi study. II Developmental differences and their significance. Z. Anat. Entwickl. Gesch. 136:125-142.

Marin-Padilla, M., 1978. Dual origin of the mammalian neocortex and evolution of the cortical plate. Z. Anat. Embryol. 152:109-126.

Mizukawa, K., McGeer, P.L., Vincent, S.R., and McGeer, E.G., 1987. The distribution of somatostatin-immunoreactive neurons and fibers in the rat cerebral cortex: light and electron microscopic studies. Brain Research, 426:28-36.

Papadopoulos, G.C., J.G. Parnavelas, and Cavanagh, M.E., 1987. Extensive co-existence of neuropeptides in the rat visual cortex. Brain Res. 420:95-99.

Price, D.J. and Zumbroich, T.J., 1989. Postnatal development of corticocortical efferents from area 17 in the cat's visual cortex. J. Neurosci. 9:600-613.

Rakic, P., 1988. Specification of cerebral cortical areas. Science 241:170-176.

Valverde, F. and Facal-Valverde, M.V., 1988. Postnatal development of interstitial (subplate) cells in the white matter of the temporal cortex of kittens: A correlated Golgi and electron microscopic study. J. Comp. Neurol. 269:168-192.

Wahle, P. and Meyer, G. J., 1987. Morphology and quantitative changes of transient NPY-ir neuronal populations during early postnatal development of the cat visual cortex. J. Comp. Neurol. 261:165-192.

INDIVIDUAL DIFFERENCES IN CONTRAST SENSITIVITY FUNCTIONS

OF HUMAN ADULTS AND INFANTS: A BRIEF REVIEW

David Peterzell, John S. Werner and Peter S. Kaplan

University of Colorado
Boulder, CO 80309-0345 U.S.A.

ABSTRACT

Even when individuals are matched for age and ocular health, their contrast sensitivity functions (CSFs) will differ. Some of these differences seem to be caused by individual differences in underlying spatial mechanisms that detect narrow ranges of spatial frequency. This is because an individual's performance at a particular frequency (i.e., one's sensitivity to a test frequency relative to the group mean at that frequency) tends to predict performance at nearby frequencies only. Attempts to use individual differences in CSFs to test quantitative models of spatial mechanisms are reviewed. Preliminary analyses indicate that mechanisms tuned to low spatial frequencies at birth may shift to higher frequencies during development.

INTRODUCTION

Since Selwyn's (1948) early study, the contrast sensitivity function (CSF) has been measured under many conditions (Graham, 1989). Human contrast sensitivity, like so many measures of visual performance, increases during early development and then declines gradually with age (see papers by Owsley and Weale in this volume). In general, one's sensitivity to low spatial frequencies grows more rapidly and then declines more slowly than one's sensitivity to higher frequencies.

Much of the research on the development and aging of the CSF focuses on group averages (e.g., mean contrast sensitivity is higher at 20 than 60 years of age). This review focuses not on the average sensitivities for various age-groups but rather upon individual differences within particular age groups. We suggest that the study of individual differences in CSFs provides important information that is usually overlooked in large-sample studies. These individual differences may provide clues to the spatial mechanisms that underlie contrast sensitivity, as well as to how these mechanisms change during development and scenescence.

NORMAL INDIVIDUAL VARIABILITY

Substantial individual differences in CSFs exist among observers with no known abnormalities, even when they are matched for age and ocular health (e.g., Owsley et al. 1983). In normal adults of any age, individuals' log contrast sensitivity values for a test spatial frequency are normally distributed, and the standard

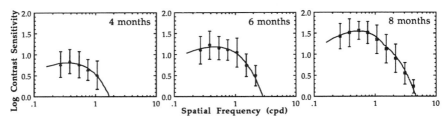

Figure 1. *Mean log contrast sensitivity as a function of spatial frequency at 4, 6, and 8 months of age. Bars denote standard deviations (from Peterzell et al. 1991b).*

deviations fall around 0.1 or 0.2 log units (Owsley et al. 1983). The CSFs of human infants also show normal variability, as shown in Figure 1. The data in the figure are from a recent study of healthy, full-term infants (Peterzell et al. 1991a,b). CSFs of eighty 4-month-old infants were measured using a preferential-looking method and the method of constant stimuli. Twenty-five were retested at 6- and 8-months. Circular sinewave gratings varied from 0.27 to 4.32 cycles per degree (cpd), contained 8 unattenuated cycles (with edges tapered to uniform gray), and rose to the desired contrast in 2 sec (mean luminance was 27 cd/m^2). The data in the figure are for the 25 infants who participated at all three ages (Peterzell et al. 1991b).

CORRELATIONAL STRUCTURE

One might expect that much of the normal variability in CSFs could be explained by random measurement error, or by individual differences in overall maturational or attentional level. If measurement error accounts for most of the variability among individuals, then an individual whose measured sensitivity is higher than average at one spatial frequency will not necessarily have higher than average sensitivity at any other frequencies. Suppose a data set lists log contrast sensitivities (or "scores") for n spatial frequencies, each recorded for s individuals. If random measurement error accounts for individual differences, then each frequency's (n) set of scores should not predict (i.e., correlate with) scores at other frequencies; there should be no significant correlations in the $n \times n$ correlation matrix.

Suppose instead that maturational or attentional level accounts for individual differences. Some observers may demonstrate especially high sensitivity at all frequencies because they are more developed (in the case of infants) or less affected by senescence (in the case of older people) than the average individual in their age group. Or, some observers may pay more attention or cooperate more than others, and therefore demonstrate higher sensitivity at all frequencies. If varying levels of maturity or attention account for most individual differences, then each frequency's set of scores should correlate uniformly and highly with scores at other frequencies; the same maturational or attentional factor that causes higher than average performance at one frequency will, in general, cause higher than average performance at all other frequencies.

Owsley et al. (1983), in a study of aging and contrast sensitivity, discovered neither uncorrelated nor equicorrelational structure in their data. Instead, scores for patterns that were close in spatial frequency tended to correlate more highly and positively than those that were farther apart. In other words, an individual's relatively high or low score at one spatial frequency was a good predictor of his or her score (relative to the mean) at nearby spatial frequencies only. Billock and Harding (1991) have recently replicated these findings, and have found that variables that are close in temporal as well as spatial frequency tend to correlate more highly than those that are farther apart in either temporal or spatial frequency.

Table 1
Correlations (r) among spatial frequency variables
(log contrast sensitivities for 4,- 6-, and 8-month-olds from Peterzell et al. 1991b).

4-MONTHS

	0.27 cpd	0.38 cpd	0.54 cpd	0.76 cpd	1.08 cpd	1.53 cpd	2.16 cpd	3.06 cpd
0.38 cpd	0.72							
0.54 cpd	0.37	0.42						
0.76 cpd	0.20	0.24	0.76					
1.08 cpd	0.23	0.22	0.67	0.79				

6-MONTHS

	0.27 cpd	0.38 cpd	0.54 cpd	0.76 cpd	1.08 cpd	1.53 cpd	2.16 cpd	3.06 cpd
0.38 cpd	0.71							
0.54 cpd	0.62	0.60						
0.76 cpd	0.52	0.25	0.47					
1.08 cpd	0.42	0.26	0.44	0.45				
1.53 cpd	0.13	0.03	0.32	0.79	0.45			
2.16 cpd	-0.09	-0.05	0.09	0.47	0.51	0.60		

8-MONTHS

	0.27 cpd	0.38 cpd	0.54 cpd	0.76 cpd	1.08 cpd	1.53 cpd	2.16 cpd	3.06 cpd
0.38 cpd	0.79							
0.54 cpd	0.79	0.67						
0.76 cpd	0.48	0.42	0.44					
1.08 cpd	0.52	0.35	0.35	0.76				
1.53 cpd	0.15	0.04	0.41	0.33	0.38			
2.16 cpd	-0.06	-0.02	0.03	0.42	0.40	0.49		
3.06 cpd	0.09	0.11	0.04	0.37	0.51	0.50	0.72	
4.32 cpd	0.20	0.24	0.27	0.26	0.43	0.17	0.52	0.59

The correlational structure found in adults is also found in infants, as shown in Table 1 (Peterzell et al. 1991a,b). Table 1 is from the same data set as the means in Figure 1. In Table 1, variables close in spatial frequency do not always correlate more highly than those that are farther apart, perhaps because of small sample size and measurement error. We have found similar correlational structure in CSFs reported by Banks and Salapatek (1981) for 1-, 2-, and 3-month-olds (Peterzell et al. 1991a).

IMPLICATIONS FOR MODELS OF SPATIAL MECHANISMS IN ADULTS

Considerable psychophysical and physiological evidence suggests that multiple spatial mechanisms, which detect narrow bands of spatial frequency and orientation, determine the contrast sensitivity function (CSF) of the human adult (Graham, 1989). If individual differences in the contrast sensitivity of spatial mechanisms cause some of the individual differences in CSFs, then appropriate models of spatial mechanism tuning may be able to explain the correlations among spatial frequency variables described above. Moreover, such correlations may provide a tool for studying spatial mechanism tuning, and how it develops.

The correlational structure described above is consistent with a multiple mechanism hypothesis. To understand this, consider again the hypothetical n (spatial frequency) by s (individual) data matrix of log contrast sensitivities, and its resulting $n \times n$ correlation matrix. At each of the n frequencies, each of the s individuals' scores may be determined by the relatively high or low sensitivity of an underlying mechanism (assuming that each independent spatial mechanism exhibits normal variablility among individuals). Each frequency's set of scores should therefore correlate with scores at other frequencies that are also detected by that mechanism, but not scores at frequencies that are determined by separate mechanisms. It follows that if individual differences in contrast sensitivity are caused by individual differences in the sensitivity of a single mechanism, then all variables in the data set would be expected to correlate highly and equally. On the other hand, patterns that are close in spatial frequency could correlate more highly and positively than those that are farther apart. This alternative structure within the $n \times n$ correlation matrix is expected if multiple mechanisms underlie the data.

If one accepts the conclusion that individual differences in CSFs are attributable to individual differences in underlying frequency-tuned mechanisms, then one can use the underlying correlational structure from empirical data to test quantitative models of spatiotemporal mechanisms. Sekuler et al. (1984) have used the four-mechanism model of Wilson and Bergen (1979) to try to account for individual differences in adult CSFs (Owsley et al. 1983). Sekuler et al. used Monte Carlo procedures, which use random numbers to test pre-specified quantitative models, to test the model of Wilson and Bergen. Although Sekuler et al. do not report the correlations that would be predicted based on the 4-mechanism model, the results from their subsequent structural modeling analyses indicate that the model predictions resembled the empirical correlations of Owsley et al. (1983).

IMPLICATIONS FOR MODELS OF THE DEVELOPMENT OF SPATIAL MECHANISMS

Can individual differences in the CSFs of human infants provide clues to how spatial mechanisms develop? Although multiple spatial mechanisms clearly exist in infants after 3 months (Van Sluyters et al. 1990), how they develop is not well known. Does a single spatial mechanism (or homogeneous group of mechanisms) determine the CSF prior to age 3-months, with mechanisms tuned to higher frequencies developing later (Banks & Ginsburg, 1985)? Or, do multiple mechanisms exist at birth, and then shift their tuning to higher spatial frequencies (Wilson, 1988)? The two figures in Figure 2 show how mechanism tuning might change from infancy to adulthood. In the example of unshifting mechanisms, a mechanism whose peak spatial frequency is 1 cpd during infancy remains tuned to 1 cpd. With age, this mechanism grows in sensitivity, and new mechanisms emerge at higher frequencies. In the shifting model, multiple mechanisms exist in infancy and shift to higher frequencies as they grow in sensitivity.

Three recent findings may imply such a shift. First, the shapes of infants' CSFs change little with age, except for rigid shifts up (in sensitivity) and to the right (to higher frequencies) on log-log coordinates (Movshon & Kiorpes, 1988). This result may imply that underlying spatial mechanisms also shift to the right. Second, mechanisms in infants that detect low spatial frequencies have the same narrow bandwidths as those in adults that detect higher frequencies (Fiorentini et al. 1983), implying a developmental shift. Third, cones migrate to the fovea during development and become densely packed (Yuodelis & Hendrickson, 1986). If spatial

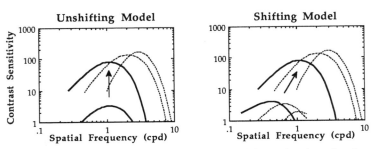

Figure 2. Unshifting and shifting models of spatial mechanism development.

mechanisms receive input from a fixed set of cones, then this packing causes shifts in mechanism tuning to higher frequencies (Wilson, 1988).

The correlations found in Table 1 may be more consistent with the shifting than the unshifting mechanism hypothesis. To understand this, the reader must be aware that adaptation and masking studies indicate that the lowest spatial frequency showing a symmetric tuning curve is near 1 cpd in the adult (Greenlee et al. 1988; Tolhurst, 1973). These results imply that one mechanism only detects patterns below 1 cpd in the adult. It follows that if spatial mechanisms remain stationary (and in this sense, adultlike) during development, then equicorrelational structure should be obtained below 1 cpd from CSFs of both adults and infants. If they shift during development from low to high frequencies, then such equicorrelational structure below 1 cpd should not be obtained from infants.

Studies of sensitivity below 1 cpd have not yet been performed on adults to determine whether equicorrelational structure exists below 1 cpd. However, such structure clearly does not exist in the data from infants. Moreover, Monte Carlo simulations of a quantitative model that shifts spatial mechanisms to higher frequencies with age (Wilson, 1988) reproduced results for 4-, 6-, and 8-month-olds, but simulations of adultlike, unshifting mechanisms did not (Peterzell et al. 1991a,b). We conclude that the results in Table 1 are consistent with the hypothesis that spatial mechanisms shift to higher frequencies during development.

ACKNOWLEDGEMENTS

This research was supported by the NICHD grant HD19143 to P.S. Kaplan and J.S. Werner. The first author's participation in the NATO ASI in Viterbo, Italy was made possible by NATO and by the National Science Foundation (USA).

REFERENCES

Banks, M. S. & Ginsburg, A. P., 1985, Infant visual preferences: a review and new theoretical treatment, *Advances in Child Development and Behavior*, **19**: 207.

Billock, V. A. & Harding, T. H., 1991, The number and tuning of channels responsible for the independent detection of temporal modulation, *Invest. Ophthalmol. Vis. Sci. Suppl.*, **32**: 840.

Fiorentini, A., Pirchio, M. & Spinelli, D., 1983, Electrophysiological evidence for frequency selective mechanisms in adults and infants, *Vis. Res.*, **23**: 119.

Greenlee, M. W., Magnussen, S. & Nordby, K., 1988, Spatial vision of the achromat: spatial frequency and orientation-specific adaptation, *J. Physiol.*, **395**: 661.

Graham, N., 1989, *Visual Pattern Analyzers.*, Oxford University Press, New York.

Movshon, J. A. & Kiorpes, L., 1988, Analysis of spatial contrast sensitivity in monkey and human infants, *J. Opt. Soc. Am. A*, **5**: 2166.

Owsley, C., Sekuler, R. & Siemsen, D., 1983, Contrast sensitivity throughout adulthood, *Vis. Res.*, **23**: 689.

Peterzell, D. H., Werner, J. S. & Kaplan, P. S., 1991a, *Sources of individual differences in the contrast sensitivity functions of human infants*, Submitted for publication.

Peterzell, D. H., Werner, J. S. & Kaplan, P. S., 1991b, Sources of individual differences in CSF development, *Invest. Ophthalmol. Vis. Sci. Suppl.*, **32**: 963.

Sekuler, R., Wilson, H. R. & Owsley, C., 1984, Structural modeling of spatial vision, *Vis Res.* **24**: 689.

Selwyn, E. W. H., 1948, The photographic and visual resolving power of lenses, Part I. Visual resolving power, *The Photographic Journal B*, **88B**: 6.

Tolhurst, D., 1973, Separate channels for the analysis of the shape and movement of a moving visual stimulus, *J. Physiol.*, **231**: 385.

Van Sluyters, R. C., Atkinson, J., Banks, M.S., Held, R.M., Hoffmann, K.-P., & Shatz, C.J., 1990, The development of vision and visual perception, *in* L. Spillmann & J. S. Werner, Eds., *Visual Perception: The Neurophysiological Foundations*, Academic Press, San Diego.

Wilson, H. R., 1988, Development of spatiotemporal mechanisms in infant vision, *Vis. Res.*, **28:** 611.

Wilson, H. R. & Bergen, J. R., 1979, A four mechanism model for spatial vision, *Vis Res.*, **19:** 19.

Yuodelis, C. & Hendrickson, A. E., 1986, A qualitative and quantitative analysis of the human fovea during development, *Vis. Res.*, **26:** 847.

A NEURAL NETWORK MODEL FOR STRIPE FORMATION IN PRIMATE VISUAL CORTEX

Wm. Cowan

Departments of Psychology and Computer Science
University of Waterloo, Waterloo, Ontario, Canada

M. J. Zuckermann

Department of Physics, McGill University
3600 University Street, Montreal, Quebec, Canada

INTRODUCTION

Spontaneous stripe formation occurs in many physical and biological systems[1], for example, the formation of a striped pattern of ocular dominance columns on layer 4, area 17, of the visual cortex, observed in sections parallel to the surface of the cortex. The ocular dominance of a cortical neuron measures the difference in excitation of the neuron when each eye is stimulated separately. In primates it begins to develop shortly before birth. When both eyes experience a normal visual environment or are deprived of pattern vision (binocular deprivation) ocular dominance forms in parallel stripes[2]. This development is disturbed, however, when a single eye is deprived of pattern vision (monocular deprivation) in which case the stripes are spaced less regularly. They also thin, or 'corrode' into patterns with broken stripes[3]. These ocular dominance patterns are symptoms of changes in the strength of synaptic connections between cortical neurons and the neurons in the lateral geniculate from which they receive their input. A summary of the theory of synaptic development and an overview of experiments performed on animals with normal visual experience can be found in our previous work[4,5].

Here we present this theory and continue its development for the formation of the occular dominance stripes. It consists of a neural net having structure based on known physiology of the primate visual system and synaptic strengths that change according to the rules of Hebbian learning[6]. A novel feature of this theory is essential for stripe formation: input correlations that exist in the visual environment are received by the photoreceptors and filtered by retinal circuitry. Thus, the correlations that are induced on the visual cortex, which are responsible for the creation of ocular dominance stripes, are determined by aspects of retinal connectivity that are well-understood and easily measurable. The physiological aspects of the theory are presented in this section and the theory is formally developed in the next section.

Visual inputs into the network are the light intensity patterns, $I_{L,R}(x',t)$, on the right and left retinas, produced by an arbitrary visual scene at time t, with x' a two-dimensional retinal coordinate. This input produces a signal of intensity $J_{L,R}(x,t)$, at the retinal ganglion cells. The signal is a convolution of $I_{L,R}$ with a function,

The Changing Visual System, Edited by P. Bagnoli and
W. Hodos, Plenum Press, New York, 1991

$W(x - x')$, representing the centre–surround receptive field of the ganglion cell,

$$J_{L,R}(x,t) = \int W(x - x)' I_{L,R}(x',t)\, dx'. \tag{1}$$

Signals from the ganglion cells pass via the optic nerve and the lateral geniculate nucleus to cortical cells in layer IV, area 17 of the visual cortex. Each cortical cell receives input from both eyes. The input, $K_0(x,t)$, to the cortex from direct stimulation by retinal ganglion cells can be expressed as a weighted sum over the input intensities

$$K_0(x,t) = V_L(x,t) J_L(x,t) + V_R(x,t) J_R(x,t). \tag{2}$$

Here $V_R(x,t)$ and $V_L(x,t)$ are the strengths of the synaptic coupling between retinal and cortical cells for input from the right and left eyes at time t. The difference between the couplings is the ocular dominance, and the ocular dominance pattern is created by variation in the strength of ocular dominance at different points on the cortex. Note that a retinotrpic map is implicitly assumed in (2), since spatial coordinates on the retina map onto corresponding coordinates on the cortex. Hence the same coordinate notation can be used for both types of cell, except that the cortical magnification factor[7] must be considered when making quantitative calculations. Because of anisotropy in the cortical magnification factor, retinal receptive fields are not radially symmetric when projected onto the visual cortex. The anisotropy varies systematically across the cortex, accounting for long range order in the striped pattern. The total response, $K(x,t)$, of a cortical cell depends on the activities, $K_0(x',t)$, of neighboring cells. This effect is formally expressed by an intra-cortical interaction, $U(x - x')$, that couples each cortical cell to its neighbours,

$$K(x,t) = \int U(x - x') K_0(x',t)\, dx'. \tag{3}$$

The above equations can be regarded as a neural network, with $J_{L,R}(x,t)$ as the input and $K(x,t)$ the output. This network learns by changing the synaptic strengths $V_{L,R}(x,t)$, which develop into the ocular dominance pattern. Synaptic strengths evolve according to Hebbian learning rules during the critical period. Our formulation of these rules[6] changes the synaptic strength proportionally to the product of the input and the output of the cortical cell,

$$\frac{d}{dt} V_a(x,t) = A K(x,t) J_a(x,t) + \text{non-linear terms}. \tag{4}$$

where $a = L, R$. The "non-linear terms" ensure that the synaptic strength functions saturate at a finite value. Eqs. (1) to (4) give the basic physiological relationships of our theory. In these equations, the neural inputs depend on time and the equations cannot be solved unless these inputs are specified.

DERIVATION OF THE LANGEVIN EQUATION

From Eqs. (1) to (4) we obtain an integral equation for the synaptic strengths

$$\begin{aligned} \frac{d}{dt} V_{L,R}(x,t) =\ & J_{L,R}(x,t) \int U(x - x') \times \\ & \times [V_L(x',t) J_L(x',t) + V_R(x',t) J_R(x',t)]\, dx' \\ & + \text{non-linear terms}. \end{aligned} \tag{5}$$

This equation can be integrated using specific retinal inputs $J_{L,R}$, but a more general solution is constructed by separating the time dependence into short and long time scales. The long scale, t_p, defines the time constant over which the stripes evolve while the short scale, t_v, is the time constant of changes in the visual stimulation. Since t_p is of the order of weeks and t_v the order of seconds, $J_{L,R}(x,t) J_{L,R}(x',t)$ can be replaced by its average over t_p

$$F_{ab}(x - x') = \langle J_a(x,t) J_b(x',t) \rangle_t. \tag{6}$$

Then Eq. (5) becomes using Eq. (6)

$$\frac{d}{dt}V_a(x,t)/dt = \int U(x-x') \times$$
$$\times [F_{a,L}(x-x')V_L(x',t) + F_{a,b}(x-x')V_R(x',t)]\,dx'$$
$$+ \text{non-linear terms.} \qquad (7)$$

The ocular dominance is the difference in synaptic coupling from the two eyes, $V_-(x,t) = V_R(x,t) - V_L(x,t)$. The dynamical equation for this quantity is

$$\frac{d}{dt}V_-(x,t) = J_-(x,t)\int U(x-x') \times$$
$$\times \{V_-(x',t)J_-(x',t) + V_+(x',t)J_+(x',t)\}\,dx'$$
$$+ \text{non-linear terms.} \qquad (8)$$

where $V_\pm(x,t) = V_R(x,t) \pm V_L(x,t)$ and $J_\pm(x,t) = J_R(x,t) \pm J_L(x,t)$. Thus, the time evolution of ocular dominance depends on two averages:

$$\langle J_-(x,t)J_-(x',t)\rangle_t = F_{RR}(x-x') + F_{LL}(x-x')$$
$$- F_{LR}(x-x') - F_{RL}(x-x') \qquad (9)$$

and

$$\langle J_-(x,t)J_+(x',t)\rangle_t = F_{RR}(x-x') - F_{LL}(x-x'). \qquad (10)$$

The behaviour of these terms depends on the visual environment of the two eyes. Under conditions characteristic of the mature visual system in an ideal viewing environment (all structured information in the same depth plane, both eyes pointed to the same point in that plane) there is perfect right-left symmetry, $J_R(x,t) = J_L(x,t)$. Then both terms vanish and the time derivative of the ocular dominance is zero. Under more normal viewing conditions the two eyes see the same visual environment, but imperfect eye-pointing occurs: in immature visual systems the mechanisms that control eye direction are not yet fully developped; and even in mature visual systems structure in the visual environment occurs in different depth planes and exact correspondence in all planes is not possible. In this case there is symmetry in the correlation functions: $F_{RR}(x-x') = F_{LL}(x-x')$ and $F_{LR}(x-x') = F_{RL}(x-x')$, but $F_{RR}(x-x') \neq F_{RL}(x-x')$. The second term in the time evolution equation is zero, but the first is non-zero. When calculated in detail the non-zero term is found to have a three-lobed structure that leads to ocular dominance stripes[5].

Similar conditions apply in embryo, after the visual system is well-enough established for spontaneous firing in retinal cells to excite the visual cortex. Ocular dominance columns begin forming in the *rhesus* monkey twenty days before birth when no visual input is available. A recent model suggests that the ocular dominance columns form initially via spontaneous firing of retinal cells, since toxic blocking of retinal activity prevents their formation. The visual environment subsequently refines the columns after birth. The formalism presented above can be applied to spontaneous firing of retinal cells in embryo. The light intensity patterns, $I_{L,R}(x,t)$, are random, and the correlation functions, $\langle I_{L,R}(x,t)I_{L,R}(x,t)\rangle_t$, which are averages over the time constant related to the evolution of the stripes, have the same functional form as for random eye pointing.

The third case occurs when the two eyes experience different visual environments, a condition that can occur naturally as a result of abnormal development of one eye or that can be produced artificially by eyelid suture or similar treatment. In this case both terms are non-zero, the first between ocular dominance at different sites on the cortex, the second mediating an interaction between the ocular dominance at one site and the total synaptic strength at other sites. Unfortunately, suitable models for the development of the total synaptic strength are unavailable: our earlier work did not require them because it was confined to the second case, in which coupling to the total synaptic strength is zero. A reasonable approximation takes the total synaptic strength to be constant; future work will relax that constraint. With the total synaptic strength constant the second term is a bias field the strength of which depends on the degree of assymmetry between the two eyes. The first term, on the other hand, is an interaction term of the same form as that treated in our earlier work. Thus, in this approximation the provides an adequate generalization to handle the case where the two eyes are treated assymmetrically.

The full Langevin equation can then be written in terms of the bias field, H, from Eqs. (8) to (10):

$$\frac{d}{dt}V_-(x,t) = \int T(x - x')V_-(x',t)\,dx' + H + \text{non-linear terms.} \tag{11}$$

where
$$T(x - x') = F^0_{RR}(x - x') - F^0_{LR}(x - x'). \tag{12}$$

and the superscript zero indicates quantities for which both eyes see the same visual environment. $T(x)$ is the three–lobed function, which is a convolution of the product of two retinal receptive fields, $W(x)$.

In reference 5 we reported preliminary results of numerical simulations of Eq. (11) for $H = 0$. In the simulations, the "non-linear terms" represent biological constraints of unknown form that confine the function, $V_-(x,t)$, between $+1$ (right eye dominance) and -1 (left eye dominance). Since an abrupt cutoff can lead to anomalous behaviour near saturation, a local cubic term, $V^3_-(x,t)$, is added to the right hand side of Eq. (11). This term ensures ensures a smooth mechanism for saturation. The model is analogous to theories that are used to describe phase separation and the resulting non-linear equation for the cortical synaptic strengths,$V(x,t)$ can be identified with a type of Langevin equation often used in statistical physics[8].

DISCUSSION AND CONCLUSION

The linear Langevin equation was solved numerically; for perfect left-right symmetry it was also solved using a perturbative approximation[9]. The results are described in reference 10. For anisotropic forms of the function, T(x), of Eq. 12 (see reference 10) a regular striped pattern was found for left–right symmetry ($H = 0$).

Several extensions to the model are worth considering. For example, ocular dominance is frozen at the end of the critical period. This may result either from central control of the plasticity of neural connections in the cortex or from a natural termination of the developmental process. Some physiological evidence[11] indicates the former; further investigation of evolution models will determine whether the action of non-linear terms can be excluded as a contrary explanation. Finally, several different mathematical expressions of Hebbian learning exist, all possesssing the same qualitative features: input activity that results in similar output activity strengthens the input connection; other input activity weakens it. It is important to investigate the robustness of simulation results as the mathematical form of learning function varies. We are also using a generalised version of this model to study orientational selectivity.

The benefit of investigating models of this type is suggested by two robust predictions. First, combining the size of retinal receptive fields with the cortical magnification factor produces a quantitative prediction of the period of stripes on the cortex with no model-dependent factors. The predicted period is 350 μm, which lies in the range of measured stripe periods. Second, since stripe orientation is controlled by receptive field anisotropy, the anisotropy of the cortical magnification factor can be used to predict the global pattern of orientation stripes throughout area 17, again with no model-dependent factors. Observed patterns are in qualitative agreement with this prediction. The second prediction suggests that it is possible to create a complete model of area 17, including boundary conditions, and observe its global development. The separation of time scales used in this model makes economical simulation of such a system possible. Thus, we believe that models based on the ideas presented here form an important adjunct to the experimental tools of neuroanatomy and neurophysiology.

ACKNOWLEDGEMENTS

This work was supported by by the NSERC of Canada, and by le Ministere des Affaires Intergouvernementales du Quebec. One of us (MJZ) wishes to thank Angela Brown, Barbara Chapman, Rodney Cotterill, John Hertz, Dale Hogan, Leslie Holden and Roger Ward for extremely interesting discussions. Both authors wish to express their gratitude to Diane Koziol for manuscript preparation.

REFERENCES

1. J. D. Murray, "Mathematical Biology", Springer Verlag, Berlin Heidelberg (1989), pp. 372–592.
2. S. LeVay, M. Connoly, J.D. Houde, and D.C. Essen "The Complete Pattern of Ocular Dominance Stripes in the Striate Cortex and Visual Field of the Macaque Monkey", *J. Neurosci.*, 5:486 (1985).
3. T.N. Wiesel, Nobel Lecture, "The Postnatal Development of the Visual Cortex and the Influence of Environment", *Biosci. Reports* 2:351 (1982).
4. J.R. Thomson, "Co-operative Models for Pattern Formation in Primate Visual Cortex: Simulation of Phase Behavior", M.Sc. Thesis, McGill University, 1989; J.R. Thomson, Wm Cowan, M.J. Zuckermann and M. Grant *in* "Lectures on Thermodyanamics and Statistical Mechanics: Proceedings of the XVIII Winter Meeting on Statistical Physics" (ed. A.E. Gonzalez, M. Medina-Noyola and C. Varea), World Scientific, Singapore, (1989), pp. 38–51.
5. J.R. Thomson, Z. Zhang,Wm Cowan,M. Grant, J.A. Hertz and M.J. Zuckermann, "A Simple Model for Pattern Formation in Primate Visual Cortex in the Case of Monocular Deprivation", *Physica Scripta* T33:102 (1990).
6. D.O. Hebb, "Organisation of Behavior", John Wiley and Sons, New York (1949).
7. B.M. Dow, R.G. Vautin R. and Bauer, "The Mapping of Visual Space onto Foveal Striate Cortex in the Macaque Monkey", *J. Neurosci.* 324:221 (1982).
8. J.D. Gunton and M. Droz, M, "Introduction to the Theory of Metastable and Unstable States", Springer Verlag, Heidelberg (1983).
9. K.R. Elder and M. Grant, "Singular Perturbation Theory for Phase Front Dynamics and Pattern Selection", *J. Phys. (London)* A23:L803 (1989).
10. J.R. Thomson, K.R. Elder, G. Soga, Z. Zhang, Wm Cowan, M. Grant and M.J. Zuckermann, "Neural Networks with Constrained Inputs as Models for Primate Visual Cortex", *Phys. Rev. A*, (submitted).
11. W. Singer, F. Tretter and R. Vinon, "Central Gating of Developmental Plasticity in Kitten Visual Cortex", *J. Neurosci.*, 5:890 (1985).

STEREO MATCHING USING RELAXATION LABELING

BASED ON EDGE AND ORIENTATION FEATURES

Jesse S. Jin

Department of Computer Science
University of Otago, Dunedin
New Zealand

INTRODUCTION

For humans, the most reliable sources of depth information come from vision. The ability to judge relative depth binocularly is called stereopsis. Binocular neurons in the visual system perform two of the operations necessary for stereopsis; feature matching and disparity computation [Poggio & Fischer 1977, Ferster 1981]. Julesz [Julesz 1960] showed by means of random-dot stereograms that binocular disparity is a sufficient cue for stereoscopic depth perception. The matching operation, though performed so well by the human visual system, raises a major problem in computer vision. In this paper we develop a model of binocular vision, which uses both binocular cues and monocular cues in stereo matching.

In our model we map images of two views to a Gaussian sphere. The mapping combines monocular features, like edge and orientation, with binocular features like fixation axis and the ratio of stereo offset and visual distance. One problem in stereo matching using edges and orientations is that orientations and edges require different coordinate systems. The results depend critically upon the scale used to measure each coordinate. We cope with this problem by using probabilities. The mapping to the Gaussian sphere defines a relation between two images and the visual world. So, the probability distribution of orientations in two images is the probability distribution of orientations in the real world with a scale factor of the determinant of the Jacobian of the mapping.

We use relaxation labeling to search for a consistent mapping between the two stereoscopic images [Rosenfeld 1977]. A consistent labeling of units in a compatibility model of the images has to satisfy the conditions:

$$0 \le p_i \le 1, \quad \sum_{k=1}^{m} p_i(\lambda_k) = 1$$

where $p_i(\lambda_k)$ is the probability of unit i being labelled as λ_k. We give a formula for the probability of a mapping satisfying the above conditions. The formula is used to set the initial probability of a labeling under a given percentile of reliability. It is also used to modify the acceleration factor of the relaxation process.

FEATURE EXTRACTION

We recognize objects by extracting features of them. It is known [Marr et al. 1979] that image structure is represented initially by zero-crossings, after the image has been

The Changing Visual System, Edited by P. Bagnoli and
W. Hodos, Plenum Press, New York, 1991

bandpass filtered at multiple scales by neural receptive fields whose two dimensional profiles resemble the Laplacian of a Gaussian function(LoG). Zero-crossings are rich in information of physically meaningful structures such as edges and occlusion boundaries. However, some simple information processing operations that are apparent in human pattern vision can be shown to be impossible in the representation of zero-crossings, because the bandpassed signals do not capture the necessary of information and there are no such zero-crossings in the signal after LoG filtering at any scale [Daugman 1988]. Later models of information processing in biological visual system have proposed that simple cells of the striate cortex in the visual cortex fire responding to phase, frequency and orientation. Watson [1983], Daugman [1985], and Caelli *et al.* [1987], among others, have used the Gabor function to model this stage of visual processing.

The Gabor function is formed from the product of a sine and a Gaussian function. By changing the phase and frequency of the sine, as well as the width of the Gaussian function, and the orientation and the ratio of spatial and spectral of the sine in the Gaussian function, a family of Gabor functions can be generated. A Gabor function with a specific set of parameters is also called a Gabor filter. They can extract frequency, phase and orientation information, which is very useful in texture discrimination, motion and pattern detection.

The general form of the 2D Gabor function is given by:

$$g(x, y) = \exp\{-k(x^2+y^2)/w^2\} \exp\{-2\pi fi[(x\cos\theta+y\sin\theta) + \phi]\}$$

where k is a scale factor and w is the width of the Gaussian function, and f is the frequency, θ is the orientation and ϕ is the phase of the sinusoidal wave inside the Gaussian function. We have $k=4\ln2$ if width is the diameter of the Gaussian function at half height and the frequency bandwidth σ of the Gabor function has a relation $\sigma=4\ln2/(\pi w)$ with the spatial width w. Psychophysical data show that frequency bandwidths for simple striate cells range from one half to 2.5 octaves [Watson 1983]. We use one octave bandwidth to comprise the range, which gives $w=1.324/f$. Eight one-octave functions cover approximately the human visual sense ranging from 0 to 60 cycles/degree. The angle interval of the function is 36°. Fig.1 shows a Gabor function and its Fourier Transform.

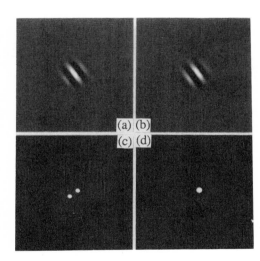

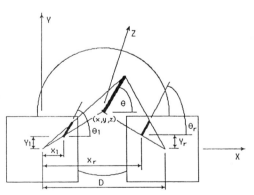

Fig.1. Gabor function and its Fourier Transform: (a) Real part of the Gabor function; (b) imaginary part of the Gabor function; (c) the Fourier Transform of (a); (d) the Fourier Transform of the Gabor function.

Fig.2. Binocular setup and Gaussian sphere model

Different choices for the values of the parameters would centre the function at different spatial locations and give it different preferred spatial-frequency and orientation responses corresponding to centroid frequency locations.

STEREO MODEL FOR MATCHING

Three steps are involved in measuring stereo disparity: (1) A particular location on a surface in the scene must be selected from one image; (2) that same location must be identified in the other image; and (3) the disparity between the two corresponding image points must be measured. Early work in stereo computer vision restricts the study to each camera separately. Feature extraction is done with information from one image only. Correlation between two cameras is not considered until matching, and even in matching, not enough attention has been paid to. Marr and Poggio [1979] developed a model of human stereopsis. In their model matching is based on zero-crossings with different scales rather than points. In humans, the two eyes look at much the same region of visual space. Within the region of binocular overlap, the two eyes view objects from slightly different vantage points, owing to the lateral separation of the eyes within the head. We develop a stereo model (see Fig.2). The origin of the system is located at the focus of the left camera and the right camera focus lies on the x axis. The two image planes are coplanar and are perpendicular to the z axis. The offset of a baseline, D, is the distance between the foci. We normalize this arrangement by using the focus f as the unit of length, i.e., f=1. This setup of the binocular model allows us to constrain the matching process to matching the features in a given left epipolar line with corresponding features in the right epipolar line. The parameters of a feature are the position and orientation of its edges.

If we represent this edge in an oriented vector in three dimensional space, it has an angle θ with the x axis and an angle φ with the z axis. By using these two angles, the edge also can be represented as a point on the surface of a unit sphere, whose origin is (x, y, z). This is known as the Gaussian sphere [Arnold & Binford 1980], and the point is located on its surface in terms of spherical coordinates θ and φ. The orientation feature represented by the point on the Gaussian sphere casts a pair of image angles, (θ_l, θ_r), on the left image and the right image. A continuous function exists for mapping the points on the Gaussian sphere, with coordinates θ and φ, to the image angles (θ_l, θ_r). Similarly, there is an inverse function P which maps points in the space $\theta_l \times \theta_r$ to points on the Gaussian sphere, $\theta \times \varphi$. There is a theorem about the probability distribution of a function of a stochastic variable,

i.e., $\psi(\theta_l, \theta_r) = |J_P| f(q(\theta, \varphi))$, where $|J_P| = \left| \dfrac{\partial(\theta_l, \theta_r)}{\partial(\theta, \varphi)} \right|$ is the Jacobian determinant of

mapping P and q is the inverse mapping function from (θ_l, θ_r) to (θ, φ).

MATCHING BY RELAXATION LABELING

We can use the probability $\psi(\theta_l, \theta_r)$ to guide stereo matching. First we extract features $(\theta_{l_1}, \theta_{l_2}, ..., \theta_{l_m})$ from the left image and features $(\theta_{r_1}, \theta_{r_2}, ..., \theta_{r_n})$ from the right image, then perform relaxation labeling on θ_{l_i} and θ_{r_j} to get the optimal matching. The updating formula is

$$p_i^{(k+1)}(\lambda) = \frac{p_i^{(k)}(\lambda)[1+q_i^{(k)}(\lambda)]}{\sum_{\lambda} p_i^{(k)}(\lambda)[1+q_i^{(k)}(\lambda)]}$$

where

$$q_i^{(k)}(\lambda) = \sum_j c_{ij} \sum_{\lambda'} r_{ij}(\lambda, \lambda') \, P_j(\lambda')$$

$$r_{ij}(\lambda, \lambda') = \frac{p_{ij}(\lambda, \lambda') - p_i(\lambda)p_j(\lambda')]}{\sigma_{p_i}(\lambda)\sigma_{p_j}(\lambda')}$$

The initial probabilities are obtained by

$$p_i = \frac{\psi_i + 2\sum_{j=i+1}^{n}\psi_j}{(\sum_{i=1}^{n}\psi_i)^2}$$

where ψ_i, $\psi_j \in \psi(\theta_l, \theta_r)$ and $\psi_i < \psi_j$ if $j < i$. Clearly $\sum_i p_i = 1$. The coefficients c_{ij} represent a possible weighting over the neighbouring objects a_i and a_j and insure that q_i is in the range $[-1, 1]$. After matching, depth is obtained from stereo disparity and surfaces of an object are interpolated by solving consistency equations.

CONCLUSION

The relaxation approach emulates the mechanisms of binocularly activated visual cortex cells like fusion and rivalry. The mechanisms of how the brain utilizes the signals from two eyes to recover the depth of objects are rather complicated. Computer emulation gives one way to explore this area.

REFERENCES

Arnold, R D & Binford, T O (1980). Geometric constraints in stereo vision. SPIE 238:281-292

Caelli, T; Rentschler, I & Scheidler, W (1987). Visual pattern recognition in humans. Biological Cybernetics 57:233-240

Daugman, J G (1985). Uncertainty relation for resolution in space, spatial frequency, and orientation optimized by two-dimensional visual cortical filters. J. Opt. Soc. Am. 2(7):1160-1169

Daugman, J G (1988). Pattern and motion vision without Laplacian zero crossings. J. Opt. Soc. Am. 5(7):1142-1148

Julesz, B (1960). Binocular depth perception of computer-generated patterns. Bell syst Tech J 39:1125-1162

Marr, D & Poggio, T (1979). A theory of human stereo vision. Proceedings of the Royal Society of London B204:301-328

Marr, D; Ullamn, S & Poggio, T (1979). Bandpass channels, zero-crossings, and early visual information processing. J. Opt. Soc. Am. 69:914-916

Poggio, G F & Fischer, B (1977). Binocular interaction and depth sensitivity in striate and prestriate cortex of behaving rhesus monkeys. J. Neurophysiol. 40:1392-1407

Rosenfeld, A (1977). Iterative methods in image analysis. In *Proc IEEE Conf on Pattern Recognition Image Processing*, pp.14-18, New York.

Watson, A B (1983). Detection and recognition of simple spatial forms. In *Physical and biological processing of images,* pp 101-114, Edited by O J Braddick & A C Sleigh, New York, Springer-Verlag

Augusti-Tocco, Gabriella
Dipartimento di Biologia Cellulare
  e dello Sviluppo
Universitá La Sapienza
P.az A. Moro
00185 Roma - Italy

Bagnoli, Paola
Facoltá di Scienze MFN
Universitá della Tuscia
Via S. Camillo de Lellis
01100 Viterbo - Italy

Bischof, Hans Joachim
Fakultat Biologie
Universitat Bielefeld
P.O. Box 8640
4800 Bielefeld 1 - Germany

Bolz, Jurgen
Friedrich-Miescher Labor
der Max Planck Gesellschaft
Spemannstrasse 37-39
7400 Tubingen - Germany

Brecha, C. Nicholas
Department of Anatomy and
  Cell Biology
VA Medical Center
Wilshire and Sawtelle Blvds.
Los Angeles, CA 90073 - U.S.A.

Brunelli, Marcello
Dipartimento di Fisiologia e
  Biochimica
Universitá di Pisa
Via S. Zeno 31
56127 Pisa - Italy

Burkhalter, Andreas
Department of Neurology
School of Medicine
Washington University
St. Louis, MI 63110 - U.S.A

Casini, Giovanni
Dept. of Anatomy and Cell Biology
VA Medical Center
Wilshire and Sawtelle Blvds.
Los Angeles, CA 90073 - U.S.A.

Chapman, Barbara
Department of Physiology
Box 0444 UCSF
San Francisco, CA 94143 - U.S.A.

Comelli, Maria Cristina
FIDIA Research Laboratories
Via Ponte della Fabbrica 3A
35031 Abano Terme (Padova) - Italy

Demircioglu, F. Ferkan
School of Medicine
Gazi University
GMK Bul.18/5 Demirtepse
06440 Ankara - Turkey

Djamgoz, B.A. Mustafa
Dept. of Pure and Applied Biology
Imperial College, Prince Consort Rd.
London SW 7 - U.K.

Domenici, Luciano
Istituto di Neurofisiologia del CNR
Via S. Zeno 51
56127 Pisa -- Italy

Engelage, Jurgen
Fakultat Biologie
Universitat Bielefeld
P.O. Box 8640
4800 Bielefeld 1 - Germany

Fite, Katherine
Department of Psychology
Massachusetts University
Amherst, MA 01002 - U.S.A.

Fontanesi, Gigliola
Dipartimento di Fisiologia e
    Biochimica
Universitá di Pisa
Via S. Zeno 31
56127 Pisa - Italy

Fritzsch, Bernd
Department of Biomedical Sciences
Creighton University
Division of Anatomy
Omaha, NE 68178 - U.S.A.

Herrmann, Kathrin
Department of Neurobiology
School of Medicine
Stanford University
Stanford, CA 94305 - U.S.A.

Hogan, Dale
Department of Anatomy and Cell
    Biology
Medical Center
Kansas University
Kansas City, KS 66103 - U.S.A.

Hodos, William
Department of Psychology
Maryland University
College Park, MD 20742 - U.S.A.

Holden, A. Leslie
Dept. of Pure and Applied Biology
Imperial College
Prince Consort Road
London SW 7 - U.K.

Jin, S. Jesse
Department of Computer Sciences
Otago University
P.O. Box 56
Dunedin - New Zealand

Karten, J. Harvey
Department of Neuroscience
California University
9500 Gilman Drive
La Jolla, CA 92093 - U.S.A.

Kuljis, O. Rodrigo
Department of Neurology
College of Medicine
Iowa University
Iowa City, IA 52242-1053 - U.S.A.

Levi, Andrea
Istituto di Neurobiologia del CNR
Viale C. Marx
00185 Roma - Italy

Owsley, Cynthia
Department of Ophthalmology
Alabama University
UAB Station
Birmingham, AL 35294 - U.S.A.

Peterzell, H. David
Infant Vision Laboratory
Department of Psychology
Colorado University
Boulder, CO 80309 - U.S.A.

Porciatti, Vittorio
Divisione Oculistica
USL 13
57100 Livorno - Italy

Rakic, Pasko
Section of Neuroanatomy
School of Medicine
Yale University
333 Cedar Street
New Haven, CT 06510 - U.S.A.

Shimizu, Toru
Department of Psychology
South Florida University
4202 E. Fowler Avenue
Tampa, FL 33620 - U.S.A.

Silva-Araujo, Antonia Luis
Institute of Anatomy
Medical School
4200 Porto - Portugal

Sturr, F. Joseph
Department of Psychology
Syracuse University
473 Huntington Hall
Syracuse, NY 13244-2340 - U.S.A.

Tavares, Maria Amelia
Institute of Anatomy
Medical School
4200 Porto - Portugal

Thanos, Solon
Max Planck Institut fur Entwicklungbiol.
Spemannstrasse 35/1
7400 Tubingen 1 - Germany

Ward, Roger
Museum National d'Histoire Naturelle
57, rue Cuvier
75005 Paris - France

Weale, Robert
Cornwall House Annex
Waterloo Road
London SE1 8TX - U.K.

Werner, Jack
Department of Psychology
Colorado University
Box 345
Boulder, CO 80309-0345 - U.S.A.

Wilm, Claudia
E. Merck Biologische Forschung
P.O. Box 4119
61 Dormstadt 1 - Germany

Zuckermann, Martin
Department of Physics
McGill University
3600 University Street
H3A 2T8 Montreal-PQ - Canada

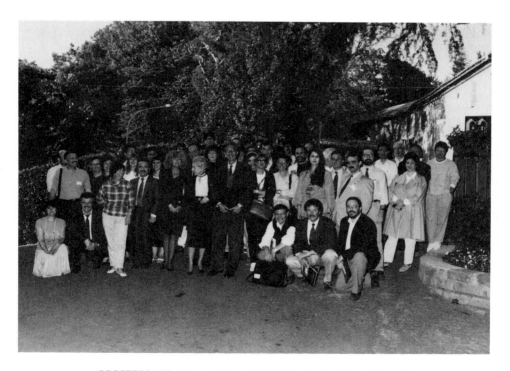

PROCEEDINGS OF A NATO ADVANCED RESEARCH WORKSHOP
ON THE CHANGING VISUAL SYSTEM
MAY 26 - JUNE 6, 1991
SAN MARTINO AL CIMINO (VITERBO), ITALY

INDEX

ABV, *see* Anomalous binocular vision
Accommodative insufficiency, 15–16
Acetylcholine, 66
Acetylcholinesterase (AChE), 312–317
AChE, *see* Acetylecholinesterase
Actin, 161, 162, 323
Actinic keratitis, 296
Actinomycin D, 180, 181
Actuarial approach, 25, 26, 28
Adaptive theory, 12
Adenosine triphosphatase (ATPase), 175, 177
Adenylate cyclase, 174, 177, 179
Afferent system, 42, 45, 62–63, 64
AFM, *see* Anomalous fusional movements
Afterhyperpolarization (AH), 175, 181
Aging, 11–19, 283–293, 303–305
    achievement peaks compared with, 14–17
    animal models of, *see* Animal models
    biomarkers and, 26–29, 30–31
    color discrimination and, 19, 30, 301–303
    contrast sensitivity and, 18, 209, 392
    HCs and, 149
    learning processes and, 171
    light and, 284–285, 287–292, 295–296,
        297–298, 299–301, 305–308, *see also*
        Ultraviolet radiation
    parabola of vision and, 17–19
    in PERG/VEP spatio-temporal patterns,
        209–216
    sensitivity losses and, *see* Sensitivity losses
    sex differences in, 285, 286, 287, 288, 289, 292,
        293
    spatial contrast sensitivity and, 119–132, *see*
        also Spatial contrast
        sensitivity
    visual acuity and, 31, 121–122, 130, 137–147,
        209
Agnosia, 51
AH, *see* Afterhyperpolarization
Alanine, 174
Amacrine cells, 38, 42, 65, 67, 71
    narrow-field, 96, 379
    wide-field, *see* Wide-field amacrine cells
Amblyopia, 15, 333, 343
Amphibians, 24, 27, 33, 34, 62, 63, 70
Andocytosis, 78
Animal models, 21–31, *see also* specific types

Animal models (*cont'd*)
    best types of, 23–25
    reasons for studying, 21–23
    relative rates of aging in, 25–26
Anisometropia, 343
Anisotropy, 398, 400
Anomalous binocular vision (ABV), 276, 277
Anomalous fusional movements (AFM), 279,
    280
Anomalous retinal correspondence (ARC),
    269–274, 276, 278–279, 280
Anophthalmia, 255–261
Anysomycin, 180
Aploscopic test, 275
Aplysia, 172–174, 175, 179, 181
Apparent latency, 213, 215–216
Aprotinin, 80
Aqueous humor, 296, 297
ARC, *see* Anomalous retinal correspondence
Astrocytes, 78, 90, 351, 352
ATPase, *see* Adenosine triphosphatase
Attenuation factor, 177
Axial optic tract, 39, 40, 45
Axons, 385, 388
    anophthalmia and, 258, 259
    in centrifugal visual system, 61, 63, 64–65
    development of, 3, 4, 5, 7
    in infant visual cortex, 250, 252
    intraocular activity blockade and,
        369
    ipsilateral projections and, 358, 359
    in learning processes, 171
    monocular deprivation and, 204, 333
    in neuronal differentiation, 311
    neuropeptides and, 187, 191
    NGF and, 347, 350, 351, 353
    ontogeny of, 38, 39, 42, 45
    of projection neurons, 234, 241, 244
    proteolytic activity blockage and, *see*
        Proteolytic activity blockage
    of tectofugal pathway, 199, 202, 204
    wide-field amacrine cells and, 105
Axotomy, 77–91, 348, 350, *see also* Proteolytic
    activity blockage

Basal optic root, 189, 191
Basal optic tract, 39

Basal telencephalon, 62, 64
Basic fibroblast growth factor (bFGF), 79, 86, 87, 88, 89, 322
BDNF, *see* Brain-derived neurotrophic factor
Behcet's disease, 365–366
bFGF, *see* Basic fibroblast growth factor
Binocular deprivation, 397
Binocular vision
    in strabismus, 275, 276, 277
    tectofugal pathway and, 201, 206
Bio-economics, 13, 14–15, 16–17
Biomarkers of aging, 26–29, 30–31
Bipolar cells, 95
Birds, *see also* specific types
    advantages of studying, 24
    biomarkers of aging in, 27, 28
    centrifugal visual system of, 61, 62, 63, 66, 67, 68, 69, 70–71
    ontogeny of, 34, 42
    reasons for studying, 22–23
    retina of, 137–147, 283–293
    in visual hierarchy, 51–58
Blindness, 51, 56, 215–216, 284
Blindsight, 56
Bloch-Sulzberger syndrome, 361–363
Blue-sensitive cones, 3, 152, 163, 302, 303
Brain-derived neurotrophic factor (BDNF), 79, 87, 88, 89, 354
Bruch's membrane, 283, 292, 304

Calendar effects, 22, 25
Callosal cells, 234–235, 236, 237, 239, 240, 258
Calpain, 80
cAMP, *see* Cyclic adenosine monophosphate
Campimetry, 275
CAT, *see* Chloramphenicol acethyl transferase
Cataracts
    spatial contrast sensitivity and, 119, 120, 123–124
    UVR and, 295, 297–298, 307
Catecholamines, 100, 107, 193, 383, *see also* specific types
Cathepsin, 80
Cats
    LGN of, 369–372
    monocular deprivation in, 206
    tectofugal pathway in, 199
    visual cortex of, 385–388
    in visual hierarchy, 57
cDNA, 320, 321, 323, 325
Central nervous system (CNS), 149, 347, 353
Central vision, 130
Centrifugal thalmic optic nucleus, 63–64
Centrifugal visual system, 61–71
    functional investigations of, 67–68
Cerebral cortex, 1, 3
cGMP, *see* Cyclic guanosine monophosphate
ChAT, *see* Choline acetyltransferase
Chloramphenicol acethyl transferase (CAT), 323, 324
Choline acetyltransfease (ChAT), 314, 315, 342
Cholinergic cells, 96, 105, 106, 110, 111, 347, 353

Choriocapillaris, 283, 284, 285, 292
Choroid, 287, 299, 304, 365
Chromaticity horizontal cells, 151, 152, 153, 154, 159, 162, 163
Chromogranin, 325, 328
Chymotrypsin, 80
Cichlid fish, 42
    ipsilateral projections in, 357–359
CNS, *see* Central nervous sytem
Color discrimination
    aging and, 19, 30, 301–303
    tectofugal pathway and, 199
    UVR and, 296
Cones, *see also* Growth cones
    aging in, 285, 301–303
        animal models of, 30
        light and, 287, 288, 289, 290, 291, 292, 299–301, 305–308, 396
        sensitivity losses and, 219–221, 222, 228, 229–230
        sites of loss in, 303–305
        spatial contrast sensitivity and, 129
        visual acuity and, 140
    blue-sensitivity, *see* Blue-sensitive cones
    contrast sensitivity and, 394
    development of, 3
    green-sensitivity, *see* Green-sensitive cones
    HCs and, 149–164, *see also* Horizontal cells
    long-wave-sensitivity, *see*
        Long-wave-sensitive cones
    middle-wave-sensitivity, *see*
        Middle-wave-sensitive cones
    red-sensitivity, *see* Red-sensitive cones
    short-wave-sensitivity, *see*
        Short-wave-sensitive cones
Conjunctivitis, 365
Contrast sensitivity, 209, 248
    individual differences in, 391–395
    monocular deprivation and, 335, 336, 339, 342
    spatial, 119–132, 248
        individual differences in, 392, 393, 394–395
        underlying mechanisms of, 122–129
        visual tasks and, 129–132
    UVR and, 18
Cornea, 140, 295, 296, 297, 299, 300, 301
Corneal scarring, 12
Cortical cells, 377, 398
    monocular deprivation and, 334, 336, 337, 342, 350
    sensitivity losses and, 222
Corticotectal cells, 234, 235, 236, 237, 238, 240, 241
Corticothalmic cells, 241
Cotrasmission, 185
Cotton-wool spots, 366
CRE, *see* Cyclic adenosine monophosphate (cAMP)-responsive element
Crocodiles, 64
Crystalline lens, 19, 215
    light and, 18, 295, 296, 297–298, 299, 301, 305, 306
    ontogeny of, 45

Crystalline lens (cont'd)
  sensitivity losses and, 221, 229
  spatial contrast sensitivity and, 119, 123–124
  visual acuity and, 140
Cyclic adenosine monophosphate (cAMP)
  HCs and, 161
  in learning processes, 173, 174, 176–177, 179, 180, 181
  VGF gene and, 322, 323, 324
Cyclic adenosine monophosphate (cAMP)-responsive element (CRE), 180, 323
Cyclic adenosine monophosphate (cAMP)-responsive element binding protein (CREBP), 180
Cyclic guanosine monophosphate (cGMP), 179
Cycloeximide, 181, 323
Cyclostomes, 61, 65, 66, 68, 69, 70, see also specific types
Cysteine, 328
Cytochalasin, 162
Cytochrome c, 334, 335, 336, 339, 342
Cytochrome oxidase, 249, 258, 259, 260, 262, 263, 264
Cytokeratin, 362, 363

Dark adaptation, 221
  centrifugal visual system and, 71
  HCs and, 155, 160, 161, 164
  sensitivity losses and, 223, 224, 226, 227, 229–230
  spatial contrast sensitivity and, 129
Darwin, Charles, 33
dbcAMP, see Dibutyryl cyclic adenosine monophosphate
Dendrites
  in centrifugal visual system, 65
  of HCs, 160
  in infant visual cortex, 252
  intraocular activity blockade and, 369–372
  ipsilateral projections and, 358
  light adaptation and, 156–158, 160
  in neuronal differentiation, 311, 317
  ontogeny of, 37, 43
  of projection neurons, 233, 234, 235, 237
  proteolytic activity blockage and, 87
  synaptic plasticity and, 152, 153, 156–158
  of tectofugal pathway, 201–202, 205
  of wide-field amacrine cells, 105
Detection thresholds, 122, 129, 224
Diabetes mellitus, 367–368
Diabetic retinopathy, 120, 367–368
Dibutyryl cyclic adenosine monophosphate (dbcAMP), 161, 324
Diencephalon, 62, 63, 193
3,3' Dihydroxy-alpha-carotene, 299
Diplopia, 271, 273–274, 276, 279
Dishabituation, 172, 173–174, 175
Disparity computation, 403
Disposable-soma theory, 12, 22, 27, 146
DNA, 22, 296, 298, 324, 329

Dolphins, 24
Dopamine
  HCs and, 160–161
  in learning processes, 174, 177, 179
  visual acuity and, 143
  wide-field amacrine cells and, 97, 107, 111, 379, 382
Dorsal raphe nucleus, 62, 64
Dorsal root ganglia (DRG), 313–315
Dorsal thalamus, 62
Dorsal ventricular ridge (DVR), 54, 55, 56, 57
DRG, see Dorsal root ganglia
Driving, 119, 129, 130–131
Drusen, 119
DVR, see Dorsal ventricular ridge

Ectopic neurons, 64, 66, 69
Ectostriatum, 200, 201, 202–203, 204–205, 206
Edinger-Westphal nucleus, 43
Efferent system, 53, 70, 235
  ontogeny of, 39, 40–42, 45, 46
EGF, see Epidermal growth factor
Electrogenic pump, 175–177
Electroretinograms (ERGs), 68, see also Flash electroretinogram; Pattern electroretinogram
Emetine, 180
Endoplasmic reticulum, 185–186, 325
Ependymal cells, 37
Epidermal growth factor (EGF), 322
EPSPs, see Excitatory post-synaptic potentials
EPTA, see Ethanolic-phosphotungstic acid
Equilibrium hues, 302
ERGs, see Electroretinograms
Estropia, 277, 279
Ethanolic-phosphotungstic acid (EPTA), 153, 156
Excitatory post-synaptic potentials (EPSPs), 67, 172, 173, 180
Extracellular unit recording, 335, 336–337
Extraocular muscles, 35, 43
Extrastriate cortex, 199, 200
  hierarchial model of, 51, 53, 55, 56, 57–58

Face identification, 119, 129–130
Factor VIII, 361–362
Feature extraction, 403–405
FERG, see Flash electroretinogram
Ferret visual cortex, 375–377
Fibrillogenesis, 181
Fish, 24, see also specific types
  ontogeny of, 34, 42
Flash electroretinogram (FERG), 137, 140
Flash-on-flash technique, 220, 223, 224, 227, 228, 229–230
Forebrain
  NGF and, 347, 353
  ontogeny of, 34–35, 36, 37, 45
Fovea, 284, 304
  contrast sensitivity and, 394
  diabetes and, 367
  light and, 299, 301

Fovea (*cont'd*)
  sensitivity losses and, 220
Foveolar hemorrhages, 367
Free radicals, 11, 284, 285, 295, 298, 299

GABA, *see* Gamma-aminobutyric acid
Gabor function, 404
Gain control, 226
Gamma-aminobutyric acid (GABA)
  in centrifugal visual system, 66
  in HCs, 158, 162
  in learning processes, 174
  in wide-field amacrine cells, 96, 97, 105, 106,
    110, 111, 379, 382
Ganglion cells, 95
  aging in, 128, 140, 222
  anophthalmia and, 259
  axotomy in, *see* Axotomy
  Bloch-Sulzberger syndrome and, 362
  in centrifugal visual system, 62, 64, 65, 66, 67,
    71
  development of, 1, 3
  HCs and, 164
  in infants, 248
  intraocular activity blockade and, 372
  ipsilateral projections and, 357, 358, 359
  in learning processes, 173, 174, 178, 179, 182
  monocular deprivation and, 204
  neuropeptides in, 186, 187, 188, 192, 194
  NGF and, 347, 348–350, 353, 354
  ontogeny of, 35, 37, 38, 39, 40, 41, 42, 44, 45
  sensitivity losses and, 222
  spatial contrast sensitivity and, 128
  stripe formation and, 397–398
  tectofugal pathway and, 200, 204, 206
  visual acuity and, 140
  wide-field amacrine cells and, 101, 103, 104,
    105, 106, 108, 109, 110, 111–112, 379, 382
Gaussian sphere model, 403, 404, 405
Genes, 13, 14, 22, *see also* specific types
GFAP, *see* Glial fibrillary acidic protein
Glaucoma, 120, 365
Glial cells, 353
Glial fibrillary acidic protein (GFAP), 361
Glutamate, 342
Glycine, 106, 111, 174, 382
GnRH, *see* Gonadotropin-releasing hormone
Gonadotropin-releasing hormone (GnRH), 66
Green-sensitivity cones, 3, 152, 153, 159, 163,
    164, 301, 302
Growth cones, 109, 188, 237, 380, 381
GTP, *see* Guanosine triphosphate
Guanosine triphosphate (GTP) gammaS, 179
Gunn's sign, 366

Habituation, 172, 173, 174, 175, 177, 181, *see also*
    Dishabituation
Haeckelian recapitulation, 36
Hagfish, 63, 64, 70
  ontogeny of, 33, 34, 38, 39, 40, 43, 45
Haloperidol, 160
HCs, *see* Horizontal cells

Hearing drop test, 270
Hebbian learning rules, 397, 398, 400
Hemophilia, 12
Heterochronic transformation, 36, 37
Histidine isoleucine immunoreactivity, 107
Horizontal canal, 43, 44, 46
Horizontal cells (HCs), 95, 149–164
  behavioral/ecological effects of, 162–164
  chromaticity type, *see* Chromaticity
    horizontal cells
  electrophysiological/ultrastructural
    correlations in, 158–160
  light adaptation and, 153–158, 160, 164
  luminosity type, *see* Luminosity horizontal
    cells
  neurochemical signals in, 160–162
Horopter techniques, 275
Horror fusionis concept, 280
5HT, *see* Serotonin
6-Hydroxydopamine (6-OHDA), 160, 174
Hypertension, 366
Hypopyon, 365
Hypothalamus, 62

IBMX, 176, 179
192-IgG monoclonal antibody, 347, 348
Indoleamine-accumulating amacrine cells, 105,
    106
Infants
  cones in, 299, 300
  contrast sensitivity in, 248, 391–395
  visual cortex of, 247–252
Inflection biomarkers, 28, 31
INL, *see* Inner nuclear layer
Inner nuclear layer (INL), 95
  NGF and, 348, 349
  wide-field amacrine cells in, 101, 103, 105,
    108, 109, 110
Inner plexiform layer (IPL), 37, 95
  proteolytic activity blockage and, 78, 81, 84
  wide-field amacrine cells in, 98, 99, 100, 101,
    103, 104, 105, 107,
108, 109, 110, 186, 379, 381, 382, 383
Intensity discrimination, 56, 68
Interleukin 6, 322
Interleukines, 90, 322
Interplexiform cells, 65, 95, 105
Int-1 oncogene, 311
Intraocular activity blockade, 369–372
Intraocular lenses (IOLs), 123–124, 295, 307
IOLs, *see* Intraocular lenses
ION, *see* Isthmo-optic nucleus
IPL, *see* Inner plexiform layer
Ipsilateral projections, 357–359
Iridocyclitis, 365
Iris, 14, 287
Isthmo-optic nucleus (ION), 63, 64, 66, 68, 69, 71

Kallikrein, 80
Kangaroos, 24
Keith-Wagener-Barker classification, 366
Keratitis, 365

Lactate dehydrogenase, 312
Lampreys, 62, 63, 66, 67
    ontogeny of, 34, 37, 38, 39, 40, 41, 42, 43, 44,
        45, 46
Langevin equation, 398–400
Laser interferometric techniques, 124, 127, 128,
    132
Latencies, 213, 214, 215–216
Lateral geniculate nucleus (LGN), 215
    anophthalmia and, 255, 256, 257
    development of, 1, 3–4
    hierarchial model of, 51
    in infants, 248
    intraocular activity blockade and, 369–372
    monocular deprivation and, 206, 333, 334
    NGF and, 333, 334, 348, 350, 353
    projection neurons and, 233, 241
    stripe formation and, 398
Lateral posterior nucleus, 234
L-dopa, 143
Learning processes, 171–183
    electrogenic pump modulation in, 175–177
    habituation in, see Habituation
    neurotransmitters in, 177–179, 181, 183
    non-associative, 172–175, 177
    sensitization in, see Sensitization
    short to long term, 179–183
Leeches, 175–177
Lens, see Crystalline lens
Leupeptin, 80, 90
LGN, see Lateral geniculate nucleus
LHRH, see Luteinizing hormone releasing
    hormone
Light, 17–19, 22, 23, 295–308
    aging and, 284–285, 287–292, 295–296,
        297–298, 299–301, 305–308, see also
        Ultraviolet radiation
Light adaptation, 221
    HCs and, 153–158, 160, 164
    sensitivity losses and, 226, 228, 229–230
Light scatter, 125, 126, 132
Lipofuscin, 283–284, 285, 292–293
    Bloch-Sulzberger syndrome and, 362
    light and, 17–18, 287, 289, 292, 305
Long-wave-sensitive (LWS) cones, 299, 300,
    301, 302, 303, 304, 305, 306, 307
Lower-field myopia, 143
Luminosity horizontal cells, 150, 151, 152, 153,
    154, 156, 158, 163
Luteinizing hormone releasing hormone
    (LHRH), 66
LWS cones, see Long-wave-sensitive cones

Macroglial cells, 78, 90, 91
Macrophages, 91
Macula, 284, 304
    diabetes and, 367
    hypertension and, 366
    light and, 301
    spatial contrast sensitivity and, 119, 120
Macular edema, 367
Macular ischemia, 367

Macula star, 366
Magno pathway, 215, 248, 250, 252
Mammals, 24, 62, see also specific types
    ontogeny of, 34
    in visual hierarchy, 51–58
Marginal optic tract, 39, 40, 189, 191, 193
Martian canal effect, 61
Medial optic tract, see Axial optic tract
Melanin, 283, 284, 287, 289, 293, 299
Melanolipofuscin, 283–284, 285
Memory, 171, 172, 179–183
Menopause, 29
Mesencephalon
    centrifugal visual system in, 61–62, 63, 69,
        70
    neuropeptides in, 188–192
Meso-diencephalic junction, 62
Met-enkephalin, 66
Methysergide, 174, 175
Microglial cells, 79, 81, 89, 90–91
Microphthalmia, 256
Middle temporal area, 56–57
Middle-wave-sensitive (MWS) cones, 299, 300,
    301, 302, 303, 304, 305, 306, 307
Miosis, 13–14, 122–123, 209, 221
Monensin, 326
Monkeys
    tectofugal pathway in, 199
    visual cortex of, 249, 250, 261–265
    in visual hierarchy, 56–57
Monoclonal antibodies, 188, 316, 347, 348, 379
Monocular deprivation, 203–206, 397
    NGF and, 333–343, 348, 350–353
        extracellular unit recording of, 335,
            336–337
        VEP in, 334, 335–336, 339, 340, 341
Monte Carlo simulations, 395
Morphogenesis, 35, 36–37, 45
Motion discrimination, 56, 57
Motoneurons, 172–173, 180, 181
mRNA
    in learning processes, 179, 180, 181
    NGF, 353, 354
    NGFR, 347, 348, 350, 353
    prosomatostatin, 187
    VGF, 320, 321, 322, 323, 328
MWS cones, see Middle-wave-sensitive
    cones
Myelin, 38, 77, 91, 203, 206, 252, 351, 352
Myopia, 143
Myosin, 317

NADPH-diaphorase, 106, 107
Naka-Rushton analysis
    of sensitivity losses, 224–226, 227, 230
    of visual acuity, 140
Narrow-field amacrine cells, 96, 379
Neocortex, 54, 55, 57
Neostriatum, 200
Neovascularization, 365
Nerve growth factor (NGF), 312, 347–354
    exogenous administration of, 350–353

Nerve growth factor (*cont'd*)
 monocular deprivation and, 333–343, 348, 350–353, *see also* Monocular deprivation
 proteolytic activity blockage and, 77, 89
 VGF gene as marker of, 319–329, *see also* VGF gene
Nerve growth factor receptors (NGFR), 347, 348–350, 353–354
N-Neuraminidase-inhibitor, 80
Neurites, 311
Neurons, 209, 283
 in centrifugal visual system, 61–63, 64, 66, 68, 69, 70
 development of, 1–7, 8
 differentiation of, 311–317
 ectopic, 64, 66, 69
 in learning processes, 171–173, 175–177, 180, 181
 monocular deprivation and, 204–206, 333, 334, 335, 338, 342, 343
 motor, *see* Motoneurons
 NGF and, 347, 353
 NPY in, 385–388
 ontogeny of, 34–35
 orientation-specific responses in, 375–377
 projection type, *see* Projection neurons
 proteolytic activity blockage and, 77, 78
 sensitivity losses and, 221
 sensory, *see* Sensory neurons
 SOM in, 385–388
 spatial contrast sensitivity and, 128
 stereopsis and, 403
 of tectofugal pathway, 199, 201, 202–203, 204–206
Neuropeptides, 185–196, *see also* specific types
 in centrifugal visual system, 61, 66, 67
 distribution of, 188–194
 role of, 186–187
Neuropeptide Y (NPY), 187, 385–388
 anophthalmia and, 259–260, 261
 distribution of, 188–191, 193, 194
Neurophagy, 78
Neurotransmitters, 1, 6, 7, *see also* specific types
 in centrifugal visual system, 61, 66, 69
 in learning processes, 177–179, 181, 183
 in neuronal differentiation, 311, 312, 313
 sensitivity losses and, 222
 wide-field amacrine cells and, 107
NGF, *see* Nerve growth factor
NGFR, *see* Nerve growth factor receptors
Non-adaptive theory, 12
Non-associative learning processes, 172–175, 177
NPY, *see* Neuropeptide Y
Nucleus rotundus, 201, 203, 204–205, 206

Octopamine, 175
Ocular absorbing molecules, 295–296
Ocular aperture, 13, 17–18
Ocular muscles, 35, 43–44, 45, 46
Oculomotor nuclei, 62
6-OHDA, *see* 6-Hydroxydopamine

Oligodendrocytes, 77
ONL, *see* Outer nuclear layer
Ontogeny, 33–46
 dishabituation and, 173
 of efferent system, 39, 40–42, 45, 46
 of retina, *see* under Retina
 of retinopetal system, 35, 39, 40–42, 45
 of telencephalic areas, 57–58
 of vestibulo-ocular motorsystem, 43–44
 of wide-field amacrine cells, 96, 107–112, 379
OPL, *see* Outer plexiform layer
Opsins, 3
OPT complex, *see* Opticus principalis thalmi complex
Optical blur, 120, 121, 141
Optical simulations, 126
Optic chiasm, 38
Optic cup, 36
Optic fiber layer, 37, 38
Optic nerve, 304
 axon regeneration following transection of, *see* Proteolytic activity blockage
 in centrifugal visual system, 61, 64–65, 66, 67, 68
 ipsilateral projections and, 357–359
 NGF and, 347, 348, 350, 351, 352
 ontogeny of, 40, 42
 SRIF and, 104
 stripe formation and, 398
 tectofugal pathway and, 200
Optic neuritis, 215–216
Optic tectum
 in centrifugal visual system, 62, 64, 67, 68–69
 hierarchial model of, 51, 53, 56, 57
 ipsilateral projections and, 357, 358
 mononuclear deprivation and, 204
 neuropeptides in, 188–192, 194, 195
 ontogeny of, 37
 tectofugal pathway and, 200, 204, 206
Optic tract, 358
 axial, 39, 40, 45
 basal, 39
 marginal, *see* Marginal optic tract
Opticus principalis thalmi (OPT) complex, 200–201
Optokinetic nystagmus, 67
Orgel's catastrophe theory, 11
Ouabain, 175, 177
Outer nuclear layer (ONL), 287, 288, 289
Outer plexiform layer (OPL), 3, 99, 104, 105, 303
Owls, 199, 200
Ozone layer, 308

Panum's area, 274, 275
Papain, 80
Papilledema, 366
Parafovea, 299
Parcellation theory, 69
Parkinson's disease, 143
Parvo pathway, 215, 248, 250, 252
Pattern discrimination, 56, 57, 68, 199

Pattern electroretinogram (PERG), 137,
140–141, 142, 143, 145–147
spatio-temporal patterns of, 209–216
Pepsin, 80
Pepstatin, 80, 90
PERG, *see* Pattern electroretinogram
Peri-aqueductal gray matter, 62
Peripheral nerve-derived growth supporting
factors, 89
Peripheral nervous system (PNS), 347
Peripheral vision, 130
Phagocytosis, 284, 306
Phorbol ester, 173, 177
Photoreceptors, 95
aging in, 19, 283, 284, 293, 301
light and, 17, 285, 287, 289, 292, 299, 306
sensitivity losses and, 222
sex differences in, 287
spatial contrast sensitivity and, 125, 128
visual acuity and, 140
anophthalmia and, 259, 261
development of, 3
HCs and, 149
Phylogeny, 51–76
Pigeons
neuropeptide functions in, 187
tectofugal pathway in, 199, 200–201
visual acuity in, 137, 138–142, 143
Pigments, 19, 22, 303, *see also* specific types
light and, 17–18, 296, 297, 299, 301
sensitivity losses and, 222, 227
spatial contrast sensitivity and, 119
PKA, *see* Protein kinase A
PKC, *see* Protein kinase C
Plasmin, 80
PMMA, *see* Polymethyl methacrylate
PNS, *see* Peripheral nervous system
Poisson probability rule, 100
Polymethyl methacrylate (PMMA), 307
Pons, 234
Potassium, 312
Presbyopia, 12, 120, 140, 143
Primates, *see also* specific types
advantages of studying, 24
visual cortex in, 248, 249
visual system development in, 1–8
Prisms, 277–278, 279, 280
Projection neurons, 233–244
anophthalmia and, 258
in-vitro studies of, 233, 237, 240–242, 244
morphological types of, 234–235
target specific morphology in, 235–237
Proline, 325, 328
Prosomatostatin, 187
Protease inhibitors, 77–91, *see also* Proteolytic
activity blockage;
specific types
Protein kinase A (PKA), 173, 180
Protein kinase C (PKC), 173, 177
Protein kinases, 161, 173, 177, 180
Proteolytic activity blockage, 77–91
axonal transport and, 87

Proteolytic activity blockage (*cont'd*)
in-vitro cell generation following, 87
measurement of retinal fibers in, 81
retrograde labeling of cells in, 81–87
Pseudo-Panum's area, 274, 275
Pseudopigment effect, 164
Pterygium, 298
Puberty, 25, 27–28
Pupil diameter, 13–14, 215, 302, 303
sensitivity losses and, 221
spatial contrast sensitivity and, 122–123
visual acuity and, 139–140
Puromycin, 181
Pyknotic cells, 110
Pyramidal cells, 233; 234, 240, 241, 244

Quail
light exposure and, 305
retinal aging in, 285–292, 292
visual acuity in, 137, 142–146

Rabbits
monocular deprivation in, 206
retina of, 95–115, 379–383
Radiation, 17–19, *see also* Light
Red glass test, 275
Red-sensitive cones, 3, 301, 302, 303
HCs and, 150, 151, 153, 154, 155–156, 163, 164
Refractive errors, 120, 121, 140
Regressed vision, 33, 39
Relaxation labeling, 403–406
Renin, 80
Reptiles, 24, 27, *see also* specific types
centrifugal visual system in, 62, 63, 65, 68, 69
ontogeny of, 34
Response compression, 226
Retina
aging in, 12, 15, 19, 22, 137–147, 209, 215,
283–293, 302, 303–304
animal models of, 30
light and, 18, 284–285, 287–292, 297–298,
299–301, 306, 307
sensitivity losses and, 221
sex differences in, 285, 286, 287, 288, 289,
292, 293
spatial contrast sensitivity and, 119, 123,
124, 125, 126, 132
Behcet's disease and, 365
Bloch-Sulzberger syndrome and, 361–363
centrifugal visual fibers in, *see* Centrifugal
visual system
development of, 1–2, 3
diabetes and, 367–368
hypertension and, 366
ontogeny of, 34–35, 38–40, 44, 45
differentiation in, 35, 36–37, 43, 45
organization in, 37–38, 46
in strabismus, 280
visual acuity and, 137–147, *see also* Visual
acuity
Retinal ablation
as anophthalmia model, 257–261

Retinal ablation (*cont'd*)
  neuropeptides and, 187, 188–194, 195
  visual cortex and, 257–261
Retinal aneurysms, 366
Retinal capillary occlusion, 366
Retinal detachment, 365
Retinal edema, 124, 367
Retinal hemorrhages, 366, 367
Retinal ischemia, 368
Retinal pigment epithelium (RPE), 36, 283–284,
    285, 293, 304
  Bloch-Sulzberger syndrome and, 361, 362,
    363
  light and, 17–18, 287, 289, 292, 299, 305, 306
  sensitivity losses and, 222
  sex differences in, 287
Retinal stripes, 397–398, 399, 400
  proteolytic activity blockage and, 79
Retinal vasculitis, 365
Retinoblastomas, 361
Retinofugal fibers, 40, 45
Retinoic acid, 36
Retinopetal system, 69, 70
  ontogeny of, 35, 39, 40–42, 45
Retino-recipient dorsal thalmic nuclei, 53
Retzius cells, 175, 177, 179
Rhodopsin, 297–298
RMI1233OA, 174, 177
RNA, 321, 323
Rodents
  anophthalmia in, 255–256
  somatosensory cortex in, 261–265
Rods, 285, 304
  animal models of, 30
  development of, 3
  light and, 288, 289, 290, 291, 292, 296, 306
  sensitivity losses and, 219, 222, 228
  sex differences in, 287
  spatial contrast sensitivity and, 129
RPE, *see* Retinal pigment epithelium
Rubeosis, 365

Saccadic eye movements, 71, 247
Salus's sign, 366
Sciatic nerve-derived exudate, 87, 88
Sclera, 45
Scleritis, 365
Scotomas, 12
SDS PAGE, 326, 328
Secretogranin, 325, 328
Selective stablization, 205, 206
Senescence, *see* Aging
Senile miosis, *see* Miosis
Sensitivity losses, 219–230, *see also* specific
    types
  mechanisms of, 221–223, 229–230
  physiology of, 223, 224–227
  psychophysical paradigm of, 223–227
  receptoral vs. post-receptoral, 228–229
  sites of, 221–223
Sensitization, 172, 173–174, 175, 177, 180,
    181

Sensory neurons
  in learning processes, 172, 173, 175–177, 180,
    181
  NGF and, 347
Serotonin (5HT), 64, 66
  in learning processes, 173, 174, 175, 176, 179,
    180
Short-wavelength light, 22, 301
Short-wave-sensitive (SWS) cones, 299, 300,
    301, 302, 303–305, 306, 307
Skin cancer, 298
Snakes, 62, 63, 64, 65
Sodium-potassium electrogenic pump, 175–177
SOM, *see* Somatostatin
Somatosensory cortex, 261–265
Somatostatin (SOM), 186, 187, 188, 385–388
  distribution of, 192, 193, 194
Somatostatin immunoreactive amacrine cells
    (SRIF), 96, 97, 186
  ontogeny of, 108–110, 111–112
  organization of, 98, 100, 103–105, 106, 107
Spatial contrast sensitivity, *see* Contrast
    sensitivity, spacial
Spinal cord neurons, 313, 314, 315
Spinules, 152, 155, 156–158, 159, 160–162
SRIF, *see* Somatostatin immunoreactive
    amacrine cells
Stereopsis
  relaxation labeling in, 403–406
  in strabismus, 270, 274, 275
Steroid hormones, 145, 146
Strabismus, 269–280
  ARC in, 269–274, 276, 278–279, 280
  monocular deprivation and, 343
  sensori-motor adaptive phenomena in,
    277–278
  suppression in, 269–274, 275, 276
Striate cortex
  development of, 1, 3
  hierarchial model of, 51, 53, 56–58
  in infants, 249, 250, 252
  lesions in, 56–57
  stereopsis and, 404
Striated glasses test, 271–274, 277
Substance P, 66, 186, 188
  distribution of, 189, 191–192, 193, 194
Sunglasses, 295, 305, 307
Superior colliculus
  anophthalmia and, 255
  hierarchial model of, 51
  in infants, 247
  ipsilateral projections and, 357
  neuropeptides in, 195
  NGF and, 348, 353
  projection neurons and, 234, 235, 237, 238,
    241
Suppression, 269–274, 275, 276
Suprasylvian gyrus, 57
Suprathreshold contrast levels, 122, 129, 132
SWS cones, *see* Short-wave-sensitive cones
Synapses, 1, 3, 5–7, 8
  in infant visual cortex, 247, 252

Synapses (*cont'd*)
  in learning processes, 172–173, 177
  monocular deprivation and, 204, 333, 334, 350
  in neuronal differentiation, 313
  stripe formation and, 397, 398, 399–400
  in tectofugal pathway, 204, 205
  in TH immunoreactive cells, 382
  visual acuity and, 143
Synaptic plasticity, 149–164, *see also* Horizontal
    cells

Tectal evoked potentials (TEP), 141–142
Tectofugal visual pathway, 53–54, 56, 57–58,
    199–206
  development of, 201–203
  plasticity of, 203–205
Tegmentum, 61–62
Telencephalon
  centrifugal visual system and, 62, 63, 64
  hierarchial model of, 57–58
  neuropeptides in, 193–194, 195
Teleosts, *see also* specific types
  centrifugal visual system in, 61, 62, 63, 66, 69,
    70, 71
  HCs of, 149–164
Temporal cortex, 51
TEP, *see* Tectal evoked potentials
Tetrodotoxin (TTX), 369–370, 371, 372, 376
TH, *see* Tyrosine hydroxylase
Thalamus, 70
Thalmofugal visual pathway, 53–54, 56, 57, 199,
    200
Threshold vs. intensity (t.v.i.) functions, 223,
    224, 225, 226–227, 230
Threshold vs. radiance functions (t.v.r.), 304, 305
TPA, 322, 324
trk oncogene, 354
Trophic effects, 171, 186
Trypsin, 80
Tryptophan, 298
TTX, *see* Tetrodotoxin
Tubulin, 181
t.v.i. functions, *see* Threshold vs. intensity
    functions
t.v.r., *see* Threshold vs. radiance functions
Tyrosine, 325
Tyrosine hydroxylase (TH) immunoreactive
    amacrine cells, 96
  development of, 379–383
  ontogeny of, 107–108, 110–112
  organization of, 97–101, 105, 106

Ultraviolet radiation (UVR), 17–19, 22, 23,
    295–296, 297–298, 299, 301,
    305–306, 307–308
Ultroser, 315, 317
Useful field of view, 130
Uveitis, 365
UVR, *see* Ultraviolet radiation

Varicosities
  sensitization and, 180, 181

Varicosities (*cont'd*)
  in wide-field amacrine cells, 98, 99, 101, 105,
    380, 381, 382
Vasoactive intestinal polypeptide (VIP)
    immunoreactive amacrine cells, 96, 97
  organization of, 98, 100, 101–103, 105, 106–107
Ventrolateral thalmic nucleus, 62, 63
VEP, *see* Visual evoked potentials
Veratridine, 313, 315
Vestibulo-ocular motorsystem, 43–44
VGF gene, 319–329
  modulation of, 320–325
  regulated secretion compartment and,
    325–328
VIP, *see* Vasoactive intestinal polypeptide
Visual acuity, 137–147, 209
  animal models of, 31
  behavioral manifestations of, 138–140,
    142–143
  hierarchial model of, 56, 57
  monocular deprivation and, 339, 340, 342
  morphological changes and, 140
  spatial contrast sensitivity and, 121–122, 130
  TEP and, 141–142
Visual cortex, 209, 255–265, 304
  animal models of, 30, 31
  anophthalmia and, 255–261
  in centrifugal visual system, 68
  development of, 1, 3, 6, 7, 8
  in infants, 247–252
  monocular deprivation and, 206, 333, 335,
    336, 338, 342, 343, 350
  NGF and, 350, 353
  NPY and, 385–388
  orientation-specific neuronal responses in,
    375–377
  projection neurons in, *see* Projection neurons
  SOM and, 385–388
  somatosensory cortex compared with,
    261–265
  spatial contrast sensitivity and, 128
  stereopsis and, 404
  stripe formation and, 397–401
  visual acuity and, 143
Visual evoked potentials (VEP), 202, 205
  monocular deprivation and, 334, 335–336,
    339, 340, 341
  spatio-temporal patterns of, 209–216
Visual hierarchies, 51–58
  assumptions for, 53
  lesion effects in, 56–57
  pathways in, 53–54
Visual streak
  SRIF and, 104, 109
  TH immunoreactive cells and, 97, 98, 99, 383
  VIP immunoreactive cells and, 102
Visual wulst, 53, 56, 57, 195, 200, 201
Vitreous humor, 38, 296, 297

Whales, 24
Wide-field amacrine cells, 95–112, 186
  development of, 379–383

Wide-field amacrine cells (*cont'd*)
    ontogeny of, 96, 107–112, 379
    organization of, 97–107
    SRIF, *see* Somatostatin immunoreactive
        amacrine cells
    TH reactive, *see* Tyrosine hydroxylase
        immunoreactive amacrine cells
    VIP reactive, *see* Vasoactive intestinal
        polypeptide immunoreactive amacrine
        cells

Withdrawal reflex, 172

Xanthophyll, 299

Yellow-sensitive cones, 302, 303

Zebra finch tectofugal pathway, 199–206